SPORTS AND PHYSICAL EXERCISE IN EARLY MODERN CULTURE

It is often assumed that a recognisably modern sporting culture did not emerge until the eighteenth century. The plethora of physical training and games that existed before 1700 tend to fall victim to rigid historical boundaries drawn between "modern" and "pre-modern" sports, which are concerned primarily with levels of regulation, organization and competitiveness. Adopting a much broader and culturally based approach, the essays in this collection offer an alternative view of sport in the early modern period. Taking into account a variety of competitive as well as non-competitive forms of sport, physical training and games, the collection situates these types of activities as institutions in their own right within the socio-cultural context of early-modern Europe.

Treating the period not only as a precursor of modern developments, but as an independent and formative era, the essays engage with overlooked topics and sources such as court records, self-narratives and visual materials, and with contemporary discussions about space, gender and postcolonial studies. By allowing for this increased contextualization of sport, the collection is able to integrate it into more general historical questions and approaches.

The volume underlines how developments in early modern sport influenced later developments, whilst at the same time being thoroughly shaped by contemporary notions of the body, status and honour. These notions influenced not only the contemporary sporting fashion but the adoption of sports in elite education, the use of sports facilities, training methods and modes of competition, thus offering a more integrated idea of the place of sport in early modern society.

Rebekka von Mallinckrodt is Professor for Early Modern History at the University of Bremen. She has worked in the field of religious studies, history of the body as well as postcolonial studies. With regard to sports and physical exercise she has published *Bewegtes Leben – Körpertechniken in der Frühen Neuzeit* (Body Techniques in the Early Modern Period), exposition catalogue Herzog August Library Wolfenbüttel (Harrassowitz 2008) as well as several articles on the cultural history of swimming, diving and running.

Angela Schattner is Max Weber 2016/17 Fellow at the University of Bremen and was Research Fellow in Early Modern History at the German Historical Institute London from 2010–2016. She specialises in the social and cultural history of Early Modern Britain and Germany and the history of the body, disability, sports, exercise and leisure. She is the author of *Zwischen Familie, Heiler und Fürsorge. Das Bewältigungsverhalten von Epileptikern in deutschsprachigen Gebieten des 16.–18. Jahrhunderts*.

Sports and Physical Exercise in Early Modern Culture

New Perspectives on the History of Sports and Motion

Edited by

REBEKKA VON MALLINCKRODT
University of Bremen, Germany

ANGELA SCHATTNER
German Historical Institute London, UK

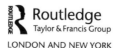

Routledge
Taylor & Francis Group

LONDON AND NEW YORK

First published 2016
by Routledge
2 Park Square, Milton Park, Abingdon, Oxon OX14 4RN

and by Routledge
711 Third Avenue, New York, NY 10017

Routledge is an imprint of the Taylor & Francis Group, an informa business

British Library Cataloguing in Publication Data
A catalogue record for this book is available from the British Library

Library of Congress Cataloging-in-Publication Data
Names: Mallinckrodt, Rebekka v. (Rebekka von), 1971– | Schattner, Angela, 1981–
Title: Sports and Physical Exercise in Early Modern Culture. New Perspectives on the History of Sports and Motion / edited by Rebekka von Mallinckrodt and Angela Schattner.
Description: Surrey, UK England ; Burlington, VT : Ashgate, [2015] | Includes bibliographical references and index.
Identifiers: LCCN 2015019033 | ISBN 9781472411945 (hardcover)
Subjects: LCSH: Sports—Europe—History. | Physical education and training—Europe—History.
Classification: LCC GV603 .S67 2015 | DDC 796.094—dc23
LC record available at http://lccn.loc.gov/2015019033

ISBN: 9781472411945 (hbk)
ISBN: 9781315610443 (ebk)

Typeset in Garamond Premier Pro
by Apex CoVantage, LLC

Contents

List of Figures and Table

Figures

Table

List of Contributors

Alessandro Arcangeli is Associate Professor of Early Modern History at the University of Verona (Italy). His main research interests and publications concern the cultural history of early modern dance and leisure, and cultural history itself as a way of doing history. He is the author of *Cultural History: A Concise Introduction* (Routledge 2011) and *Recreation in the Renaissance: Attitudes Towards Leisure and Pastimes in European Culture, c. 1425–1675* (Palgrave Macmillan 2003).

Wolfgang Behringer is Professor of Early Modern History at Saarland University (Germany). His main research interests lie in the cultural history of the early modern period. He has published widely on witchcraft in early modern Germany, the cultural history of climate change and sports history. His latest publications include *A Cultural History of Climate* (Polity Press 2009), *Kulturgeschichte des Sports. Vom antiken Olympia bis zur Gegenwart* (A Cultural History of Sports: From Ancient Olympia to the Present) (C.H.-Beck 2012), and *Tambora und das Jahr ohne Sommer. Wie ein Vulkan die Welt in die Krise stürzte* (Tambora and the year without a summer. How a volcano plunged the world into crisis) (C.H.-Beck 2015).

Sandra Cavallo is Professor of Early Modern History at the Royal Holloway University of London and specializes in the history of medicine, gender and the home. Her latest publications include *Artisans of the Body in Early Modern Italy* (Manchester University Press 2007), *Spaces, Objects and Identities in Early Modern Italian Medicine* (Blackwell 2008), *Domestic Institutional Interiors in Early Modern Europe* (Ashgate 2009) and *A Cultural History of Childhood and the Family*, vol. 3 (Berg 2010), co-authored with Tessa Storey, *Healthy Living in Late Renaissance Italy* (Oxford University Press 2013). From 2009 to 2012 she led the Wellcome Trust Project Grant 'Healthy Homes and Healthy Bodies in Renaissance and Early Modern Italy' and looked at the construction of the healthy domestic environment and the healthy body in the late Renaissance.

David Day is Reader in Sports History in the Department of Exercise and Sport Science at Manchester Metropolitan University where his research interests focus on the history of coaching practice and training and the biographies of nineteenth- and early twentieth-century coaches. He was contributor to, and editor of, *Sporting Lives*, which brought together some of Britain's leading sports historians and biographers and his chapter on nineteenth-century 'London Swimming Professors: Victorian Craftsmen and Aquatic Entrepreneurs' was published in Neil Carter (ed.), *Coaching Cultures* (Routledge 2011). His monograph *Professionals, Amateurs and Performance: Sports Coaching in England, 1789–1914* was published by Peter Lang in 2012 and his *A History of Sports Coaching in Britain* was published by Routledge in 2015.

Martin Dinges is Deputy Director of the Institute for the History of Medicine at the Robert Bosch Foundation, Stuttgart and Adjunct Professor of Modern History at the University of Mannheim. His main research interests are the modern history of health and gender history. Recent publications include: Geschlechterspezifische Gesundheitsgeschichte: Warum nicht einmal Männer...?, *Medizinhistorisches Journal*, 50, 1 and 2 (2015) (Guest-editor); *Medical Pluralism and Homoeopathy in India and Germany (1810-2010)* (Franz Steiner Verlag, 2014); *The Transmission of Health Practices (1500–2000)* (Franz Steiner Verlag 2011); *Männlichkeit und Gesundheit im historischen Wandel ca. 1800 – ca. 2000* (Manliness and Health in Historical Perspective ca. 1800 – ca. 2000) (Franz Steiner Verlag 2007).

Tomasz Gromelski is Research Fellow in Humanities at Wolfson College, Oxford, and Postdoctoral Researcher on the ESRC-funded project 'Everyday life and fatal hazard in sixteenth-century England'. His research interests are in the social and cultural history of Tudor England and of sixteenth-century Europe. He has also published articles and book chapters on political thought and political culture in late medieval and early modern Poland-Lithuania.

Steven Gunn is Fellow and Tutor in History at Merton College, Oxford. His research interests are in the political, social, cultural and military history of England and its continental neighbours from the mid-fifteenth to the later sixteenth century. He is the editor of *The Court as a Stage: England and the Low Countries in the Later Middle Ages* (Boydell P. 2006) with Antheun Janse and *Arthur Tudor, Prince of Wales: Life, Death and Commemoration* (Boydell P. 2009) with Linda Monckton. He is currently writing a book on Henry VII's 'New Men' and directing a project on everyday life and accidental death in sixteenth-century England. He has used material from coroners' inquests in his article 'Archery Practice in Early Tudor England', *Past and Present*, 209 (2010): pp. 53–81.

Christian Jaser is a postdoctoral research assistant at the chair of Late Medieval History at Humboldt University Berlin. He is currently working on his second book about fifteenth-century Italian and upper-German horse-racing in comparative perspective. His latest publication is *Ecclesia maledicens. Rituelle und zeremonielle Exkommunikationsformen im Mittelalter* (Ecclesia maledicens: Forms of Ritual Excommunication in the Middle Ages) (Mohr Siebeck 2013).

Benjamin Litherland is a lecturer in journalism and media at the University of Huddersfield. He has recently completed his PhD, *The Field and the Stage: Pugilism, Combat Performance and Professional Wrestling in England, 1700 – 1980* and is currently editing a special edition for *Sport in History* assessing the relationship between sport and other leisure industries. Overall, his research is located on the borders and boundaries of sport, the theatre and the media and is concerned with how these cultural forms are socially and culturally reproduced.

Rebekka von Mallinckrodt is Professor of Early Modern History at the University of Bremen. She has worked in the field of religious studies, history of the body as well as postcolonial studies. From 2015 to 2020 she leads the ERC Consolidator Grant Project 'The Holy Roman Empire of the German Nation and its Slaves'. With regard to sports and physical exercise she has published *Bewegtes Leben – Körpertechniken in der Frühen Neuzeit* (Live on the Move – Body Techniques in the Early Modern Period), exposition catalogue Herzog August Library Wolfenbüttel (Harrassowitz 2008) as well as numerous articles on the cultural history of running, swimming and diving as for example 'Exploring Underwater Worlds. Diving in the Late Seventeenth-/ Early Eighteenth-Century British Empire' in *Empire of Senses. Sensory Practices and Modes of Perceptions in the Atlantic World* (Brill forthcoming).

Angela Schattner is Research Fellow in Early Modern History at the German Historical Institute London. She specializes in the social and cultural history of Early Modern Britain and Germany and the history of the body, disability, sports, exercise and leisure. She is the author of *Zwischen Familie, Heiler und Fürsorge. Das Bewältigungsverhalten von Epileptikern in deutschsprachigen Gebieten des 16.-18. Jahrhunderts* (Franz Steiner Verlag, 2012).

Tessa Storey is a research associate with Prof. Sandra Cavallo on the Wellcome Trust funded project, 'Healthy Homes and Healthy Bodies in Renaissance and Early Modern Europe' (2009–2012) and co-authored with Sandra Cavallo, *Healthy Living in Late Renaissance Italy* (Oxford University Press 2013). Her research interests are in the social, cultural and gender history of early modern Italy, with special reference to prostitution and material culture. Her book *Carnal Commerce in Counter Reformation Rome* was published by Cambridge University Press in 2008. She worked together with Professor David Gentilcore (Leicester University) on a database of early modern Italian recipe books as part of the Wellcome Trust funded strategic award, 'The Cultures and Practices of Health'. This database, available online at https://lra.le.ac.uk/handle/2381/4335, contains 3,033 recipes concerned with medicine, hygiene and cosmetics drawn from a wide range of Italian 'Books of Secrets'.

B. Ann Tlusty is Professor of History at Bucknell University in Pennsylvania, USA. Her publications include *The Martial Ethic in Early Modern Germany: Civic Duty and the Right of Arms* (Palgrave Macmillan 2011), *Bacchus and Civic Order: The Culture of Drink in Early Modern Europe* (University Press of Virginia 2001) and numerous articles concentrating on gendered behaviours including drinking, duelling, gambling and the culture of weapons. Tlusty's current work examines the use of handwriting by non-professional writers as a context for understanding the development of language 'from below'.

Michael Wert is a Japanese and East Asian historian at Marquette University. His book addresses the historical memory of 'losers' of the Meiji Restoration (1868) from the nineteenth century to the present: *Remembering Restoration Losers: Memory and Tokugawa Supporters in Modern Japan* (Harvard Asia Center Press, January 2014). He has worked on his second project, physical and martial culture in early modern Japan, especially among the non-samurai, since 2001. His most recent publication on this topic is the short essay, 'Bakumatsu Fencing Schools and Nationalism in Japan', in *Japan at War: An Encyclopedia* (ABC-CLIO 2013).

Acknowledgements

This volume arises from the conference 'Sport in Early Modern Culture' which was jointly organised and sponsored by the international network of the German Research Foundation (DFG) 'Body Techniques in the Early Modern Period' (MA 4520/2–1) and the German Historical Institute London in November 2011. We would like to thank both sponsors for their generous help which also enabled the production of this volume. With her perfect organisation, Carole Sterckx made sure that the conference ran smoothly: thanks so much for that.

Moreover, we would like to thank Ashgate for publishing this volume and especially Tom Gray for his ongoing support and pleasant collaboration, Gemma Hayman for her wonderful organisation and Gail Welsh for her support in proof-reading the text. We also found the feedback of anonymous peer-reviewers very helpful. Our thanks, too, to all the contributors for their hard work and text revisions as well as Lisa Städtler and Kai Gräf for checking footnotes and formalities. Jane Rafferty and Angela Davies from the German Historical Institute London have kindly translated, proofread and edited parts of the contributions and helped us to (hopefully) avoid any serious mistakes for which we would like to express our deepest gratitude. Any remaining errors, however, are our responsibility alone.

Last but not least our thanks go to the members of the international network of the German Research Foundation (DFG) 'Body Techniques in the Early Modern Period': Wolfgang Behringer (Saarbrücken), Pascal Brioist (Tours), Martin Dinges (Stuttgart), Mariacarla Gadebusch Bondio (München), Jonathan Kohlrausch (Lübeck), Ulrike Krampl (Tours), Kristin Marek (Bochum/Karlsruhe), Ulrich Rehm (Bochum), Herman Roodenburg (Amsterdam), Lyndal Roper (Oxford), Ulinka Rublack (Cambridge), Georges Vigarello (Paris) and Janina Wellmann (Berlin/Tel Aviv). Even though not all members could contribute to this volume, the regular network meetings and discussions that took place in 2010 and 2011 in Berlin, Saarbrücken, Paris and London not only enriched our own research but were also very pleasant occasions.

Therefore, we hope that this will not be the last collective publication on this topic emerging from this group of Early Modernists.

Rebekka von Mallinckrodt
University of Bremen

Angela Schattner
German Historical Institute London

Introduction

Rebekka v. Mallinckrodt and Angela Schattner

Ball, comprising airy spirits
That form and move it:
Fateful apple, which Mars contests
Amongst deceit and fraud,
and which Fortune turns:
Globe, which like a canonball, flung by a strong hand cleaves the air,
Spherical cloister, enclosed with difficulty,
it quietens and keeps silent,
And between strikes and challenges, it stops and pauses:
Narrow-minded and ignoble world, which flees and deceives,
And which distributes and grants for equal reward,
Odes, indignation, blows, humiliation and fury
To winners and losers.[1]

Like Capradosso, who, in his praise of *calcio* dating from 1630, wrote about Florentine football as an allegory of life, others in the early modern period were moved by the passions of sport. Despite the need to observe Sunday, English men and women in the sixteenth century loved to play sport on the first day of

---

[1] Agostiniano Capradosso, *Il Calcio, Poesia, All'Illustrissimo Signor Pietro Bardi, Conte di Vernio*, 2 February 1630, Biblioteca Nazionale Centrale, Florence, Palat. 298, fol. 8v–9r, cited in Horst Bredekamp, *Florentiner Fußball: Die Renaissance der Spiele* (Berlin, 2nd revised edn 2006), p. 179, endnote 328:
'Palla, ch'entro racchiude
Aereo spirto, che l'informa, e muove:
Pomo fatal, che sotto insidie, e frodi
Marte il contende, e la fortuna il gira:
Globo, che qual bombarda,
Tocco da forte man l'aria divide:
Rotondo Chiostro, ove racchiuso à sforza
Ecolo cede, e tace,
E fra gl'urti, e l'offese ha posa, e pace:
Angusto Mondo, e vile,
Che fugge, e inganna, e sol comparte, e dona
Per egual merto à' Vinti, e Vincitori:
Ode, Sdegni, Percosse, Onte e Furori'.

the week. And, although it led to conflicts, their favourite place for this was the churchyard. There were also many commercial sports facilities, and not only in England.[2] In 1598 a member of the papal legation counted more than 250 indoor tennis courts in Paris, the capital of early modern *jeu de paume* (a precursor of real tennis). These courts were open to artisans as well as burghers and the aristocracy; the existence of 70 of them can definitely be attested in other sources; and women as well as girls also played *jeu de paume*.[3] In just two years (1573–4) the Bavarian dukes William and Ferdinand ordered no fewer than 11,000 balls and 50 racquets from Hans Fugger.[4] In Venice from the late fifteenth century, peasant women from the surrounding areas regularly took part in rowing races.[5] From the eighteenth century the rural elite in Japan practised fencing as a sport.[6] In the same century, numerous learn-to-swim brochures describing swimming and diving techniques were published on the European continent, forming part of a tradition of writings that, since the sixteenth century, had codified the rules of sports and games. They were read in many countries and in many languages.[7]

All these examples demonstrate the great importance, but also the wide social and geographical spread and diversity, of voluntary physical activity, games, sports and physical exercise in the early modern period. Still, early modern sports and physical exercise are a rather neglected topic despite the inspiring work by some advocates of early modern sports in the last decades. This is not due to a general lack of interest in sports history: In the past few decades a number of significant works have been published on the cultural history of sport and its connection to society. However, these studies concentrated on developments in the nineteenth and twentieth centuries. The early modern period, if included at all, has often received only marginal attention. This is due to the fact that in the beginning of the historiography of sports, advanced in the 1970s by pioneers of the field such as Allen Guttmann, sports were conceptionalized as part and parcel of modernization[8] which proved to be counterproductive for research on

---

[2]   See the contributions by Steven Gunn and Thomasz Gromelski and Angela Schattner in this volume, Chapters 2 and 3, pp. 76–79.

[3]   See Chapter 4 by Christian Jaser in this volume.

[4]   Wolfgang Behringer, 'Arena and Pall Mall: Sport in the Early Modern Period', *German History*, 27/3 (2009): pp. 331–57, at p. 344.

[5]   See Chapter 7 by Alessandro Arcangeli in this volume, pp. 161–63.

[6]   See Chapter 12 by Michael Wert in this volume.

[7]   See Chapter 11 by Rebekka v. Mallinckrodt in this volume.

[8]   Allen Guttmann, *From Ritual to Record: The Nature of Modern Sports* (OE 1978, New York, 2004); Norbert Elias and Eric Dunning (eds), *Quest for Excitement: Sport and Leisure in the Civilising Process* (OE 1986, Dublin, 2008). The modernization thesis is uphold by Guttmann to the present day: Allen Guttmann, *Sports: The First Five Millennia* (Amherst, 2004), pp. 68–76; Guttmann, 'Afterword. From Ritual to Record: A Retrospective Critique', in *From Ritual to Record: The Nature of Modern Sports* (New York, 2004), pp. 163–74. This

the early modern period (here understood as covering the years 1500 to 1800). Although since the 1970s we have seen the publication of important case studies on the rise and culture of various individual sports,[9] and large-scale surveys of games and pastimes in various countries in the early modern period,[10] the study of sport and physical exercise has remained limited largely to its connection with courtly society (tournaments, hunting and dancing).[11] One exception

---

argument has been picked up and continued in current sports historiography. Christiane Eisenberg links the beginnings of modern sport with the rise of betting on sport and British society's highly developed competitive thinking in the early industrial period (Christiane Eisenberg, *'English Sports' und deutsche Bürger. Eine Gesellschaftsgeschichte 1800–1939* (Paderborn, 1999); Eisenberg, 'Towards a New History of European Sport?', *European Review*, 19/1 (2011): pp. 617–22). Most recently, Stefan Szymanski has linked the rise of modern sport with that of assocations which, in his view, were only possible in eighteenth-century Britain, and has identified sports clubs as the crucial factor in a definition of sport (Stefan Szymanski, 'A Theory of the Evolution of Modern Sport', *Journal of Sport History*, 35/1 (2008): pp. 1–32).

[9] See e.g. Heiner Gillmeister, *Tennis: A Cultural History* (Leicester, 1997); Michael Flannery and Richard Leech, *Golf through the Ages: Six Hundred Years of Golfing Art* (Fairfield, 2004); Horst Bredekamp, *Florentiner Fussball – Die Renaissance der Spiele* (Berlin, 2006); Cees de Bondt, *Royal Tennis in Renaissance Italy* (Turnhout, 2006).

[10] See e.g. Carlo Bascetta, *Sport e giochi. Trattati e scritti dal XV al XVIII secolo* (2 vols, Milan, 1978); Jean-Michel Mehl, *Les Jeux au Royaume de France du XIIIe au début du XVIe siècle* (Paris, 1990); Nancy L. Struna, *People of Prowess: Sport, Leisure and Labour in Early Anglo-America* (Chicago, 1996); Alessandro Arcangeli, *Recreation in the Renaissance: Attitudes Towards Leisure and Pastimes in European Culture* (Basingstoke, 2003).

[11] See e.g. for hunting and riding: Phillipe Salvadori, *La chasse sous l'Ancien Régime* (Paris, 1996); Martin Knoll, *Umwelt – Herrschaft – Gesellschaft. Die landesherrliche Jagd Kurbayerns im 18. Jahrhundert* (St. Katharinen, 2004); Werner Rösener, *Die Geschichte der Jagd. Kultur, Gesellschaft und Jagdwesen im Wandel der Zeit* (Zürich, 2004); Karen Raber and Treva J. Tucker (eds), *The Culture of the Horse: Status, Discipline and Identity in the Early Modern World* (New York and Basingstoke, 2005); Emma Griffin, *Blood Sport – Hunting in Britain since 1066* (New Haven, 2007). For martial arts and tournaments: Alan R. Young, *Tudor and Jacobean Tournaments* (London, 1987); Maria Vittoria Baruti Ceccopieri (ed.), *La civiltà del torneo (sec. XII–XVII). Giostre e tornei tra Medioevo ed età moderna* (Narni, 1990); C. Gillmor, 'Practical Chivalry: The Training of Horses for Tournaments and Warfare', *Studies in Medieval and Renaissance History*, 13 (1992): pp. 5–29; Helen Watanabe-O'Kelly, *Triumphall Shews: Tournaments at German Speaking Courts in their European Context 1560–1730* (Berlin, 1992); Helen Watanabe O'Kelly, 'Tournaments in Europe', in Helen Watanabe O'Kelly and Pierre Béhar (eds), *Spectaculum Europaeum: Theatre and Spectacle in Europe (1580–1750)* (Wiesbaden, 1999), pp. 593–639; Sydney Anglo, *The Martial Arts of Renaissance Europe* (New Haven and London, 2000); Helen Watanabe O'Kelly, 'Early Modern Tournaments and their Relationship to Warfare: France and the Empire Compared', in Karin Friedrich (ed.), *Festive Culture in Germany and Europe from the Sixteenth to the Twentieth Century* (Lewiston, 2000), pp. 233–44; Pascal Brioist, *Croiser le fer. Violence et*

is the history of sport in Britain, which has given an important boost to the investigation of early modern sport in connection with popular recreations and pastimes,[12] individual sports such as cricket, boxing and horse-racing in Britain,[13] and individual sporting events.[14] Most of these studies, however, focus on developments in England in the eighteenth century which, according to the pioneers of sports historiography, was viewed as a take-off phase for later developments, while, apart from Dennis Brailsford's excellent study, the earlier period has largely been ignored.[15] This lack of interest in early modern sport was based on the common assumption of a strong discontinuity between 'premodern' and 'modern' sport and the belief that sport only attained real social relevance, and is thus worth investigating, from the second half of the nineteenth century.[16]

culture de l'épée dans la France moderne (XVIe–XVIIIe siècle) (Seyssel, 2002); Alessandro Marcigliano, *Chivalric Festivals at the Ferrarese Court of Alfonso II d'Este* (Oxford, 2003); G. Hanlon, 'Glorifying War in a Peaceful City: Festive Representation of Combat in Baroque Siena (1590–1740)', *War in History*, 11/3 (2004): pp. 249–78; Braden K. Frieder, *Chivalry and the Perfect Prince: Tournaments, Art, and Armor at the Spanish Habsburg Court* (Kirksville, 2008). For dancing: Rudolf Braun and David Gugerli, *Macht des Tanzes – Tanz der Mächtigen. Hoffeste und Herrschaftszeremoniell 1550–1914* (Munich, 1993); Marie-Thérèse Mourey, 'Galante Tanzkunst und Körperideal', in Rebekka von Mallinckrodt (ed.), *Bewegtes Leben. Körpertechniken in der Frühen Neuzeit* (Wiesbaden, 2008), pp. 85–103.

[12]　See esp. Robert Malcolmson, *Popular Recreations in English Society 1700–1850* (Cambridge, 1973); Emma Griffin, *England's Revelry: A History of Popular Sports and Pastimes, 1660–1830* (Oxford, 2005).

[13]　See e.g. for cricket: Christopher Brookes, *English Cricket: The Game and its Players through the Ages* (London, 1978), pp. 45–66; Michael Harris, 'Sport in the Newspapers Before 1750: Representations of Cricket, Class and Commerce in the London Press', *Media History*, 4/1 (1998): pp. 19–28; Derek Birley, *A Social History of English Cricket* (London, 1999), pp. 12–25; David Underdown, *Start of Play: Cricket and Culture in Eighteenth-Century England* (London, 2000). For boxing: Nat Fleischer, *The Heavyweight Championship: An Informal History of Heavyweight Boxing from 1719 to the Present Day* (London, 1949); Dennis Brailsford, *Bareknuckles: A Social History of Prize-Fighting* (Cambridge, 1988); Dennis Brailsford, *British Sport: A Social History* (Cambridge, 1992); Dennis Brailsford, *A Taste for Diversions: Sport in Georgian England* (Cambridge, 1999); Dave Day, 'Entrepreneurial Pugilists of the Early Eighteenth-Century', in Dave Day (ed.), *Sporting Lives* (Manchester, 2011), pp. 167–79. For horse-racing: Wray Vamplew and Joyce Kay, 'A Modern Sport? "From Ritual to Record" in British Horseracing', *Ludica*, 9 (2003): pp. 125–39.

[14]　Martin Polley, *The British Olympics: Britain's Olympic Heritage, 1612–2012* (London, 2011); Conrad Brunström, Tanya M. Cassidy and Martha K. Zebrowksi (eds), 'Olympic Special Issue', *Journal for Eighteenth-Century Studies*, 35/2 (2012): pp. 159–248.

[15]　Dennis Brailsford, *Sport and Society, Elizabeth to Anne* (London, 1969).

[16]　A recent example which again emphasizes the perception that sport was only socially relevant from the late nineteenth century can be found in contributions by Paul Ward, 'Last Man Picked? Do Mainstream Historians Need to Play with Sports Historians?', pp. 11–2 and Matthew L. McDowell, 'Sports History: Outside of the Mainstream? A Response to

Sociologists and specialists in modern sport have frequently presented the early modern period as merely a forerunner to nineteenth- and twentieth-century developments. The many different forms of physical training and games with a physical emphasis that existed at that time were and are often denied the status of 'sport' altogether. In many cases early modern sport is presented as popular and folkloric, or as shaped by courtly ritual, [17] because, as John McClelland has pointed out: 'Modern sport can only exist if early modern sport does not.'[18]

Since the 1980s, however, Guttmann's definition of sport – as characterized by secularization, equal opportunity in competition and with regard to the terms and conditions of competition, specialization of roles and functions, rationalization, bureaucratic organization, quantification, and the quest for records – has been criticized. Arnd Krüger, John McClelland and John Marshall Carter challenged this antithetical juxtaposition in 1984 and again in 1990. They pointed out that attempts to rationalize, standardize and quantify sport could already be found in medieval English tournaments and during the Italian Renaissance. They also rejected the view that early modern sport was entirely ritualistic, and underlined the ritual aspects of modern sport.[19] Yet ultimately this only resulted in a clarification of Guttmann's argument. In his response to the criticism of Krüger and Carter, Guttmann accepted that quantification, records and other features of his definition of sport appeared sporadically in premodern times. He emphasized, however, that it is how these characteristics interact systematically that makes them modern.[20] Wolfgang Behringer, John McClelland, Brian Merrilees and Rebekka von Mallinckrodt took up the conceptual debate again. In 2004 and 2008 Mallinckrodt argued that the sports paradigm should be conceptually expanded. It seemed to her that, in relation to current as well as historical phenomena, it was too restricted to cover the culture of movement of a society in its entirety.[21] In their edited volume of essays on

Ward's "Last Man Picked"', p. 18 in the special issue 'What is the Future of Sport History in Academia?' of *The International Journal of the History of Sport*, 30/1 (2013).

[17] See for example Eisenberg, 'Towards a New History of Sports?', p. 620: 'Here, one thinks of the remnants of a few individual early-modern folk games in remote geographical areas, such as soule, the ballgame played in parts of Normandy and Brittany; or of fencing as part of the corporate culture of guilded artisans, students or aristocrats.' See also John McClelland, 'Introduction', in John McClelland and Brian Merrilees (eds), *Sport and Culture in Early Modern Europe* (Toronto, 2009), pp. 23–40, here pp. 24, 32.

[18] McClelland, 'Introduction', p. 36.

[19] Arnd Krüger and John McClelland (eds), *Die Anfänge des modernen Sports in der Renaissance* (London, 1984); John Marshall Carter and Arnd Krüger (eds), *Ritual and Record: Sports Records and Quantification in Pre-Modern Societies* (Westport, 1990).

[20] Guttmann, 'Afterword', p. 172.

[21] Rebekka von Mallinckrodt, 'Bewegte Geschichte – Plädoyer für eine verstärkte Integration und konzeptuelle Erweiterung der Sportgeschichte in der frühneuzeitlichen

continental Europe from the twelfth to the seventeenth centuries, published in 2009, McClelland and Merrilees argued not only that the term 'sport' should be applied to early modern 'autotelic ludic physical contests' on the basis of their rule orientation, organization and other features of 'modern' sport,[22] but also that modern sport had never assumed such an unambiguous, monolithic and immutable form as supporters of the sports paradigm claimed.[23] In the same year, Behringer went a step further and declared the early modern period as formative for the history of sport as demonstrated by contemporary developments like the 'sportification' of tournaments and popular games, the inclusion of physical exercise in school curricula and behaviour manuals since the Renaissance, the building of permanent sports facilities, the codification and printing of rules, commercialization and professionalization.[24]

This volume builds on these works by adding further supportive evidence and new perspectives to the history of early modern sports and exercise. Along with McClelland and Merrilees, we share a desire to research the early modern culture of movement *as sport* as this has the advantage of distinguishing a set of competitive, playful physical activities which were characterized by their own rules and social norms from other recreational activities and pastimes like cards and dice, music or theatrical performances which have up until now been the focus of research on leisure and pastimes. However, we also believe that restricting ourselves to competitive sport would narrow the perspective so much that it would be inappropriate for an investigation of the culture of movement, either today or in the early modern period. This volume therefore includes competitive sport along with non-competitive forms of physical exercise, education and games in a wider investigation of 'movement cultures' in early modernity. This is not to deny that there are differences in the concepts, aims, organization and practices of 'sport', 'exercise' and other forms of physical movement. However, Martin Johnes, Tony Collins, Dion Georgiou and Benjamin Litherland are among those who have recently questioned how meaningful a singular concept of 'sport' can be as a conceptual framework for the analysis of very different physical activities as socio-cultural phenomena. They have stressed the permeability of boundaries between sport and other physical activities.[25] By including and

Geschichtswissenschaft', *Historische Anthropologie*, 12/1 (2004): pp. 134–9, at p. 135; Mallinckrodt, 'Einführung. Körpertechniken in der Frühen Neuzeit', in Rebekka von Mallinckrodt (ed.), *Bewegtes Leben. Körpertechniken in der Frühen Neuzeit* (Wolfenbüttel, 2008), pp. 1–14, p. 7.

[22]   Guttmann, *From Ritual to Record*, pp. 3–4.

[23]   McClelland, 'Introduction', pp. 25, 28, 36.

[24]   Behringer, 'Arena and Pall Mall', pp. 331–57; Wolfgang Behringer, *Kulturgeschichte des Sports. Vom antiken Olympia bis zur Gegenwart* (Munich, 2012), pp. 19–20, 408–9.

[25]   Tony Collins, 'Work, Rest and Play: Recent Trends in the History of Sport and Leisure', *Journal of Contemporary History*, 42 (2007): pp. 397–410, at p. 399; Martin Johnes,

comparing different forms of physical activity and considering their differences and commonalities we can understand more fully the boundaries of the concept of 'sport' and its relationship with 'exercise' and other physical activities. The focus of this volume lies on human sports and exercise while animal sports like coursing, horse-racing or animal baiting have largely been excluded. Instead, we wanted to highlight sports like ball games as well as physical exercise activities which have not yet received the appropriate attention in the context of early modern sports, such as, for example, swimming.

To take these different types of sport and physical exercise seriously as institutions in their own right, they need to be explored in their socio-cultural context in the early modern period. The chapters, therefore, make closer connections with social and cultural history approaches, and with current trends, such as women's and gender history, the spatial turn and global history, in order to integrate the history of early modern sport more strongly into general history, as has already been done for modern sports history. For it seems to us that the history of early modern sport can provide, as Michael Wert puts it in his chapter,[26] a lens through which to observe historical change.

While much of the research on early modern sports to date has utilized normative source materials (e.g. treatises, sports manuals, legislation) and has thus concentrated on a viewpoint based on elite discourses, the chapters in this volume focus on practices of sports and exercise and their relationship to these discourses. They investigate court records, self-narratives and visual materials among other things to expand the source basis with regard to early modern practices in particular. In contrast to the volume edited by McClelland and Merrilees, which ends in the seventeenth century, we feel it is important to look at the whole of the early modern period (1500–1800) in our volume, in order to be able to grasp continuities and changes. Therefore, we did not urge contributors to make cuts on the time span they cover if they felt it necessary for their topic to go back to late medieval times or forward into the nineteenth century as long as their focus was on the early modern period. In the sources we investigated, we could find no confirmation of McClelland's thesis that sport declined in the seventeenth and eighteenth centuries.[27] This may be due to the frequently observed discrepancy between prescriptive texts and early modern practices.

We advocate the proposition formulated with regard to modern sports by Tomlinson and Young of an investigation of the 'diversity and commonalities' of movement cultures in and beyond Europe, and a more detailed analysis of

---

'British Sports History: The Present and the Future', *Journal of Sport History*, 35/1 (2008), pp. 65–71, at p. 69; Dion Georgiou and Benjamin Litherland (eds), *Special Issue: Sport's Relationship with Other Leisure Industries*, Part I: *Sites of Interaction, Sport in History*, 34/2 (2014): pp. 186–7.

[26] Wert, Chapter 12 in this volume.

[27] McClelland, 'Introduction', pp. 34–5.

these patterns, how they changed over time and their embeddedness in regional contexts and traditions.[28] For us, it seemed important to localize sports practices and diversify the existing research by expanding the geographical coverage. The chapters in this volume look at evidence from England, Italy, France, the Holy Roman Empire and even from beyond Europe (Japan). Although not primarily comparative in their approach, the chapters highlight interconnections between regional sporting cultures and show the existence of European sport networks as demonstrated by the example of *jeu de paume*. Starting from France, this competitive sport spread throughout Europe from the Middle Ages before England was also gripped by tennis fever. Equipment was despatched across borders, and pamphlets encouraged the spread of the game and imposed consistency within it. There were various trends in early modern Europe in which particular sports and exercise fashions spread, that need to be studied in future.

Similarly, we endorse the plea made by Tomlinson and Young, following Peter Burke, for a historiography that works less with dichotomies. This volume investigates the early modern period not pre-eminently as a precursor of modern developments, but as an independent and at the same time formative period in the history of sports. The chapters in our volume show that, for example, with respect to the professionalization of sportsmen and their trainers, economization, the construction of sports facilities and the codification, standardization and scientization of sport, lines of development can be traced far back into the early modern period, and that these cannot be adequately grasped by an antithetical juxtaposition between premodern and modern sport.[29] McClelland even points to continuities going back to the Middle Ages.[30]

The current volume is based on the papers given in 2011 at the conference 'Sport in Early Modern Culture', organized by the German Historical Institute London in collaboration with the international network 'Body Techniques in the Early Modern Period' (financed by the German Science Foundation). The chapters presented here combine different approaches and perspectives to explore early modern physical culture. Jaser, Litherland, Day, Tlusty, Mallinckrodt and Wert use the example of one specific sport (tennis, boxing, fencing, shooting, swimming), and in Behringer's case, a subgroup of sports (ball games), to explore wider developments in early modern sport, such as commercialization,

---

[28]   Alan Tomlinson and Christopher Young, 'Towards a New History of European Sport', *European Review*, 19/4 (2011): pp. 487–507, at pp. 491–8.

[29]   Peter Burke, 'The Invention of Leisure in Early Modern Europe', *Past and Present*, 146 (1995): pp. 136–50; Tomlinson and Young, 'Towards a New History of European Sport', p. 497.

[30]   McClelland, 'Introduction', pp. 30–31 mentions professional jousters as early as the twelfth century and points out that standardized rules and scoring systems for jousting had been codified and published by the mid-fifteenth century.

sportification and scientization. Gunn and Gromelski, Schattner, Arcangeli, Cavallo and Storey, and Dinges use specific source materials (coroners' inquest reports, health and education guides) or a specific methodological approach (spatial arrangements) to analyse the context, aims and concepts of sport and physical exercise more generally. While Benjamin Litherland and David Day focus on professional sportsmen, most of the chapters in this volume look at amateur sportsmen and sport as a recreational and sociable activity. The texts are organized into four thematic groups:

1. What Sports? Tracing Early Modern Sports Practices;
2. Sport for Money and Glory? Commercialization and Professionalization;
3. Promoting Health or Danger? Physical Exercise under Scrutiny; and
4. Enhancing or Endangering Status and Identity?

The chapters in the first part contextualize European sport in the early modern period and ask basic questions such as where, when, how and by whom sporting activities and exercise were undertaken. They consider new source material for research on sport, such as coroners' inquest reports, and test the benefit of using existing theories such as sportification and methodological approaches such as space to explore developments in early modern sport. The chapters in this section reveal a rich sporting culture at all levels in England and continental Europe from the sixteenth century. Sport was a recreational everyday activity quite detached from the ritualistic forms so often assumed for early modern sport.

Wolfgang Behringer investigates the Europe-wide 'sportification' of early modern ball games from the sixteenth century. Since the Renaissance, ball games had become increasingly popular among the European nobility. During the sixteenth century ball games superseded martial sports, such as the tournament, at the courts of Europe. As sporting competitions without a military drill, they posed a much lower risk of injury. Increasingly praised by educationalists and physicians as an ideal of healthy and noble exercise which conveyed to aristocratic youth an elegant and gentlemanly ideal of the body, ball games became a fixed part of aristocratic education. In addition to riding, fencing, dancing and hunting, aristocratic young people now routinely studied the rules and practice of popular ball games as part of an aristocratic lifestyle. The Europe-wide dissemination of these games, which were played by Italian nobles and French and English courtiers as well as at small courts like those of the Palatine princes, meant that ball games such as *jeu de paume* and *pallone*, i.e. their rules, techniques and equipment, were standardized. This was reflected in the increased number of manuals that were sold all over Europe and translated into various languages, the institutionalization of facilities for ball games at princely courts and the many playing partners of European princes.

But it was not only the aristocracy who had a rich sporting culture and practised martial and non-martial sport, as the contribution by Steven Gunn and Tomasz Gromelski shows. In their chapter they explore the practice of early modern sport and recreational activities in sixteenth-century England, as reflected in inquest reports on sudden deaths submitted by coroners. Although coroners' reports have their limitations as they only record 'dangerous' sports and exercises, they provide reliable statistical evidence of times, places, performers, spectators and sporting habits. Their detailed descriptions of the circumstances of accidents sometimes confirm, sometimes amplify or contradict what legislation, litigation and treatises suggest about early modern sporting cultures and practices. Their evidence shows that early modern sport was practised nearly all year round and far more regularly than previously assumed, when Sunday was regarded as the usual day for sport. Various sports were played by all levels of society, from poor day labourers to the king, and largely on communal grounds. While archery was the most inclusive exercise undertaken by men of all ranks in communities all over England, coroners' reports confirm that hunting was the most exclusive recreational activity and that at least these 'dangerous' sports and exercises were a man's world, promoting notions of manliness and reducing women to the role of spectators.

An equally rich English sporting culture across all levels of early modern society from the fifteenth to the seventeenth centuries is revealed in Angela Schattner's contribution. Testing a spatial approach as an analytical tool for a history of sport and exercise, the chapter analyses three different types of places and how they were constituted by different social groups as a space for their sports. This approach allows a more detailed contextualization of sports practices by comparison with other leisure and social practices, and shows changes in the use of sporting spaces over time. Communal spaces such as churchyards and commons offered places where parish, village and quarter communities could meet and engage in social activities and sport, thus strengthening community identities. These spaces, however, were never uncontested and conflicts, especially about the use of churchyards, arose between parishioners and church officials. Successful campaigns banning sport from the churchyard in rural areas and the growing pressure of population growth on public spaces in cities encouraged the setting up of new commercialized, semi-public sporting grounds attached to drinking establishments from the end of the sixteenth century. These, in turn, changed the social mode of sport and exercise, favouring new constellations. In the meantime, aristocrats and guilds strengthened their status and group identities by creating their own sporting grounds and limiting access to specified individuals from the fifteenth century, thus underlining their exclusivity.

The chapters in the first section trace early modern sports practices in a variety of source materials, such as diaries, account books, ground plans, court records and coroners' inquest reports to uncover their social and cultural contexts.

While these source materials also have drawbacks and only reveal a part of the rich history of early modern physical culture, they can help to correct and enrich the stereotypical ideal conceptions of contemporary normative discourses. They also show that the early modern period had different sporting cultures which existed side by side and in exchange with each other, and suggest that future research might need to differentiate between a pan-European aristocratic culture of sport and exercise and various regional sporting cultures at the level of the middling and lower ranks. We will also have to differentiate more clearly between developments in rural areas (although these are difficult to grasp as there is a lack of source material) and those in urban and metropolitan areas.

While the chapters in the first part explore a rich early modern sporting culture on a community-supported but also private, non-commercial basis, the second part focuses on a strong commercial interest in sport that can be traced throughout the early modern period. Studies of the socio-economic aspects of early modern sport have so far concentrated on sport as a consumer good for spectators, and especially on aristocratic patronage and the process of professionalization in spectator sports such as boxing, cricket and horse-racing in the eighteenth century.[31] However, the early modern period saw also other forms of commercialization and consumption of sport apart from spectator events. Publicans have long been identified as early leisure and sports entrepreneurs who provided space and provision for both amateur and professional sportsmen in their establishments.[32] This development started much earlier than has been realized, and publicans were not the only entrepreneurs to make a profit from providing sporting spaces. In England and France, a lively urban market for purpose-built, commercially run sports facilities for non-professional sportsmen developed from the fifteenth century.[33] Paris, for example, was Europe's capital of tennis with dozens of commercially run tennis courts catering for the

---

[31] See e.g. David Underdown, *Start of Play: Cricket and Culture in Eighteenth-Century England* (London, 2000), pp. 79–80, pp. 88–90; Vamplew and Kay, 'A Modern Sport?', pp. 125–39; Ruti Ungar, 'A Fashionable and Commercial Amusement: Boxing in Georgian England', in Christiane Eisenberg and Andreas Gestrich (eds), *Cultural Industries in Britain and Germany, Sport, Music and Entertainment from the Eighteenth to the Twentieth Century* (Augsburg, 2012), pp. 23–35.

[32] See e.g. Rowland Bowen, *Cricket: A History of its Growth and Development throughout the World* (London, 1970), p. 262; Dennis Brailsford, *British Sport: A Social History*, pp. 27–8, pp. 77–80; Neil Tranter, *Sport, Economy and Society in Britain 1750–1914* (Cambridge, 1998), pp. 14–15; Brailsford, *A Taste for Diversions*, pp. 108–13; Tony Collins and Wray Vamplew, *Mud, Sweat and Beers: A Cultural History of Sport and Alcohol* (Oxford and New York, 2002), pp. 5–6, 27.

[33] Angela Schattner, '"For the Recreation of gentleman and other fit persons of the better sort": Tennis Courts and Bowling Greens as Early Leisure Venues from Sixteenth- to Eighteenth-Century London and Bath', *Sports in History*, 34/2 (2014): pp. 198–222.

sporting tastes of the nobility and artisans alike. These played a crucial role in the institutionalization of sport in the early modern period and venues like these also provided space for the rising spectator sports events of the seventeenth century.[34] Eighteenth-century developments are therefore not just a take-off phase for what happened in the nineteenth and twentieth centuries, but already have a long tradition.

In his chapter, Christian Jaser uncovers the urban tennis culture of late medieval and early modern Paris, where the tennis court as a commercial venue played a crucial role. Tennis was firmly established in contemporary urban leisure culture. Around 70 tennis courts are traceable between 1300 and 1600; most of them, unsurprisingly, in the noble and university quarters where aristocrats and students were their best customers, but also in artisan quarters which had developed their own tennis culture. While princely ball houses were private institutions reserved for members of the court and invited guests, the largest part of this impressive infrastructure of tennis courts was supported by private initiatives pursuing commercial interests. As sites of leisure, ludic competition, sociability, consumption and betting for players and spectators, commercial tennis courts were also an important real estate investment for wealthy elites in the fifteenth-century building boom, and a source of income for their owners. Proprietors rented playing areas and sports equipment to their customers, and the French guild of ball and racquet manufacturers made enormous profits from the Parisian tennis boom. This business and the Parisians' enthusiasm for the sport could not even be curbed by the city magistrates' attempt to suppress it and to promote military-style exercise such as archery and crossbow-shooting as alternative leisure pursuits.

Another sort of leisure and sports entrepreneur provides the focus of Benjamin Litherland's chapter on boxing celebrities in London in the first half of the eighteenth century. From the end of the seventeenth century, pugilism was transformed from a sideshow at animal sports events to a nationwide spectator sport as a result of the declining interest in animal sports, a rise in London wages and a growing consumer culture. Contemporary boxing stars such as James Figg, George Taylor and Jack Broughton profited from a growing audience of spectators for sport from all ranks. This allowed them to maintain their own amphitheatres where they fought and staged fights as independent sports entrepreneurs. The emergence of a nationwide press meant that these professional boxers could create their own celebrity status and themselves become marketable products. Using newspaper advertisements, press conferences and trade cards, these individuals turned their names and those of their self-run sports venues into nationwide brands by emphasizing their prowess as boxers and the high

---

[34]   Schattner, "'For the Recreation of gentleman and other fit persons of the better sort'", pp. 215–16.

entertainment value of their prizefights, thus becoming a recognizable factor in this early boxing industry. Their celebrity status in turn gave them more opportunities to sell their own promotional materials and to profit from their professed superior boxing skills by successfully establishing and promoting their own schools-at-arms in their amphitheatres.

A number of these professional boxers extended their careers beyond active participation in the sport. As professional trainers they not only taught gentlemen amateurs in their schools-at-arms, but also promoted boxing talent from the lower ranks and prepared professionals for important fights, as David Day shows in his chapter on the development of concepts of training in eighteenth-century Britain. The commercialization of the sport and the huge role of betting in it meant that there was a lively interest in optimizing the performance of the combatants. At the same time, the Enlightenment was promoting a belief in self-improvement and incipient industrialization was setting in motion an interest in streamlining work processes. Boxing manuals disseminated these new views in the eighteenth century. Professional trainers sought out talent, but emphasized that regular practice could compensate for weaknesses. The authors of these manuals spoke of a science of boxing and, in line with the most recent findings of mechanics, included anatomy and physiology in their treatises. In them, they addressed what have remained the key essentials of training to the present day: diet, exercise, psychology and technique. This made boxing acceptable to the upper classes. It also influenced other sports, such as running, which drew on methods of training developed for boxing.

All three chapters show that the consumer and printing revolutions, industrialization and growing mobility promoted the spread and economic exploitation of spectator sports and the professionalization of sportsmen and coaches alike. But this was not a sudden change from early modern developments, which had already been under way since the fifteenth and sixteenth centuries.

Despite, or perhaps because of, the existence of well-developed infrastructure and practice, sport itself was not uncontroversial. Sport and exercise featured in various contemporary discourses: theological–moral, educational and medical,[35] which offered contemporaries an interpretative framework for classifying sporting activity and its usefulness in everyday life, but also employed it for their own agendas. While the moral discourse sought to reform contemporary sporting practice in regard to Christian values,[36] educational and medical discourses discussed sport and fitness in terms of their pedagogical and health benefits as

[35]   Brailsford, *Sport and Society*, see e.g. chapters 'Sport and The Puritans', pp. 122–43, 'The Motion of Limbs', pp. 158–97; Burke, 'The Invention of Leisure in Early Modern Europe', pp. 136–150; Arcangeli, *Recreation in the Renaissance*, see e.g. chapters 'The Medical Discourse', pp. 18–45, 'The Moral Discourse', pp. 46–72.

[36]   See e.g. Angela Schattner, 'Theologies of Sport: Protestant Ideas on Bodily Exercise, Sports Practise and Christian Lifestyle in the Declaration of Sports Controversy in

physical exercise. Exercise was interpreted according to contemporary medical knowledge based on ancient Galenic dietetics, but discussions about beneficial and detrimental motion also considered social status and clearly differentiated between ages, genders and social classes/estates. Analyses of self-narratives make it clear just how frequently athletic activities were undertaken, and how varied they were. Considering contemporary semantics and agendas, the chapters in the third part, 'Promoting Health or Danger? Physical Exercise under Scrutiny', focus on the framework for interpreting sport and exercise constructed in contemporary discourses on gender, education and (public) health, and reflect mutual relationships between practices and discourses.

In his chapter entitled 'Exercise for Women' Alessandro Arcangeli establishes that according to the doctrine of humours, their moist temperament meant that sport was even more important for women than for men in achieving a balance. Against this, however, was the (largely male) view of women in terms of their reproductive function as mothers and wet-nurses, and moral objections. Exercises prescribed for women therefore always involved a smaller range of motion, and were to be carried out more gently and with less physical effort than those for men. Contemporaries also noticed large social differences. It was denied that upper-class women needed any time for recovery because of their 'inactivity', yet their leisure, enforced by social convention, was regarded as a health hazard. Women from the lower rank, by contrast, did not need to worry about a lack of movement. Yet it was often working-class and elite women who ignored these rules of conduct, which suggests that as far as sport was concerned, class/ rank was more significant than gender.

In their chapter, Sandra Cavallo and Tessa Storey show how medical and social ideas influenced and competed with each other. Their study of medical literature and family letters in sixteenth- and seventeenth-century Italy reveals a change in tone regarding exercise in the course of the sixteenth century. In calling for more moderation in exercise, medical health guides and educational literature not only considered health aspects but also reflected the re-shaped lifestyles, values and aspirations of a courtly and urban aristocratic culture. Estate had become an additional category by which the human body could be medically described. Contemporary advice literature increasingly recommended gentler and more 'decorous' exercise befitting the gentleman's or gentlewoman's status that would not overstrain their bodies, which were not used to hard labour. *Pallamaglio* was recommended not only because of its health benefits but also because it was played with clean hands; and walking had become the preferred exercise of men and women in noble families. Hunting as a conventionalized expression of 'noble' identity and warrior–noble masculinity remained important to male as

Seventeenth-Century England', *Archiv für Reformationsgeschichte/Archive for Reformation Studies*, 105 (2014): pp. 353–82.

well as female rulers until the end of the seventeenth century, but the non-ruling nobility pursued it in line with new notions of restrained and decorous gentility.

Martin Dinges investigates health advice dispensed in the German-speaking area in the eighteenth and early nineteenth centuries. Following the ancient tradition of *res non naturales*, a balance between rest and movement was seen as especially beneficial to health. In order to counter alleged degeneration since the Middle Ages, Enlightenment doctors such as Johann Peter Frank prescribed a form of secularized and personalized preventative health care in the context of the state's population and public health policies. It was claimed that the middle classes and aristocracy harmed their children by coddling them but, as in earlier writings, it is striking how many warnings were issued against unconditional participation in sport. In addition, most recommendations were made for boys and young men up to the age of 25, implicitly perpetuating gender and age-specific roles. On the other hand, German-language ego-documents reflect a wide range of forms of movement, many of which, such as riding, running and going for walks, formed a natural part of everyday life. Gymnastics, by contrast, was spread by a deliberate process that stimulated controversial discussion. This new programme provided its own language and framework for interpretation.

All three chapters refer to prescriptive medical and educational sources. At the same time, by presenting examples of sporting *practices* they make clear that contemporary normative discourses, as in other areas of life, only partially shaped the behaviour of people in the early modern period. The (heuristic) difficulty arises, however, of how these physical practices can be grasped beyond a prescriptive literature, as the treatises always also provide a contemporary framework of interpretation.

In the medical treatises of the time, the idea that athletic activities and physical exercise might endanger a person's social status was raised only indirectly, but issues of class and standing are of central importance in Part IV, 'Enhancing or Endangering Status and Identity?'. Many sports were seen as being more problematic with regard to standing in the early modern period than in the nineteenth and twentieth centuries. A closer look at the sources, however, often shows that this did not mean that a specific sport was not practised at all, but only by some groups and not by others (or not in public). Swimming, for instance, despite its usefulness, was initially slow to catch on in bourgeois and aristocratic circles, since it was considered an activity of the lower ranks. In other instances, notions of male honour were at stake. This section also shows how specific sports switched from one social group to another, changing techniques and meaning at the same time. For example, in early modern Japan the social decline of rural samurai brought about a change in sword fighting: once an expression of aristocratic culture, it now became a competitive sport among wealthy peasants.

In the German-speaking lands of the Holy Roman Empire, by contrast, the opposite development could be observed, as B. Ann Tlusty shows in her chapter. From the Middle Ages to the sixteenth century the sword was a weapon carried by all male nobles, burghers and artisans as a sign of their personal honour, but also of their ability to defend the community. By the mid-eighteenth century, however, wearing a sword had become a privilege limited to soldiers, students and nobles. This increasingly restrictive practice emphasized not only the privileges of this elite, but also the authorities' monopoly of power. In an analogous process, shooting fraternities and festivals lost the support of the authorities in the early modern period. From the Middle Ages to the early seventeenth century they had represented towns and provided military training, but these functions were increasingly being replaced by the drill of standing armies. At their peak, *Schützenfeste* had brought together nobles, artisans and burghers who, by participating, had demonstrated their capacity for self-defence, their courage and economic independence.

Taking the example of swimming, by contrast, Rebekka von Mallinckrodt in her chapter traces the social rise of a body technique in eighteenth-century France. Contemporary sources describe swimming as a practice common among the lower ranks, sailors and boatmen. Learning to swim cost very little or nothing, which made it unsuitable to confer social distinction. Enlightenment writers used these egalitarian connotations in formulating their political criticism of the *ancien régime* and to present the ruling elite as 'effete' and 'degenerate'. They also, however, tried to ennoble swimming by integrating it into dietetic and utilitarian frameworks and erudite discourses, by scientific investigation and methodological instruction, thus elevating their own social and economic status as scientific writers. The founding of Paris's first swimming school in 1785 as a relatively exclusive institution and the social rise of some authors writing about swimming show that this strategy was successful. In the long term the influence of these writers was so great that the modern historiography of swimming generally only begins with this textualization. Thus this contribution links up with the discussion of the source basis in the first section of the volume.

In his chapter, Michael Wert shows that Allen Guttmann's paradigm of the development of modern sport cannot adequately describe historical processes in Japan. First, the sportification of swordsmanship, which he takes as his example, took place before the impact of Western influence, and independently of it. Secondly, this process was much more complicated in relation to the social groups involved than Guttmann's paradigm allows. In the seventeenth century, Japanese swordsmanship developed into a cultural art that was less a martial art than a form of physical and mental exercise that was originally open only to the Samurai elite. In the eighteenth century rural commoners who had been ennobled copied this practice to demonstrate their membership of the Samurai. At the same time they developed fencing, which was more competitive and spread among non-warrior practitioners. The need for self-defence in rural areas resulted in the rapid dissemination of fencing in the nineteenth century which even legal prohibitions could not stop. Thus Japanese swordsmanship can be seen, thirdly, as an example of how an art originally without a practical purpose developed into a useful fighting technique.

All three chapters show that it is necessary to differentiate between those who wrote about sport and those who practised it. We furthermore need to look more closely at how shifts occurred in this field and how specific sports were taken over and transformed by different social groups.

We therefore finish this introduction not with a new definition of sport, but with a plea for early modern practices in sport to be investigated in a more differentiated way that takes greater account of their contemporary logic. As the contributions to this volume show, they existed in great variety and numbers. A flexible approach to presenting them seemed more appropriate than a schematic one, as most of the examples discussed here, classified as 'not yet fully developed sports', would miss the most interesting aspects. The real anachronism lies therefore in using a nineteenth-century tool to unlock a period reaching from the sixteenth to the eighteenth century, one that had its own logic and a rich culture of movement. While developments in early modern sport, such as the scientization of sports skills and the professionalization and commercialization of sport build a bridge to later developments, early modern sporting practice was also heavily shaped by contemporary notions of the body, status and honour. These notions influenced not only contemporary sporting fashions but also the incorporation of sport into elite education, the use of sports facilities, training methods and modes of competition. To this extent the early modern period was not only a formative period for later developments, but also an independent one that can be fully understood only when viewed not from nineteenth- and twentieth-century perspectives and criteria, but in the social and cultural context of early modern society.

PART I
What Sports?
Tracing Early Modern Sports Practices

Chapter 1

The Invention of Sports: Early Modern Ball Games

Wolfgang Behringer

That the ball game is the most prominent among all sports, can be seen in all places and more notable towns, and by the example of all Christian princes in particular, who erect separately respectable and large buildings for that nice and sensual exercise.[1]

Hippolytus Guarinonius, 1610

In 1610 the physician Hippolytus Guarinonius (1571–1654)[2] published a massive volume on the physical and spiritual dangers of his period: *Die Grewel der Verwüstung Menschlichen Geschlechts* (The Abominations of Desolation of Humankind). The massive volume, dedicated to Emperor Rudolf II (1552–1612, r. 1576–1612), is divided into seven books, each partitioned

---

[1]   Hippolytus Guarinonius, *Die Grewel der Verwüstung Menschlichen Geschlechts* (OE 1610, 2nd edn Ingolstadt, 1616), pp. 1208–9: 'Daß aber Das Ballspiel das Hauptspiel unter allen Spielen sey, zeigen alle Oerter und namhaffte Stätt/ insonderheit alle Potentaten der Christenheit an/ welche zu Erhaltung dieser schönen und lustigen Ubung/ besonders gelegne und ansehnliche grosse Gebäw führen/ und darzu mit aller Nohtwendigkeit/ auch mit darzu bestimpten und beywohnenden Ballmeistern versehen/ und ihre Jugend/ meistens die Edle Knaben besonders fleß darinnen abrichten lassen.'

[2]   Guarinonius was son of the Imperial court physician Bartholome Guarinoni and Catharina Pellegrini from Trient. He was born in Trient (today Trento in Italy), capital of a prince-bishopric dependent on the dukes of Tyrol. His parents could not marry, and his birth was therefore illegitimate. After his childhood in Trento, in 1583 he followed his father to Vienna, and soon after to Prague, where he attended the Jesuit College until 1593. From 1593–1597 he studied in Padua, where he obtained doctorates in the arts and in medicine. In 1598 he was ordained physician in Trento, and soon after employed by the City of Hall in Tyrol as town physician. In 1607 he was appointed court physician of the Habsburg princesses Maria Christina (1574–1621) and Eleonora (1582–1620), daughters of Archduke Charles II of Innerösterreich (Graz), in the local *Damenstift*. In 1618 Guarinoni's birth was declared legitimate by Pope Paul V, see Jürgen Bücking, *Kultur und Gesellschaft in Tirol 1600 – Des Hippolytus Guarinonius 'Grewel der Verwüstung Menschlichen Geschlechts' (1610) als kulturgeschichtliche Quelle des frühen 17. Jahrhunderts* (Lübeck and Hamburg, 1968); Klaus Amann and Max Siller (eds), *Hippolytus Guarinonius. Akten des 5. Symposiums der Sterzinger Osterspiele 'Die Greuel der Verwüstung menschlichen Geschlechts'. Zur 350. Wiederkehr des Todesjahres von Hippolytus Guarinonius (1571–1654)* (Innsbruck, 2008).

into two parts, covering firstly the positive and secondly the dangerous aspects. Book six, *On Exercise*, is the most extensive publication on sports in German in the early modern period, and – most surprisingly – Guarinonius looks upon most sports very favourably, including all kinds of running, jumping, wrestling, fencing, dancing, jousting, climbing, mountaineering, throwing, swimming, hunting, hawking, fishing, riding, tilting at the ring and similar games, driving carts and sledges, walking, etc. Only their abuse seems dangerous, as for instance exercising excessively, exercising after meals, dancing while pregnant, tightrope walking, and of course any kind of games of chance. However, particularly dangerous is the opposite of sports: idling or loafing.[3]

Two chapters in his book *On Exercise* are treating ball games: Chapter 15 reports *Of Seven Different Forms and the Usage of Ball Games*,[4] followed by chapter 16 where some additional ball games are discussed, such as *pallamaglio*, shuttlecock and bowling. The reason for treating these games separately seems to be that these were considered either games for elderly men (pall mall), or for women, though of all estates, even princesses (shuttlecock), or for common people (throwing stones or pieces of iron, and bowling, which Guarinonius really seems to dislike strongly, although he admits that there were also more refined ways of bowling).[5] Chapter 15 groups together the more demanding ball games. His 'Seven Different Forms' were (1) the *Raggetenspiel*, that is tennis played with rackets, the game with the small ball, formerly played with the hand (e.g. *palma, paume, jeu de paume*), which was still in use in parts of Italy. But there, as well as in France or in Germany, the game was meanwhile usually being played with rackets, either in a ballhouse with a tiled floor, or outdoors on a court. (2) Handball, with a larger ball, widely in use in Italy, but also in Germany, (3) the game with a medium-sized, hard leather ball, struck with a striking device, much in use in Bohemia, but not in Italy, (4) an unnamed, very competitive version of dodgeball, which Guarinonius seems to prefer to all other ball games, (5) an unnamed, rather funny game, where balls had to be pushed into holes, and unsuccessful players should be pitched by the opposite party, (6) another kind of tennis with wooden rackets (*britschen* or *pallets*), but with large inflated balls, played in the imperial ballhouse in Prague, and finally (7) the game with the large ball (*pallone*), inflated with air ('wind'), and struck with the

---

[3]   Guarinonius, *Grewel der Verwüstung*, Book 1: On God; 2: On Human Nature; 3: On the Air; 4: On Nutrition; 5: On Depletion of the Body; 6: On Exercising; 7: Of Sleep, 'Das sechst Buch. Betreffend den sechsten neben natürlichen und unvermeidlichen Hauptpuncten/ Nemblich die Leibsbewegung oder Ubung', pp. 1155–266; 'The other part of book 6', pp. 1235–66.

[4]   Guarinonius, *Grewel der Verwüstung*, Book 6, chapter 15, pp. 1208–13: 'Von siebenerley underschiedlichen Förm und Nutzbarkeit des Ballenspiels', represents the only systematic treatment of ball games in German before the eighteenth century.

[5]   Guarinonius, *Grewel der Verwüstung*, Book 6, chapter 16, pp. 1213–15.

bracciale.[6] Due to his education, Guarinonius understands that the ball games of his time were different from those played in Greek and Roman Antiquity. None of the games with the four ancient kinds of balls – *follis, paganica, trigonalis* and *harpastum* – were comparable to the recent games.[7] Modern ball games had developed into 'the most prominent of all sports',[8] a claim that had not even been made by Antonio Scaino (1524–1612), author of the most important early modern book on ball games. When Scaino refers to 'this game of ours which is to be placed before all other games' in his concluding remarks, this is mostly for medical reasons.[9]

'The Most Prominent among all Sports'

Guarinonius opens his chapter on ball games by noticing that they were 'age-old', and that they were 'common among all people'.[10] Among the Greeks and the Romans ball games were so popular that already Pliny had tried to determine who had been the originator. But his claim that a certain Pythone had invented the games and had started this wonderful and healthy exercise, seems hardly credible. Guarinonius does not mention that already Homer had mentioned ball games, and that Caesar and Augustus counted among the most prominent enthusiasts in ancient Rome.[11] As a medical doctor it was important for Guarinonius that already the 'medicines' king', Galen, the famous doctor of a school of gladiators in Pergamon, whose medical teachings were taught at European universities well into the eighteenth century, had written a booklet on exercise by ball games, and that already this example of erudition had proven

---

[6]   Guarinonius, *Grewel der Verwüstung*, pp. 1209–13. Surprisingly Guarinonius mentions neither *scanno*, nor *calcio*/football, although these ball games were treated by Scaino and other authors. Sometimes misleading classifications are provided by: Erwin Mehl, 'Von siebenerley unterschiedlichen Förm und Nutzbarkeit des Ballenspiels', *Die Leibeserziehung* (1957): pp. 200–207.

[7]   Guarinonius, *Grewel der Verwüstung*, p. 1207: 'inmassen dann das Ballspielen zu unsern Zeiten ... auch ohne Zweifel weit fürtrefflicher und kunstreicher als damals/ also haben wir auch deren Spiel weit mehr Weiß und Fürmen/ als sie hetten'.

[8]   Guarinonius, *Grewel der Verwüstung*, p. 1208.

[9]   Giorgio Nonni (ed.), Antonio Scaino, *Trattato del giuoco della palla* (OE Venice, 1555, Reprint Urbino, 2000): 'che sia degno esser antposto a tutti altri esercitii de'giuochi'. In English quoted from: W. Kershaw and P.A. Negretti (eds and trans.), Antonio Scaino, *Treatise on the Game of the Ball* (OE Venice, 1555, London, 1984), p. 191.

[10]   Guarinonius, *Grewel der Verwüstung*, p. 1208: 'Das Ballspiel ist nicht weniger uhralt/ als allen Völckern bishero annehmlich'.

[11]   Rolf Hurschmann, 'Ballspiele', in *Der Neue Pauly. Enzyklopädie der Antike*, vol. 2, pp. 426–7.

that the game with the little ball was of the utmost usefulness for the exercise of all parts of the body. Galen's text on ball games had indeed been printed in Milan in 1562, and reprinted afterwards, and it was this publication Guarinonius was referring to.[12] Here the claim of prominence was supported by *anciennité* as well as the ball games' particular importance for health. The reference to Galen was of course commonplace, already Scaino had placed it most prominently in his booklet, in the dedication, as well as in the foreword, in the last part of the book (chapter 3) and again in his concluding remarks.[13] But since Galen was at the heart of the medical curriculum, authors throughout the fifteenth century had referred to his remarks on the ball game, for instance Leon Battista Alberti (1406–1472).[14] And Hieronymus Mercurialis (1530–1606), court physician of Emperor Maximilian II, professor of medicine in Padua, and subsequently in Bologna and in Pisa, had treated the ancient ball games in his path-breaking six books on gymnastics, first published in Venice in 1569 and frequently reprinted afterwards.[15]

Guarinonius's second argument is that in all European towns large separate buildings had been constructed for the ball sports, equipped with ball masters for the training of the youth. Princes of all European territories had erected ballhouses in the course of the sixteenth century, and we shall see that this had been a recent development indeed. All these ballhouses were not just designed and built, but had to be maintained, which meant permanent expenses for refurbishment, equipment and salaries.

His third reason why ball games were deemed the most prominent of all sports, emphasizes an aspect quite contrary to the former: that for those willing to play the costs were low. Virtually everybody, even the poor, could start playing, as soon as they were able to buy a ball, or to make one themselves. Ball games could be played by everybody, just for fun, or in order to tire oneself out. One could even play ball alone, if no fellow players were available, as Guarinonius explains, by jacking the ball up in the air, or shooting it against a wall.[16] The

---

[12]   Galen, *Il libro dell' esercitio della palla* (Mailand, 1562).

[13]   Kershaw and Negretti, Scaino, *Treatise on the Game of the Ball*, pp. 24, 191.

[14]   Leon Battista Alberti, *I primi tre libri Della Famiglia* (OE 1440, Reprint Florence, 1946), pp. 104–6.

[15]   Hieronymus Mercurialis, *De Arte Gymnastica libri sex, in quibus exercitationum omnium vetustarum genera, loca, modi, facultates et quidquid denique ad corporis humani exercitationes pertinent, diligenter explicatur* (OE Venice, 1569, Venice, 1587), pp. 83–95. Mercurialis taught at Padua from 1569 to 1587, but when Guarinoni took up his studies there in 1593, Mercurialis had already moved to nearby Bologna, and soon after to Pisa.

[16]   Guarinonius, *Grewel der Verwüstung*, p. 1208: 'Das Ballspielen aber ist meniglichen/ und sogar den armen/ all denen befreyt/ so nur mit Balln zu kauffen/ oder selbst einen zu machen vermögen. Uber das nimpt auch mit dieser gelegenheit zu/ daß solches Ballspiel meniglich für sich selbsten allein zu gutem vergnügen/ und zu guter Müdigkeit/ wann er

importance of Guarinonius's care for the common people can be taken from the fact that previous authors on ball games, and foremost Antonio Scaino in his famous *Treatise on the Game of the Ball*, unanimously tried to portray ball games as a noble exercise, akin to noble people. But even Scaino had to admit that some of the ball games required more strength than most of the noblemen could afford. *Pallone*, for instance, to him seemed to be more suitable to craftsmen, or soldiers. King James I (1566–1625) – in contrast – mentions but a number of ball games ('playing the caitche or tennise ... palle maille & suche like other faire & plaisant field games') in his instruction to Prince Henry (1594–1612), but remains clear that 'the honorablest & most commendable games that ye can use, are on horse-back'.[17] Guarinonius seems to have missed this royal recommendation, and not even noticed its German translation, dedicated to Prince-Elector Palatine Frederick IV (1574–1610).[18]

'Playing Balloon all day long': A Case Study of Palatine Princes[19]

Not by coincidence was the British royal sports instruction dedicated to Prince-Elector Palatine Frederick IV. It was yet unknown, that King James's daughter Elizabeth Stuart (1596–1662), and Frederick's son Frederick V (1596–1632), the future 'winter king' of Bohemia,[20] would marry soon after.[21] What was manifest though was that Frederick IV counted among the most sportive princes of Europe. The Protestant hero – he founded the Protestant Union in order to propel the Calvinist cause in Central Europe[22] – was vituperated by Jakob

---

keinen gesellen hat/ sich üben kann/ wann er nun den Ballen in die Höch/ oder ein weil an ein Wand hinan schlegt/ so wird ihme der Balln gnug/ hindersich/ fürsich/ auff der Seiten/ und aller Orten im Widerschnellen/ zu schaffen geben.'

[17]   James I, *Basilikon Doron, His maiesties instructions to his dearest sonne, Henry the prince* (London, 1603), pp. 120–21.

[18]   James I, *Basilikon doron oder Instruktion und Underrichtung Jakobi deß Ersten dieses Namens in Engelandt […] an Seiner Kön. Mayr. geliebten Sohn Printz Henrichen* (Speyer, 1604), pp. 131–2. The dedication merely says 'Friedrich von der Pfalz', and it seems more likely that this refers rather to the ruling prince than to his under-age son, who as Frederick V would later marry Elisabeth Stuart, James I's daughter.

[19]   Jakob Wille (ed.), 'Das Tagebuch und Ausgabenbuch des Churfürsten Friedrich IV. von der Pfalz', *Zeitschrift für die Geschichte des Oberrheins*, 3 (1880): pp. 201–95, entry 12 March 1596: 'Haben wir mit den ballonen den ganzen Tag gespilet.'

[20]   Brennan C. Pursell, *The Winter King: Frederick V of the Palatinate and the Coming of the Thirty Years' War* (Aldershot, 2003).

[21]   Magnus Rüde, *England und Kurpfalz im werdenden Mächteeuropa. Konfession – Dynastie – kulturelle Ausdrucksformen* (Stuttgart, 2007).

[22]   Albrecht Ernst and Anton Schindling (eds), *Union und Liga 1608/09. Konfessionelle Bündnisse im Reich – Weichenstellung zum Religionskrieg?* (Stuttgart, 2010).

Wille, the editor of his diary, even 300 years later: In the prince-elector's private notations there is nothing on religion, or politics, but notes on all kinds of sports and games on a daily basis. And Frederick's expense registers confirm that picture and add more information about betting and wagers. Historian Moriz Ritter (1840–1923) wrote derogatively: 'The young prince was but an empty character, driven by an insatiable lust for hunting and tournaments, dancing and noising revelries.'[23] Even in this rejection Frederick was being stereotyped, since in his diary there is no particular enthusiasm for dancing, but rather for tilting at the ring and particularly for ball games. A peace-loving, sporting prince obviously failed to meet the expectations of nineteenth-century nationalists: They were looking for heroic warriors, not for ball players, as paragons for adolescents. But even on Sundays, and with other Protestant leaders, as the princes of Anhalt, Frederick preferred playing ball games: 'Played balloon with prince Christian and prince Bernert after sermon.'[24]

In historiography, Palatine princes have so far neither been related to sports nor to ball games in particular, although a good number of sources offer such an opportunity: First, investment in arts demonstrates their enthusiasm for sports, as for instance a large tapestry in the former residence of Prince Palatine Johann Casimir (1543–1592) at Kaiserslautern, representing a game of *pallone*.[25] Second, diaries provide insights into the minds, since among Protestant princes diaries and correspondence were recommended as a token of introspection, and like their Hessian counterparts,[26] the Palatine princes were particularly eager in keeping diaries. Third, serial sources like account books provide additional evidence. Princes would not always bother to mention physical exercises in their diaries, but expense registers are telling of their favourable treatment of travelling ball game champions, the employment of itinerant ball teachers, the purchase of sports equipment, and their expenditure for betting. Without the

---

[23]   Moriz Ritter, 'Friedrich IV', in *Allgemeine Deutsche Biographie*, 7 (1877): pp. 612–21: 'Der junge Fürst war eben eine innerlich leere Natur, von unersättlichem Hang nach Jagd und Ritterspielen, nach Bällen und lärmenden Lustbarkeiten.'

[24]   Wille, 'Das Tagebuch und Ausgabenbuch des Churfürsten Friedrich IV': entry 14 March 1596: 'Hab ich mit fürst Christian und fürst Bernert nach der bredig deß ballonnen gespilet.' Christian von Anhalt-Bernburg (1568–1630) was Frederick's governor of the Upper Palatinate; Bernhard VIII von Anhalt (1571–1596), died in the Turkish Wars some months after the Heidelberg tennis match.

[25]   Martin Dolch, *Das Ballonspiel auf dem großen Wandteppich im Pfalzgrafensaal* (Kaiserslautern, 1978). The tapestry was commissioned by Johann Casimir von Pfalz-Simmern (1543–1592), who resided in Kaiserslautern from 1559 to 1583. Johann Casimir was the second son of the Calvinist Prince Elector Palatine Fredrick III. From 1583, Johann Casimir served as guardian of his nephew Frederick IV and as administrator of the Palatinate.

[26]   Helga Meise, *Das archivierte Ich. Schreibkalender und höfische Repräsentation in Hessen-Darmstadt 1624–1790* (Darmstadt, 2002).

account books we would not know that wagering was indispensably connected with ball games, and what sums were spent.[27] And fourth, sports are mentioned in the correspondence, though in editions there is a danger that the editors cut out subjects that seemed unimportant to them, unless the correspondents were hunting with Louis XIV of France, as for instance Elizabeth Charlotte Duchesse d' Orleans, née Princess von der Pfalz, known as Lieselotte von der Pfalz in her country of birth (1652–1722).[28]

In the Palatinate, we can observe the rise of ball sports in the course of the sixteenth century. An early champion of Protestantism, Ottheinrich von der Pfalz (1502–1559), reports a four-day shooting competition held in mid-October 1523 in the bishop's residence at Bruchsal, where prince elector Ludwig V (r. 1508–1544), his Lutheran brother and successor Prince Palatine Frederic II (r. 1544–1556), Prince Palatine Wolfgang as well as the bishops of Freising and Speyer, the Catholic princes palatine Philipp (r. 1499–1541) and George (r. 1513–1529) – the latter as the host – took part.[29] What sounds like a family meeting across confessional divides, turns into a mass sporting event at the next shooting contest at Heidelberg (30 May–5 June 1524). Again all Palatine brothers and cousins turned up, but there were furthermore 652 shooters, who were being entertained at 90 tables for a whole week. Afterwards the Palatine princes attended a dance at Stuttgart, hosted by Archduke Ferdinand of Austria, who had occupied the country in the name of Emperor Charles V, then they travelled to Munich to watch the footraces at the annual St Jacob's Fair (*Jakobidult*), to see the horse races, and to participate in the dancing, hunting and shooting, organized by Duke Albrecht IV of Bavaria. Like the Palatine princes, the Bavarian dukes were members of the Wittelsbach dynasty. Travelling from the Munich games, the princes attended a hunting party in the prince-bishopric of Freising, a shooting in the Upper Palatinate, and another shooting competition in the Young Palatinate, a recently created territory around Neuburg on the Danube. From there, they went by ship to the Imperial City of Regensburg (Ratisbon), for yet another prize shooting. These sporting holidays lasted without any interruption from May to December 1524, with little reference to the Reformation, the negotiations at the Imperial diets at Speyer, Augsburg and Regensburg that same year.[30] All of these Palatine princes were young, they were enthusiastic sportsmen, but ball games were not yet of

---

[27]　Wille, 'Das Tagebuch und Ausgabenbuch des Churfürsten Friedrich IV': pp. 201–95.

[28]　Wilhelm Ludwig Holland (ed.), *Elisabeth-Charlotte, Herzogin von Orléans, Briefe aus den Jahren 1676–1722*, 6 vols (Stuttgart, 1867–1881).

[29]　Hans Rott, 'Das Tagebuch Ott Heinrichs [1521–1534]', *Mitteilungen zur Geschichte des Heidelberger Schlosses*, 6 (1912): pp. 46–133, p. 95.

[30]　Rott, 'Das Tagebuch Ott Heinrichs', pp. 98–9.

much importance. Clearly it made sense that a tournament book was dedicated to one of these princes, Johann II von Pfalz-Simmern (1492–1557).[31]

Perhaps it was the Calvinistic Palatine Prince Johann Casimir von Pfalz-Simmern – who had been educated at the courts of France and of Lorraine, and as Duke in Kaiserslautern (from 1559) had commissioned the balloon tapestry – who introduced the inclination to ball games to the Palatinate.[32] In the diaries of his charge, Prince Elector Palatine Frederick IV, almost no day lapses – except for days of travelling, of sickness and of the highest church holidays – without ball games, tilting at the ring, hunting, shooting, or at least gambling (cards, dices). In the Electoral capital Heidelberg, there were organized spaces for each of these activities, including a ballhouse next to the castle, but even outside Heidelberg the prince took every opportunity for exercising: In Amberg, capital of the Upper Palatinate, he engaged in no less sports than shooting, tilting at the ring, *pallone*, sledging, skating, throwing snow balls and fencing. In nearby Neumarkt, he insisted on playing *pallone*, tilting at the ring and sledging. In the Electoral Palatinate, he engaged in shooting with crossbows (Mannheim), rifles (Zweibrücken, Wersau), tilting at the ring (Frankental, Mannheim, Zweibrücken and Wersau) and shooting (Kaiserslautern, Ramstein, and Zweibrücken). His sporting itinerary continues in neighbouring territories, where he was playing *pallone* and tilting at the ring (Ansbach in the Margraviate, Stuttgart in Württemberg, Baden-Durlach and Baden-Baden, Nassau-Saarbrücken, Nassau-Ottweiler) and shooting with rifles (Nassau-Saarbrücken, Imperial City of Straßburg). The best sporting facilities were to be found within his residence at Heidelberg: There was a ballhouse, firing ranges and shooting galleries, facilities for shooting with crossbows and with rifles, for tilting at the ring, for *pallone* and *jeu de paume*, for fencing and wrestling, in winter for sledging, and there was a bear garden for blood sports. In both his capitals – in Heidelberg and Amberg – Frederick repeatedly noted that he had been playing ball 'all day long'.[33]

His account book – preserved from June 1599 to June 1600 – sharpens our knowledge of this prince's sporting enthusiasm. Here we can find the details

---

[31]   Georg Rüxner, *Thurnier-Buch. Von Anfang, Ursprung und Herkommen der Thurnier in teutscher Nation* [dedicated to Johann II. von Pfalz-Simmern] (Simmern, 1530, Reprint with a foreword by Willi Wagner, Solingen, 1997). This volume was reprinted many times in the sixteenth century. Johann II was the father of Prince Elector Frederick III.

[32]   Friedrich von Bezold, 'Johann Casimir, Pfalzgraf bei Rhein', in *Allgemeine Deutsche Biographie* (ADB), vol. 14 (1881), pp. 307–14. The vast edition of his correspondence was obviously purged from anything non-political: Friedrich von Bezold (ed.), *Johann Casimir von der Pfalz: Briefe des Pfalzgrafen Johann Casimir mit verwandten Schriftstücken, 1576–1592*, 3 vols (Munich, 1882–1903). Johann Casimir was a son of Frederick III, and guardian of Frederick IV.

[33]   Wille, 'Das Tagebuch und Ausgabenbuch des Churfürsten Friedrich IV. von der Pfalz': pp. 201–95, here pp. 203–243.

about the prince elector's betting losses in games against 'a French ball player in the ball house', not less than 18 fl. on 13 July, and again 53 fl. against an Italian professional on 29 and 30 July. On 23 October, the prince elector bought from an elderly Italian ball player a number of rackets, and lost against another Italian master no less than 106 fl. on 27 October. On 2 November, the prince lost 180 fl. to another Italian professional, and furthermore he bought rackets (*racketen*) again, this time for 53 fl. This was much more than a day labourer could earn in a year. Maybe the wagers served as a kind of compensation for the itinerant ball-playing masters, a kind of salary, and certainly as a recognition of their mastership. In other cases, Frederick simply sponsored itinerant Italian 'ball players', or an 'Italian ballplayer boy', maybe because he won the matches, and had to find alternative ways of compensation. French professionals were always experts of the *jeu de paume* (tennis), whereas Italians were offering *pallone* matches as well. In the diary shooting and tilting at the ring seem to prevail, but the account book reveals the importance of the ball games: Occasionally, Frederick supports a foreign fencing master, who offers a fencing school in the shooting area of Heidelberg, and on one occasion he offers his servants Fritz and Hans at Mannheim 3 fl. for their success in a footrace. But most of the payments were related to ball games.[34] Unlike the diary, the account book proves the claim of Guarinonius, that 'like in Italy, in Germany most princes and lords are not being ashamed of playing with chaps from the lower orders, if they are well enough trained in that game'.[35]

Wagering in ball matches was obviously habitual among the princes. On 8 August, Frederick IV lost 26 fl. to the Rhinegrave Johann Casimir von Salm-Kyrburg (1577–1651), on 1 November he lost to him not less than 101 fl., and the same day 400 fl. to Rhinegrave Philipp. The Rhinegraves were distant relatives of the Palatines, but their scattered small territories were comparatively poor. It seems unlikely though that Frederick felt the necessity to sponsor them like itinerant ball players. Betting was customary also with equally important princes. Later in November Frederick lost lesser sums to the Calvinist Landgrave Moritz von Hessen-Kassel (1572–1632, r. 1592–1632) (13 November),[36] who sponsored tennis halls in his territory in order to keep the youth away from alcohol and laziness.[37] Frederick also lost to the Calvinist Count Albrecht Otto von Solms-Laubach (1576–1610) (17 November),

34   Wille, 'Das Tagebuch und Ausgabenbuch des Churfürsten Friedrich IV. von der Pfalz': pp. 244–95.

35   Guarinonius, *Grewel der Verwüstung*, p. 1209.

36   Gerhard Menk (ed.), *Landgraf Moritz der Gelehrte. Ein Kalvinist zwischen Wissenschaft und Politik* (Marburg, 2000).

37   Wilhelm Streib, 'Geschichte des Ballhauses', *Leibesübungen und körperliche Erziehung*, 54 (1935): pp. 373–82, 419–32, 448–64, cit. p. 449.

whose sister Agnes (1578–1602) was married to Landgrave Moritz;[38] and to the Lutheran Duke Christoph von Braunschweig-Lüneburg (1566–1633).[39] One of the preferred domestic tennis partners of the prince elector seems to have been his 'Küchenmeister' Franz von Hammerstein, whom he owed 22 fl. in the Heidelberg ballhouse on 5 September, and another 50 fl. on 2 November. Wagering, like the sports, was just for fun, and never endangered the prince's household, nor his religious conscience. All the betting losses and purchase of sports equipment remained unimportant compared to his expenditure for textiles, jewellery, tapestry, paintings and horses, luxury goods, which amounted to about 20,000 fl. within that same year.[40]

Among the more important festivities of the period were the marriage celebrations of Duke Wolfgang Wilhelm von Pfalz-Neuburg (1578–1653, r. 1614–1653), whose succession to the territories of Jülich and Cleves in the Lower Rhine region triggered the related wars. His marriage marked a turning point in the history of European confessionalism, since in the aftermath of Henry IV's conversion he was the first Protestant prince of importance to convert to Catholicism. This was inaugurated by his wedding with a Catholic princess of Bavaria in Munich in 1613, a daughter of the Wittelsbach Duke Wilhelm V of Bavaria and Renata of Lorraine. And the celebrations were modelled on their wedding festivities of 1568, characterized by widely reported tournaments and dancing events.[41] Wolfgang Wilhelm surely enjoyed the stately noble exercises, although he had different inclinations. As a prince he had taken down notes, which allow for deep insights into his daily schedule. In many cases his routines are summarized by just one sentence: 'In the morning council, in the afternoon pallonen.'[42] The prince was playing with the big ball from noon until the break of dawn. He was another Palatine sports enthusiast.

[38]   Heiner Borggrefe, Vera Lüpkes and Hans Ottomeyer (eds), *Moritz der Gelehrte. Ein Renaissancefürst in Europa* (Eurasburg, 1997).

[39]   Wilhelm Sauer, 'Christian von Braunschweig-Lüneburg', in *ADB*, 4 (1876), pp. 162–3.

[40]   Wille, 'Das Tagebuch und Ausgabenbuch des Churfürsten Friedrich IV': pp. 244–95.

[41]   Massimo Troiano, *Die Münchener Fürstenhochzeit von 1568. Zwiegespräche über die Festlichkeiten bei der Hochzeit des bayerischen Erbherzogs Wilhelm V. mit Renata von Lothringen* (Munich, 1568, reprint Munich and Salzburg, 1980).

[42]   Friedrich Zoepfl, 'Ein Tagebuch des Pfalzgrafen Wolfgang Wilhelm von Pfalz-Neuburg aus dem Jahr 1593', *Jahrbuch des Historischen Vereins Dillingen*, 37 (1924): pp. 136–46. Friedrich Zoepfl, 'Ein Tagebuch des Pfalzgrafen Wolfgang Wilhelm von Pfalz-Neuburg aus dem Jahr 1600', *Jahrbuch des Historischen Vereins Dillingen*, 38 (1925): pp. 72–99. Friedrich Zoepfl, 'Ein Tagebuch des Pfalzgrafen Wolfgang Wilhelm von Pfalz-Neuburg aus dem Jahr 160', *Jahrbuch des Historischen Vereins Dillingen*, 39/40 (1926/1927): pp. 173–209.

Ball game enthusiasm did not end with the fall of the Calvinist Elector Palatine Frederick V, who joined the Oranien-Nassau relatives in Dutch exile.[43] The famous sketch-book by Adriaen van de Venne (1589–1662), providing marvellous illustrations of *pallone*, tennis, shuttlecock (of two ladies), *pallamaglio*, billiard and other sports, was perhaps commissioned by Frederick V, who is several times depicted in the album, as well as other members of the family, including Elizabeth Stuart, and the new Stadholder Friedrich Heinrich von Oranien-Nassau (1584–1647).[44] Frederick's son, Prince Rupert (1619–1682) in particular remained sportive until an older age,[45] and still counted among the best tennis players of the British nation when he was close to 50 years old, as we can take from Samuel Pepys's diaries (2 September 1667).[46] Rupert was the younger brother of the ruling Palatine Prince Elector Karl Ludwig (1617–1680) and of Sophie of Hannover (1630–1714), the Palatine princess, who justified the Hanoverian succession to the English throne. Also the French progeny of the Palatines remained passionate ball players. Rupert's niece Liselotte von der Pfalz (1652–1722), daughter of Karl Ludwig and spouse of the Duke of Orléans, was in deep sorrow that her son, the young Duke of Orléans, would contract serious diseases from over-passionate ball playing, swimming, and visits to his mistress.[47]

'Not retrieved from anything Ancient': A Renaissance of Ball Games?

The Renaissance, it could be argued, brought about a renaissance of the ball games. However, it is necessary to keep in mind that ball games were practised earlier, as can be seen by the famous quote from William FitzStephens (c. 1174–1183), describing the Shrove Tuesday activities in the vicinity of London:

> After lunch all the youth of the city go out into the fields to take part in a ball game. The students of each school have their own ball; the workers from each city craft are also carrying their balls. Older citizens, fathers, and wealthy citizens come on horseback to watch their juniors competing, and to relive their own youth

[43] His mother Luise Juliana von Oranien-Nassau (1576–1644) was a daughter of the Dutch national hero Wilhelm I von Oranien (born Count of Nassau-Dillenburg, 1533–1584). Her half-brother Moritz von Oranien (1567–1625) was governor of the Netherlands, followed by their half-brother Friedrich Heinrich von Oranien (1584–1647).

[44] Butt Johnson, 'Van de Venne's Album', Giornale Nuovo, 25 August 2007. Reproductions in: Martin Royalton-Kisch (ed.), *Adriaen van de Venne's Album in the Department of Prints and Drawings in the British Library* (London, 1988).

[45] Frank Kitson, *Prince Rupert: Admiral and General-at-Sea* (London, 1998).

[46] Samuel Pepys, *Die Tagebücher. Vollständige Ausgabe in neun Bänden* (Berlin, 2010), vol. 8, p. 525.

[47] Holland, *Elisabeth-Charlotte, Herzogin von Orléans*, vol. 1, p. 412.

vicariously: you can see their inner passions aroused as they watch the action and get caught up in the fun being had by the carefree adolescents.[48]

Bans on ball games started as early as 1314 because of their noisiness and troublesomeness, and in France they were banned in 1319 and 1331. Edward III of England (1312–1377) banned ball games in 1349, because they distracted manpower from archery, and in 1363 he banned handball, football and hockey together with throwing stones, and blood sports.[49] Ball games were not recognized as being politically desirable at that point. And not even the famous *Book of Sports* in the first half of the seventeenth century counts ball games among the lawful sports.[50] Most recently, Anna Maria Nada Patrone has provided a survey of the position of ball games in the Late Middle Ages, demonstrating that there have always been kinds of ball games, but that they were not particularly valued until the advent of Renaissance enthusiasm for ancient sports.[51]

So it clearly made a difference, when school reformers as Pietro Paolo Vergerio (1370–1444) from Capodistria (today Koper in Slovenia) included ball sports among the exercises for a systematic physical training of the body in order to counterbalance the exercise of the brain.[52] And it was the small Italian states that put theory into action: Commissioned by Margrave Gianfrancesco I Gonzaga of Mantua (1395–1444, r. 1407–1444), the first humanistic gymnasium – or court academy – was created by the scholar Vittorino da Feltre (1378–1446) around 1425.[53] In his *Casa Giocosa* – in addition to training in languages – the pupils were taught riding, fencing, swimming, archery and playing various ball games,[54] as was already emphasized by the Florentine chronicler Vespasiano

---

[48]   Francis Peabody Magoun, 'Football in Medieval England and Middle-English Literature', *The American Historical Review*, 35/1 (1929): pp. 33–45.

[49]   Morris Marples, *A History of Football* (London, 1954), p. 32.

[50]   Lionel Arthur Govett, *The King's Book of Sports: A History of the Declarations of James I and Charles I. as to the Use of Lawful Sports on Sundays, with a reprint of the declarations* (London, 1890).

[51]   Anna Maria Nada Patrone, 'I giochi di palla nel Piemonte del Tardo Medioevo', in Andrea Merlotti (ed.), *Giochi di palla nel Piemonte medievale e moderno* (Rocca de Baldi, 2001), pp. 43–76.

[52]   Pietro Paolo Vergerio, *De ingenuis moribus et liberalibus adolescentiae studiis* (OE Venice, 1402, Venice, 1472).

[53]   Gregor Müller, *Mensch und Bildung im italienischen Renaissance-Humanismus* (Baden-Baden, 1984), pp. 73–5.

[54]   Jean-Claude Margolin, 'Une école d'humanism et de sports au XV siècle: la "Giocosa" de Mantove', *Education physique e de sports*, 49 (1960): pp. 56–7. John Mclelland, 'Leibesübungen in der Renaissance und die freien Künste', in Arnd Krüger and John McLelland (eds), *Der Anfang des modernen Sports in der Renaissance* (London, 1984), pp. 85–110.

da Bisticci.[55] Vittorino recommended systematic training and ball games on a daily basis. And Cees de Bondt renders it likely that one of the first purpose-built tennis halls was created for the *Casa Giocosa*, adjacent to Mantua's ducal palace, in the mid-fifteenth century.[56] The second modern gymnasium was commissioned in 1429 by Margrave Niccolò III d' Este of Ferrara (1383–1441) for the education of his son Leonello (1407–1450). Its director became Guarino da Verona (1370–1460), another famous Renaissance scholar, who promoted the ball games as one of the principal exercises in the education of young noblemen. Guarino was inspired by Pliny the Younger's *Epistolae*, which he had discovered in 1419, where the game of *pila* was recommended as particularly beneficial for both body and mind. From 1436, Guarino directly influenced the architecture of the Villa Belriguardo, which was endued with a ball court, resembling Pliny's description of *sphaeristerium* courts as part of his Tusculum and Laurentine villas.[57]

It was a result of this Renaissance education programme, that a first generation of princes, as Ludovico III Gonzaga of Mantua (1412–1478),[58] Ercole I d'Este of Ferrara (1431–1505),[59] or Federico da Montefeltro (1422–1482) in Urbino, started constructing ball courts in their gardens, and tennis halls within their *palazzi*, sometimes by converting already existing halls. They represented something like a founding generation, determined to create particular architectural spaces for ball sports. The military leader Francesco I Sforza (1401–1466), who managed to usurp the duchy of Milan in 1450, and felt the necessity to acquire legitimacy, started his reign with hiring a number of tennis professionals, and with commissioning tennis courts in several castles (Villanova, Cassino, Milano). His son Galeazzo Maria Sforza (1444–1476), married to a daughter of Ludovico III Gonzaga, commissioned a famous oversized *sala della balla* in the Castello Sforzesco, where visitors like the King of Denmark were asked to watch the tennis professionals play.[60] Galeazzo started betting at the tennis court in Ferrara at the age of 13. His preserved account

---

[55]   Bernd Roeck (ed.), Vespasiano da Bisticci, *Grosse Männer und Frauen der Renaissance* (OE Florence, 1483, Munich, 1995), pp. 283–4.

[56]   Cees De Bondt, *Royal Tennis in Renaissance Italy* (Turnhout, 2006), pp. 36–7.

[57]   Eugenio Garin, *L'educazione in Europa (1400–1600)* (Bari, 1957), pp. 139–40; Renate Schweyen, *Guarino Veronese. Philosophie und humanistische Pädagogik* (München, 1973); De Bondt, *Royal Tennis*, pp. 51–2.

[58]   Eleonore Gürtler, 'Ludovico III. Gonzaga (1412–1478), 2. Markgraf von Mantua', in *Circa 1500. Leonhard und Paola – ein ungleiches Paar. De ludo globi – Vom Spiel der Welt. An der Grenze des Reiches*, Landesausstellung 2000 (Mailand, 2000), p. 78.

[59]   Thomas Touhy, *Herculean Ferrara. Ercole d'Este, 1471–1505, and the Invention of a Ducal Capital* (Cambridge, 1996).

[60]   Gregory Lubkin, *A Renaissance Court: Milan under Galeazzo Maria Sforza* (Berkeley, 1994).

books of the years 1472–1476 list the names of all his opponents and the amount of the wagers. When he visited Lorenzo de Medici in Florence in 1476, no less than 10 professional tennis players (*giochatori da balla*) accompanied him to demonstrate their skills.[61]

With respect to the Renaissance, it is worth mentioning that the contemporaries, although referring to ancient Greek and Roman authors, were emphasizing that the contemporary ball sports were indeed novel. They were no ancient remains, and they had not yet been in use in this form in the Middle Ages. When Paolo Cortese (1465–1510), apostolic secretary of a good number of popes and bishop of Urbino, provided the first detailed list of ball games in a book on *The Office of Cardinals*, he proposes explicitly that the *pallone* game had been invented two generations ago by Niccolo III d'Este. The author assures the reader that the pope – at this time Julius II (1443–1513, pope 1503–1513), to whom the publication was dedicated – agrees with the idea, that ball playing was entirely appropriate for cardinals. Cortese distinguishes between games with the large inflated ball (*pugno, lamina pugilari* [= *pallone*], *tripode* [= *Scanno*], *pedum ictu et repulse* [= Football, or *Calcio*]) on the one hand, and games with the small ball (*pila trigonali*) on the other. Senators and cardinals should avoid the big ball, since the movements required could harm their dignity. The same is true for *pallamaglio*, which may appear ridiculous. Absolutely recommendable seem the games with the small ball (*incussorium, trigonium, parietarium, funarium*). According to Martin Dolch the first three of these games did not exist at all, but the latter (lat. *funale* = cord) means *pallacorda*, that is tennis. This is what Cortese recommends without restriction, since it exercises all parts of the body and creates a lot of pleasure and recreation.[62] It seems likely that the cardinals' enthusiasm was modelled on the juvenile Cardinal Ippolito d'Este (1479–1520), who had been appointed cardinal aged 14, and had indeed commissioned a tennis hall in his Roman palazzo.[63]

[61]   De Bondt, *Royal Tennis*, pp. 41–2.

[62]   Paolo Cortese, *De Cardinalatu* (San Gimignano, 1510). The work is divided in three books: I. Ethicus, II. Oeconomicus, III. Politicus. The second book deals with economy, family and friends, chapter 6 is on healthy living (*de regimine sanitatis*). The original lacks pagination. The paragraphs on the ball games (*de ludo pilae*) are – next to a facsimile of the original – translated in: Martin Dolch, 'Paolo Corteses Bemerkungen über das Ballspiel der geistlichen Würdenträger (1510)', *Stadion*, 8/9 (1982/1983): pp. 85–97.

[63]   Ippolito was a grandson of Niccolo III, son of Ercole I. d'Este (1431–1505), and brother of Isabella d'Este, Beatrice d'Este and Alfonso I d'Este.

Antonio Scaino – who dedicated his book on the ball games to Alfonso II d'Este (1533–1597, r. 1559–1597),[64] the ambitious grandson of Ercole I d'Este[65] – explicitly states in his dedication, that 'I have taken upon myself to produce a work that is new & traced in my own colors & not retrieved from anything ancient, or drawn from anything modern'.[66] Hippolytus Guarinonius does not dismiss the idea of a possible continuity of ball games from Roman Antiquity to the Holy Roman Empire, but admits that it is difficult to understand the rules of the ancient ball games, and claims that certainly the contemporary games were much more refined and admirable than those in Roman times. Furthermore there were by far more forms and ways of playing than in Ancient Greece and Rome – this is certainly not the kind of admiration for the ancient world one could expect from a 'Renaissance' scholar.[67] Renaissance sports were new, and they were different (and better) than anything that had ever existed before.

The Process of Sportification

Sports are not usually considered to have been an essential part of European history. Not even standard accounts of court festivities mentioned them until recently.[68] But at medieval court festivities clearly the tournament took a central position, despite all attempts of the church to abolish these 'heathen' performances. Tournaments required a lot of training, as we can for instance take from the autobiography of Emperor Maximilian I (1459–1519).[69] And around 1500 tournaments still made up for most of the nobility's exercises, as we can take

---

[64] Alessandro Marcigliano, *Chivalric Festivals at the Ferrarrese Court of Alfonso II d'Este* (Bern, 2003).

[65] Ercole I was father of Alfonso I (1476–1534), whose son Ercole II (1508–1559) still ruled when the book on ball games was dedicated to his son Alfonso II d'Este in 1555. All of these Este princes were dedicated tennis players, and they were intermarried with the likewise sportive dynasties of Mantua (Gonzaga), Milan (Sforza) and Florence (Medici), but also to the Dukes of Guise, who are indeed mentioned in Scaino's book as dedicated tennis players: Scaino, *Treatise on the Game of the Ball*, p. 192.

[66] Nonni, Antonio Scaino, *Trattato del giuoco della palla*, p. 8: 'havendo io presso a formar un lavoro non rinovato, o da forma alcuna antica, ò moderna tolta, ma di nuovi, & miei propri colori figurati'.

[67] Guarinonius, *Grewel der Verwüstung*, p. 1208: 'auch ohne Zweifel weit fürtrefflicher und kunstreicher als damals'.

[68] Roy Strong, *Feste der Renaissance, 1450–1650. Kunst als Instrument der Macht* (Freiburg, 1991).

[69] Joseph Kurzböck (ed.), *Der Weiß Kunig. Eine Erzehlung von den Thaten Kaiser Maximilian des Ersten. Von Max Treitzsaurwein aus dessen Angeben zusammengetragen, nebst den von Hannsen Burgmaier dazu verfertigten Holzschnitten* (OE Wien, 1775, reprint Leipzig, 2006).

from the tournament book of the same emperor.[70] Tournaments were almost as dangerous as war, or the fights of ancient Roman gladiators. And despite attempts to minimize the danger of mortal accidents, jousting remained an extreme sport with fatal accidents. The fatal blow that Henry II of France – an enthusiastic tennis player[71] – received in a joust, celebrating the Peace of Cateau-Cambrésis and a French–Spanish double marriage in 1559, showed the mortal danger to all dynasties in Europe. Even more so, as the king's sudden death destabilized the French monarchy, sparked off the French Wars of Religion, and eventually brought the Valois dynasty to an end. Tournaments were fun, good 'sports', but the price was simply too high. After the fatal accident we can observe a sharp decline of jousting and its substitution by harmless exercises such as tilting at the ring, where young nobles could demonstrate their skills without bloodshed.[72] Guarinonius is hinting at this accident in his chapter on tournaments, where he concludes that this exercise 'nowadays, praised be God, has disappeared, which has been neither Christian, nor healthy/ since the danger was inherent, if one of the fighters had to be cast to the ground'.[73] And again, at the end of his chapter on the ball games: 'Among other benefits of the ball games is not the least, as Galen says, that there is no particular danger inherent in playing it.'[74]

It is not by coincidence that Baldassare Castiglione (1478–1529) in his famous book *Il Cortegiano* recommends ball games as the ultimate exercise for young gentlemen, since here they can demonstrate all the virtues required at a civilized court. Castiglione, himself as Count of Novilara a member of the Italian aristocracy, had received his education at the court of Ludovico Sforza in Milan, and afterwards served as a courtier at the courts of Francesco Gonzaga in Mantua, and Guidobaldo da Montefeltro in Urbino, three hotspots of early ball games, before joining the court of Emperor Charles V, a practising sports fan. In his *Libro del Cortegiano* Castiglione argues that ball games better than

---

[70]   Quirin von Leitner, *Freydal. Des Kaisers Maximilian I. Turniere und Mummereyen*, 2 vols (Wien, 1880/1882); W.H. Jackson, 'The Tournament and Chivalry in German Tournament Books of the Sixteenth Century and in the Literary Works of Emperor Maximilian I', in Christopher Harper-Bill and Ruth Harvey (eds), *The Ideals and Practice of Medieval Knighthood* (Woodbridge, 1986), pp. 49–73.

[71]   Pierre de Bourdeille, Seigneur de Brantome, *Mémoires* (Amsterdam, 1722), p. 46.

[72]   The locus classicus for that change is of course: Norbert Elias, Über den Prozess der Zivilisation. Soziogenetische und psychogenetische Untersuchungen, 2 vols (Frankfurt/ Main, 1978), vol. 1, pp. 283–301. But in my eyes it is unnecessary to invoke a mystical 'civilization process' to understand why the ruling elites withdrew from the dangerous exercise of jousting.

[73]   Guarinonius, *Grewel der Verwüstung*, p. 1223.

[74]   Guarinonius, *Grewel der Verwüstung*, p. 1213: 'Unter anderen Nutzbarkeiten des Ballnspielens ist nicht eine geringe/ wie Galen sagt/ daß bey solchem kein sondere Gefahr zu förchten ist.'

any other sports are training not just speed and power, but also *sprezzatura* and elegance.[75] This was what any courtier needed. And, as we know, Castiglione's ideas were soon received everywhere in Europe, and his book was translated into vernacular languages, into French and German as well as English,[76] and was initiating a wave of similar publications, advertising the rules of politeness and education as well as their physical preconditions.

The term 'sportification' is meant to cover the process of transforming both military exercise as well as popular games into the form of a sportive contest. Eichberg uses the term 'sportification' synchronously to 'industrialization', and as a consequence of this economic transformation.[77] In my eyes it makes no sense to perceive sports as a kind of superstructure to economic change. To me it seems that the process of sportification in Europe started with the Renaissance. As Scaino – trained in Aristotelian philosophy and later indeed becoming professor of philosophy, and commentator of Aristotle[78] – points out in his chapter 'definition of the ball game', a ball game 'is a contest between at least two players who, place one at one side, the other on the other as adversaries, do battle together with a solid and round instrument made from the skin of an animal, capable of bounding, so called ball'.[79] This definition reminds of the twentieth-century sociologist of sport, Norbert Elias (1897–1990), who defined sport as 'an organized group activity centred on a contest between at least two parties. It requires physical exertion of some kind and is fought according to fixed rules'.[80] Scaino explains that ball games, like other arts, were 'at first [performed]

[75]   Fritz Baumgart (ed. and trans.), Baldassare Castiglione, *Das Buch vom Hofmann*, translation (Munich, 1986), pp. 46–9.

[76]   Baltazar de Castillon, *Les quatres livres du Courtisan*, trans. Jacques Colin (Lyon, 1537); Baldassare Castiglione, *The Courtier*, trans. Thomas Hoby (London, 1561); Walthaser Castiglion, Hofmann, *In Welsch der Cortegiano genant, ein schön holdselig Buch*, trans. Lorenz Kratzer (Munich, 1565); Baltasar Castellon, *El cortesano*, trans. Juan Boscán (Salamanca, 1581); Baldessaris Castilionii, *De Aulico libri IIII*, trans. Johannes Riccius (Frankfurt, 1584). Except for the Latin translation, each of these versions had many reprints.

[77]   Henning Eichberg, 'Vom Fest zur Fachlichkeit. Über die Sportifizierung des Spiels', *Ludica*, 1 (1995): pp. 183–200.

[78]   Erwin Mehl, 'Antonio Scaino "Trattato del giuoco della palla" (Venedig 1555)', *Leibesübungen und körperliche Erziehung*, 19/20 (1937): pp. 437–45; 21 (1937): pp. 490–96. Antonio J. Papalas, 'The *Trattato del Giuco della Palla* di Messer Antonio Scaino da Salo and the Ferrarese Cultural Ideology in the Time of Alfonso II (1559–1597)', in Patricia Castelli (ed.), *Francesco Patrizi filosofo platonico nel crepuscolo del Rinascimento* (Florence, 2002), pp. 315–21.

[79]   Kershaw and Negretti, Scaino, *Treatise on the Game of the Ball*, p. 93.

[80]   Norbert Elias, 'An Essay on Sport and Violence', in Norbert Elias and Eric Dunning (eds), *Quest for Excitement: Sport and Leisure in the Civilising Process* (Oxford, 1986), pp. 150–74, at p. 159.

without laws and fixed rules', but at a later stage, 'through the agency of wise men ... reduced to proper order and thereby acquired the name of art'.[81]

Fixing the rules is one step in the process of institutionalization, but there are earlier ones: Making ball games part of the curriculum had the consequence that every noble boy – and later every student – had to learn how to play ball games, not only in Italy, but the same was true for noble or ambitious middle-class children in Spain, Germany, Austria, Hungary, Bohemia, Poland, Scandinavia and Britain. They could learn them at a local college, or at a court, at an academy,[82] or at a university. A famous illustrated advertisement of the Tübingen College is usually being taken as an example for early modern tennis – but additional copper engravings show the shooting range, the fencing hall and the *pallone* court.[83] Young nobles could also learn the ball games at some point on their Grand Tour, for most Europeans in Italy, but for the English also in France or in the Netherlands.

The growing market for sports had consequences at several levels: first of all there was a demand for teachers. In addition to fencing, riding and dancing masters, courts and universities were now in need of masters of the ball games. So one consequence was a degree of professionalization: a new profession emerged across Europe. However, as in music, most professional teachers came from Italy (*pallone, pallamaglio*), or from France (*jeu de paume*).

Second, there was a demand for equipment. According to recent estimates several dozen balls were required to finish one tennis game. From around 1500, when the *jeu de paume* was no longer played with the hand, but with a glove and later with a racket, these devices were needed in great numbers. For the *pallone* large inflatable balls were needed, together with valves and air-pumps and the *bracciale* for striking the big ball. For *calcio* and football inflatable medium-sized balls were required. Almost all authors describe the different kinds of balls required for different ball games, but only Scaino provides exact measurements and technically detailed illustrations in order to standardize the form, size and weight of these devices.[84] For the *pallamaglio* – in English reduced to *pall mall* – a wooden hammer (*maglio*) was required to hit the wooden ball (*palla*), and furthermore a little iron gate as a target. The demand for equipment led to the rise of specialized industries, for instance for tennis balls and rackets in Paris, as well as in Northern Italy. As we can take from the correspondence of Hans Fugger (1531–1598), the Bavarian court in Munich ordered hundreds of

---

[81]   Kershaw and Negretti, Scaino, *Treatise on the Game of the Ball*, p. 11.

[82]   Norbert Conrads, *Ritterakademien in der Frühen Neuzeit. Bildung als Standesprivileg im 16. und 17. Jahrhundert* (Göttingen, 1982).

[83]   Ludwig Ditzinger and Johann Christoph Neyffer, *Illustrissimi Wirtembergici Ducalis Novi Collegii quod Tubingae qua situm qua studia qua exercitia Accurata Delineatio* (Tübingen, 1626).

[84]   Kershaw and Negretti, Scaino, *Treatise on the Game of the Ball*, pp. 99–107.

rackets, and tens of thousands of tennis balls within less than a year, which were shipped (presumably from Paris) via Antwerp and Nuremberg to Munich. The devices for *pallone* and *pallamaglio* were likewise ordered from Italy, via Milan, and presumably produced in the kingdom of Naples.[85]

Maybe most important, a demand for dedicated spaces for ball games emerged. This was first supplied with improvised playgrounds, such as castle courtyards, former tournament grounds or public playgrounds. In a second step, tennis courts were built, and as we learn from Christian Jaser's contribution to this volume (Chapter 4), Paris had a leading role in this process. No other town in Europe offered so many opportunities for playing the *jeu de paume*, and these public sports facilities added considerably to the attraction of the French capital. Wherever the French king travelled to in the sixteenth century, the tennis courts had to be prepared in advance.[86] The French example appeared to be so convincing that Scaino included the measurements of the Louvre tennis court, commissioned by King Henri II, as a model for a large tennis court (*steccato maggiore*) into his rule book, whereas the smaller court (*steccato minore*) was obviously perceived as an indigenous invention.[87] Whether ball-playing halls in castles are indeed an Italian invention,[88] ought to be discussed more carefully. The Este dynasty had outdoor and indoor courts in all their castles in and around Ferrara, as well as in Rome, Fontainebleau and in Paris, but taking Jaser's exploration of the Parisian tennis culture into account, one would hesitate to still describe the court of the Estes as the 'cradle of the game of tennis'.[89]

Another marked innovation in the history of ball games was the invention and construction of free-standing, purpose-built ballhouses. This step seems to have been something like a generation project. And we are talking of a generation of sports fans and ball game enthusiasts all over Europe. In 1492 a villa at Marmirolo was designed for the pleasure of Granfrancescio II Gonzaga (1466–1519, r. 1484–1519), containing facilities for diversions such as tennis. We know from letters of his wife Isabella d' Este (1474–1539), a passionate tennis player herself, that Marmirolo was repeatedly the venue of tennis tournaments, performed for the ducal family. One of the most dramatic settings for the construction of a ballhouse occurred in Mantua, where Federico II Gonzaga (1500–1540) was

---

[85]   Wolfgang Behringer, 'Fugger als Sportartikelhändler. Auf dem Weg zu einer Sportgeschichte der Frühen Neuzeit', in Wolfgang E.J. Weber and Regina Dauser (eds), *Faszinierende Frühneuzeit. Reich, Frieden, Kultur und Kommunikation 1500–1800. Festschrift für Johannes Burkhardt zum 65. Geburtstag* (Berlin, 2008), pp. 115–34.

[86]   Jaqueline Boucher, *Le jeu de paume et la noblesse francaise aux XVIe et XVIIe siècles*, in P. Arnaud and G. Garrier (eds), *Jeux et sports dans l'histoire*, vol. 2 (Paris, 1992), pp. 9–25.

[87]   Kershaw and Negretti, Scaino, *Treatise on the Game of the Ball*, pp. 107–9.

[88]   De Bondt, *Royal Tennis*.

[89]   Cees de Bondt, 'The Court of the Estes, Cradle of the Game of Tennis. Trattato del giuoco della palla (1555) di Antonio Scaino', *Schifanoia*, 22/23 (2002): pp. 81–102.

aiming at being appointed duke by Emperor Charles V. In order to provide a congenial environment he hired one of the most talented artists, Giulio Romano (1499–1546),[90] and started designing the famous Palazzo del Te in the 1520s. All rooms of the castle were painted with a coherent picture programme, climaxing in the 'Hall of the Giants', which was meant to adulate the emperor. Directly attached to this hall was the tennis house, since it was well-known that Charles was a passionate player. When Charles visited Mantua in March 1530 the palazzo was still a large building site, but parts of the frescoes and the tennis court were finished already. Emperor Charles engaged in a tennis double that lasted four hours.[91]

In France it was King Francis I (1494–1547, r. 1515–1547) who added ballhouses to the already existing tennis courts, in England Henry VIII (1491–1547, r. 1509–1547) wished to find tennis courts at all his castles during the annual summer round trip, and given the English climate this could only be indoor tennis courts.[92] Whereas Emperor Maximilian I had rather been a supporter of tournaments, of hunting and mountaineering, his son Philip I of Burgundy, King of Castile (1478–1506), was already said to have died after an extensive tennis match. His grandson Charles (1500–1558), Duke of Burgundy, King of Spain and elected Emperor of the Holy Roman Empire, was an able and enthusiastic tennis player. Charles's brother Ferdinand (1503–1564), from 1521 Archduke of Austria, 1531 German King and from 1556 Roman Emperor, started his reign in Austria with constructing a *Ballhaus* in the Viennese castle in the 1520s. Further ballhouses were erected within the area of the *Hofburg* – *Ballhausplatz* No. 1 is today the address of the President of Austria, and *Ballhausplatz* No. 2 is the address of the Federal Chancellor (prime minister) of Austria.[93]

In Germany clearly the princes introduced the ballhouses, and their construction seemed so extraordinary to the contemporaries that in many cases the reason for their construction was recorded. In Augsburg, for instance, a wealthy free imperial city, the merchant class had obviously no inclination to ball games. When the Imperial Diet convened there in 1548, a ballhouse was

---

[90]   Ernst H. Gombrich, '"That rare Italian master … ". Giulio Romano, Court Architect, Painter and Impresario', in David Chambers and Jane Martineau (eds), *Splendours of the Gonzaga* (London, 1981), pp. 77–85; Raffaelo Tamalio, *Federico Gonzaga* (Paris, 1994).

[91]   Livio Galafassi, 'I diversi giuochi di palla praticati nella Mantova Gonzaghesca', *Civiltà Mantovana*, 110 (2000): pp. 69–78.

[92]   David Best, *The Royal Tennis Court: A History of Tennis at Hampton Court Palace* (Oxford, 2002).

[93]   Alfred Kohler, *Ferdinand I. 1503–1564. Fürst, König und Kaiser* (München, 2003); Harald Tersch, 'Freudenfest und Kurzweil. Wien in Reisetagebüchern der Kriegszeit (ca. 1620–1650)', in Andreas Weigl (ed.), *Wien im Dreißigjährigen Krieg* (Wien, 2001), pp. 155–249.

constructed on demand of Fernando Alvarez de Toledo (1507–1582), the Duke of Alba and Spanish Viceroy of Naples, a confidant and lieutenant of Emperor Charles V.[94] When Emperor Maximilian II (1527–1576, r. 1564–1576) shifted his residence from Vienna to Prague in 1568, a ballhouse had to be constructed on the Hradschin. When – in the same year – the young Bavarian Prince Wilhelm V (1548–1626, r. 1579–1597) took residence in Landshut, a former brewery was converted into a ballhouse on the grounds of the castle Trausnitz.[95] When Archduke Ferdinand II of Tyrol (1529–1595, r. 1564–1595) married the beautiful Philippine Welser (1527–1580) from Augsburg, he ordered the construction of a ballhouse in the area of Castle Ambras near Innsbruck in 1572.[96] Throughout the sixteenth and seventeenth centuries ballhouses were constructed all over Germany, Austria and Bohemia. In general, even small residential towns as Heidelberg, Zweibrücken or Saarbrücken had at least one ballhouse attached to the castle, and mostly another one in town.[97]

Students, Players and Fans

As far as institutionalization was concerned, no town could be compared to Paris, where several hundred tennis halls were said to have existed around 1600, and the Swiss traveller Felix Platter (1536–1614) confirmed this cautiously during his stay in Paris in 1599.[98] Even if no exact numbers are available – not least because ball courts, ball rooms and detached ballhouses are constantly being conflated – it is clear that Paris was absolutely outstanding. Other northern capitals such as London or Antwerp had only approximately 15 ballhouses.[99] In Rome – where even the younger cardinals were playing tennis – there were merely 18, in Florence 12, in Ferrara 10 tennis courts.[100] Brussels, the capital

[94] Karl L.P. Tross (ed.), *Wolrad von Waldeck: Des Grafen Wolrad von Waldeck Tagebuch während des Reichstags zu Augsburg 1548*, vol. 59 (Stuttgart, 1861, reprint Hildesheim and New York, 1980), pp. 53, 107, 110.

[95] Berndt Ph. Baader, *Der bayerische Renaissancehof Herzog Wilhelms V. (1568–1579). Ein Beitrag zur bayerischen und deutschen Kulturgeschichte des 16. Jahrhunderts* (Leipzig, 1943), p. 67.

[96] Matthaeus Merian, *Topographia Provinciarum Austriacarum* (Frankfurt am Main, 1649), pp. 142–4.

[97] Günther G. Bauer, 'Das fürstliche Salzburger Hofballhaus 1620/25–1775', *Homo Ludens*, 6 (1996): pp. 107–48.

[98] Rut Keiser (ed.), *Thomas Platter der Jüngere, Beschreibung der Reisen durch Frankreich, Spanien, England und die Niederlande 1595–1600* (Basel, 1968), p. 594.

[99] Wilhelm Streib, 'Geschichte des Ballhauses', *Leibesübungen und körperliche Erziehung*, 54 (1935): pp. 373–82, 419–32, 448–64, at p. 375.

[100] De Bondt, *Royal Tennis*, p. 221.

of the Spanish Netherlands, had probably less ballhouses than Ferrara, and the same is presumably true for any other town outside France.[101] In Padua, where Mercurialis had taught and Scaino and Guarinonius had studied, there were but five ballhouses.[102]

On the other hand there was a densely woven network of ballhouses all over Western Europe. The university towns followed their princes' examples in order to attract more ambitious students. Larger towns such as Augsburg, Regensburg, Nuremberg or Strasbourg had their tennis courts and ballhouses for a variety of reasons: out of competition for Imperial meetings, as an incentive for foreigners, for students, or for more ambitious inhabitants. Not all of these buildings were commissioned by the authorities. Basel, for instance, a former Imperial City that had joined the Swiss Confederation, had one built for commercial reasons in 1604.[103] In the small residential town of Coburg, where a famous high school was aiming at regional as well as foreign students, the owner advertised his ballhouse in a stylish newssheet, with a copper engraving designed by the Frankfurt artist Matthaeus Merian.[104] In Nuremberg, an Imperial City without university or residence, a commercial ballmaster offered his service, in his own ball court, as a teacher and trainer.[105] In the eighteenth century instructions for constructing ballhouses were still part of architecture handbooks.[106]

Ballhouses usually meant tennis halls, but some of these halls, for instance one ballhouse recently reconstructed in Neugebäude Castle near (and today in) Vienna, commissioned by Emperor Maximilian II (1527–1576), were so large that they could be used for almost anything, for instance *pallone*, which required more space than tennis. Guarinonius mentions that sometimes he had seen the *pallone* performed in Prague in the 'large Ballhouse', where the noble boys of the Imperial household were exercising.[107] For other ball sports obviously no buildings were required at all. Guarinonius mentions a kind of dodgeball game between two teams of about 12 players, which he used to play while studying

---

[101]   See for Brussels, Antwerp, London, Windsor and Richmond: Keiser, *Thomas Platter der Jüngere*, pp. 657–8, 682, 788–9, 844 and 867.

[102]   Guarinonius, *Grewel der Verwüstung*, p. 1210.

[103]   F.K. Mathys, *Spiel, Sport und Turnen im alten Basel* (Basel, 1957), pp. 33–4.

[104]   Norbert Nail, '"ganz ruinieret und zum Ballspielen untauglich gemacht". Zur Geschichte des Marburger Ballhauses', in Claudia Mauelshagen and Jan Seifert (eds), *Sprache und Text in Theorie und Empirie. Festschrift für Wolfgang Brandt* (Stuttgart, 2001).

[105]   Manfred Zollinger (ed.), 'Johann Georg Bender, Kurtzer Unterricht deß lobwürdigen, von vielen hohen Stands-Personen beliebten Exercitii deß Ballen-Spiels, denen so Lust haben, solches zu erlernen, sehr nützlich gestellet durch Johann Georg Bender, Ballen-Meister in Nürnberg, Nürnberg 1680', *Homo Ludens*, 6 (1996): pp. 271–9.

[106]   Johann Friedrich Penther, *Ausführliche Anleitung zur Bürgerlichen Baukunst* (Augsburg, 1748), vol. 4, p. 101.

[107]   Guarinonius, *Grewel der Verwüstung*, p. 1212.

in the Jesuit College in Prague, in springtime, summer and autumn, on a daily basis, and sometimes even twice a day. Obviously this game was played on a lawn within the walls of the college. This – he says – was the most exciting ball game, because all parts of the body were being exercised, no money was involved, and there was a lot of fun and *gutter kurtzweil*, this was the translation of 'sports' in contemporary dictionaries. Guarinonius was sure that this was the game Galen had been talking about.[108]

Tennis is a convincing example for sportification, since the scoring remained the same from the fifteenth century up to now,[109] and by far the most ball courts and ballhouses were built for it. Maybe there were more secular buildings for ball sports than for riding, fencing, dancing and for blood sports (arenas for bull fighting, bear baiting, etc.). Tennis, or as it was called in French *jeu de paume*, clearly received the most printed rule books in the early modern period. Soon after Scaino's first description of *pallacorda*,[110] tennis books became a French domain. In the first French description Jean Gosselin recommended this game, as had Scaino, as the game most fitting for the nobility.[111] The next author was Jean Forbet L'Aisne, who already in the book title advertises the healthiness of this sport, and it was up to him to provide the most detailed rules of the game hitherto.[112] Particularly interesting is Charles Hulpeau, who reprinted all earlier French rule books in 1632 and eventually labelled tennis as the French *Royal Game*.[113] Tennis was considered to be 'the Royal Game', and a good number of European dynasties – the Valois, the Este from Ferrara, the Wittelsbachs from Bavaria, etc. – would have subscribed.

However, some other dynasties would have disagreed. The Medici were staunch supporters of football.[114] Rule books on Florentine football, starting with a *Discorso sopra il Giuoco del Calcio Fiorentino* from 1580, are closely related to the government of the Grand-Dukes of Tuscany. The most important of these

---

[108] Guarinonius, *Grewel der Verwüstung*, pp. 1211–12.

[109] Heiner Gillmeister, 'Fifteen Love: The Origin of Scoring by Fifteens in Tennis', in L.S. Butler and P.J. Wordie (eds), *The Royal Game* (Stirling, 1989), pp. 88–99.

[110] De Bondt, 'The Court of the Estes': pp. 81–102. Antonio Scaino, 'Excerpts [= Appendix II]', in De Bondt, *Royal Tennis*, pp. 209–20.

[111] Jean Gosselin, 'Déclaration de deux doubtes qui se trouvent en comptant dans le lieu de la paume, lesquelles meritent d'estre entendues par les homes de bon esprit (1579)', in Charles Hulpeau (ed.), *Le Ieu Royal de la Paulme* (Paris, 1632), pp. 1–9.

[112] Jean Forbet L'Aisne, *L'utilité qui provient du jeu de la paume au corps et à l'esprit, avec les régles du jeu de prix* (Paris, 1592).

[113] Jean Forbet, 'Les formes tenues & observes par les anciens Maistres du Royal & honorable ieu de la Paume, lors qu'il se ioue un prix', in Charles Hulpeau (ed.), *Le Ieu Royal de la Paulme* (Paris, 1632), pp. 21–4.

[114] Horst Bredekamp, *Florentiner Fußball: Die Renaissance der Spiele* (Frankfurt, 1993, 2nd revised edn Berlin, 2001).

books was indeed written by the ducal courtier responsible for the organization of court festivities: Giovanni de' Bardi (1534–1612) was a famous humanist scholar and a playwright, a member of the Florentine Academy alongside other courtiers such as Galileo Galilei.[115] The book on football is dedicated to Francesco I de' Medici, Grand-Duke of Tuscany (1541–1587, r. 1574–1587).[116] It was reprinted once every generation until the end of the seventeenth century.[117] The design of the game was visualized by a copper engraving of Alessandro Cecchini, and at first glance it seems to resemble a form of ballet rather than a ball sport, since all the 27 players on each side started from their prescribed position, and the performance took place in the majestic theatre of the Piazza di Santa Croce, with the huge church building and town houses providing a lofty scenery. However, in the publication of Pietro di Lorenzo Bini, another Florentine courtier, we can also find an abstract tableau of players' positions in their football teams on a formalized field. Similar abstract tableaus we can find in TV broadcasts of modern football matches.[118]

Unlike tennis, where the galleries of the ballhouses allowed merely for a small audience, *calcio* and *pallone* were spectator sports. Outdoor events attracted large crowds, as for instance a Florentine *calcio* in 1584, when about 40,000 attended a game.[119] And even Scaino – the admirer of tennis – admits that football in Padua, where he had studied in the 1540s, or in Ferrara the *pallone*, usually attracted much larger crowds of enthusiastic male and female audiences in the streets than the *pallacorda*.[120] Over 300 years we have numerous representations and descriptions of the game of *pallone*, which was a kind of popular sport in some regions of Italy, as for instance in the Piedmont,[121] or maybe in large parts of Northern Italy. Johann Wolfgang von Goethe mentions in his travel report, *Italienische Reise* (Italian Journey), that he watched a contest of the local team at Verona (16 September 1786) with one from neighbouring Vicenza with about

---

[115] Mario Biagioli, *Galilei, der Höfling. Entdeckung und Etikette. Vom Aufstieg der neuen Wissenschaft* (Frankfurt a.M., 1999).

[116] Giovanni de' Bardi, *Discorso sopra il giuoco del calcio fiorentino* (Florence, 1580); reprint in: Carlo Bascetta (ed.), *Sport e Giuochi. Trattati e Scritti dal XV al XVIII secolo* (Milan, 1978), vol. 1, pp. 127–62.

[117] Giovanni de' Bardi, Discorso sopra il giuoco del calcio fiorentino (Florence, 1615); Giovanni de' Bardi, 'Discorso sopra il giuoco del calcio fiorentino (1580)', in Pietro di Lorenzo Bini, *Memorie del Calcio Fiorentino* (Florence, 1689), pp. 1–29; Giovanni de' Bardi, *Discorso sopra il giuoco del calcio fiorentino* (Florence, 1673).

[118] Plate: 'Planta et ordinanza delle due squadre come stanno in atto di principiare il gioco', in Pietro di Lorenzo Bini, *Memorie del Calcio Fiorentino* (Florence, 1689).

[119] Bredekamp, *Florentiner Fußball*, p. 115.

[120] Nonni, Antonio Scaino, *Trattato del giuoco della palla*.

[121] Andrea Merlotti (ed.), *Giochi di palla nel Piemonte medievale e moderno* (Rocca de Baldi, 2001).

5,000 enthusiastic spectators.[122] Like the Dukes of Savoy[123] – it seems – that the Palatine branch of the Wittelsbach were supporters of the *pallone*. But why were there no supporters of football in Germany? Again Guarinonius may offer an answer:

> The seventh ball game is the most respectable, manliest, most courageous and most serious, to the peasants and the simple-minded it seems most extraordinary, and firstly terrifying, when they see the mighty globe, or machine with much noise flying over their heads. This ball game is customary in Germany, particularly at the courts already for many years now, and the German nobility is excessively trained in it. This ball is usually called 'der Ballon', that is, the large ball.

The *pallone* was being struck with the *bracciale* – as in Italy. But Guarinonius continues: 'This game is not nimble, but requires much strength, quick running, bending down, kicking with the feet, and a good number of players prefers to kick the ball with their foot in the air, etc.'[124] Maybe there was no football in Germany, because *pallone* was football.

An Early Modern Period of Ball Games

In conclusion, there are good arguments for claiming that there was a distinct early modern period of sports, different from all earlier periods in European history, different from other civilizations, and different from the later modern period.

First of all, due to changes in the society we have the overall process of sportification of martial arts, as well as of popular games. This is where ball games come in, and as Paul Grendler has remarked, juxtaposing them to other physical activities: 'These were truly sports and recognized as such.'[125] *Second*, we have programmatic sports education for the first time since antiquity, in schools as well as in academies, and again: ball games are important as

---

[122] Stefan Größing, 'Pallone – ein aristokratisches Ballspiel', *Homo Ludens*, 6 (1996): pp. 79–107.

[123] Duke Emanuel Filiberto (1528–1580) used to play ball games every day (prope quotidie ... pila ludebat): Andrea Merlotti, 'Introduzione', in Merlotti, *Giochi di palla*, pp. 21–42, pp. 28–32.

[124] Guarinonius, *Grewel der Verwüstung*, p. 1213: 'Und ist solches Spiel zwar nit behend/ aber es bedarff guter Kräfften/ guten Zulauffs/ buckens/ Füß Stoßens/ wie dann mancher Spieler mit dem Fuß den Balln lustig uber sich treibt/ etc.'

[125] Paul Grendler, 'Fencing, Playing Ball, and Dancing in Italian Renaissance Universities', in John McClelland and Brian Merrilees (eds), *Sport and Culture in Early Modern Europe. Le Sport dans la Civilisation de L'Europe Pré-moderne* (Toronto, 2009), pp. 293–316, here p. 306.

non-military, harmless games that nevertheless provided an all round exercise of the body. *Thirdly*, we have a new ideal of gentlemanlike behaviour, emphasizing commandment of the body and elegance of movement, and ball games are at the core of this ideal. This is why some dynasties try to get identified with certain ball games. *Fourth*, dynastic propaganda and the rules of the games were spread Europe-wide by printed books and reports: Early modern ball games certainly benefited from the printing revolution, as well as from new habits of travelling, or the communications revolution in general. All of these ball games were at least potentially European, although we can clearly identify regional preferences. And *fifth*, particular sports facilities were constructed during the early modern period, like outdoor sports fields, indoor sports halls, and detached ballhouses. Or in the words of Guarinonius: 'That the ball game is the most prominent among all sports, can be seen in all places and more notable towns, and by the example of all Christian princes in particular, who erect separately respectable and large buildings for that nice and sensual exercise.'[126]

As far as outdoor games are concerned, there were purpose-built *tennis courts* and *pallamaglio* lanes.[127] The latter were long, plane, artificially constructed stretches, fenced off from their surroundings and usually accompanied by a planted alley of trees to provide shadow in the summer. *Pallamaglio* alleys were later converted into *pall malls*, areas for walking, for building expensive houses, or for establishing stores: they became shopping malls. The generic term *mall* for a large shopping area can be traced back to an early modern ball game. A similar transformation happened to the ballhouses. Like the amphitheatres for blood sports, the early modern arenas, they were constructed roughly from the late fifteenth century onwards, and were converted mostly in the course of the eighteenth century, sometimes also used as theatres and ballet stages, sometimes turned into theatres.[128] Some were converted into stables, fencing halls, barns, but in the small Italian town of Casale Monferrato in the Piedmont, once belonging to the Gonzaga of Mantua, the ballhouse constructed in 1597 was converted into a synagogue.[129] The most famous ballhouse was of course that

---

[126] Guarinonius, *Grewel der Verwüstung*, p. 1208.

[127] The pall mall had rule books of its own: Bartolomeo Ricci, 'Lettera sulla pallamaglio, 1553–1554', in Carlo Bascetta (ed.), *Sport e giuochi. Trattati e scritti del XV al XVII secolo* (Mailand, 1978), vol. 2, pp. 261–9; Vincenzo Giustiniani, 'Discorso sopra il giuoco del pallamaglio (1626)', in Bascetta, *Sport e Giuochi*, vol. 2, pp. 326–32; Michael Flannery, 'The Rules for Playing Pall-Mall (c. 1655)', in McClelland and Merrilees, *Sport and Culture*, pp. 183–98.

[128] Jason Scott-Warren, 'When Theaters were Bear-Gardens; Or, What's at Stake in the Comedy of Humours', *Shakespeare Quarterly*, 54 (2003): pp. 63–82.

[129] Cees de Bondt, 'Ballhaus', in Werner Paravicini (ed.), *Höfe und Residenzen im spätmittelalterlichen Reich* (Ostfildern, 2005), pp. 205–7; De Bondt, *Royal Tennis*, pp. 165–86.

of Versailles, where the Third Estate of 1789 swore to resist any attempts of the monarchy at dissolving them: *le serment du jeu de paume*. So, early modern ball games were not just at the beginning of modern sports, but served as a starting point to political revolution.[130]

---

[130] Wolfgang Behringer, *Kulturgeschichte des Sports. Vom antiken Olympia bis ins 21. Jahrhundert* (München, 2012), pp. 244–247.

Chapter 2

Sport and Recreation in Sixteenth-Century England: The Evidence of Accidental Deaths

Steven Gunn and Tomasz Gromelski

Most of our evidence about sport and recreation in early modern England comes from sources generated by attempts to prohibit, control or reform such activities. At the national level, parliament legislated against pastimes that distracted people from work or military exercises, while religious, social and educational theorists wrote about the benefits of some kinds of activity and the dangers of others. At the local level, church courts, manor courts and borough courts acted to regulate some activities and facilitate others, for example banning the playing of football on Sundays, punishing servants for playing tennis, or ordering individuals to purchase bows and practise archery. Such sources are illuminating about many aspects of recreational activities, but have a number of weaknesses. They tend not to record activities which were uncontroversial or pursued under uncontroversial circumstances, for example on days other than Sunday. They supply details – of participants, techniques, equipment, locations, days and times of play – only when these are relevant to the purpose for which the record was created.[1]

This chapter presents findings from a different kind of source, the inquest reports on sudden deaths submitted by coroners to the assize justices for filing at the court of King's Bench. Some 9,000 of these dealing with accidental deaths alone – not including murders or suicides – survive from the sixteenth century. While the majority of the accidents they record involved work or travel, a significant minority, about 6 per cent, to judge from those surviving from the 1550s, shed light on leisure activities. As we shall see, they too have their limitations, but they enable us to investigate aspects of sports, games and

---

[1] David Underdown, *Revel, Riot and Rebellion: Popular Politics and Culture in England 1603–1660* (Oxford, 1985), pp. 75–6, 94; Marjorie McIntosh, *Controlling Misbehavior in England, 1370–1600* (Cambridge, 1998), pp. 96–107; Steven Gunn, 'Archery Practice in Early Tudor England', *Past and Present*, 209 (2010): pp. 57–9; John McClelland, *Body and Mind: Sport in Europe from the Roman Empire to the Renaissance* (London and New York, 2007), pp. 44–59.

leisure that are otherwise poorly recorded, and sometimes their evidence can be compared and integrated with that of prescriptive sources such as educational treatises and legislation that aimed to control the use of leisure time.[2]

More than half the accidents caused by leisure activities involved children. Usually what they were doing was just described as playing, though sometimes it is recounted in poignant detail: making mud pies, playing with foals, using vaulting horses, picking flowers or looking at their reflections in water.[3] In the adult half of the sample, sports and pastimes are more precisely identifiable, and it is this material that provides new ways to examine such activities. They range from what we would normally think of as competitive sports or games – football, wrestling, throwing sports – through physical activities with aspects of both recreation and martial training – archery, sword-play, staff-play – to other pastimes involving more or less physical exertion – swimming, hunting, bell-ringing, dancing, walking and watching or participating in various kinds of performance. Most would have fallen within the definition of 'sports' or 'games' current in sixteenth- and early seventeenth-century England, a category broader and looser than those of the modern history of sport. The 'unlawful games' condemned by proclamations such as those of 1526, 1538 and 1572 included not only football, tennis, bowls and quoits, but also dice and cards.[4] The 'lawful sports' or 'lawful recreations' envisaged in James I's and Charles I's Declarations of Sports of 1618 and 1633 included not only archery, vaulting and leaping, but also dancing, May-games, Morris dances, Whitsun-ales and rush-bearing, while the 'games' they still counted unlawful on Sundays included bear-baiting, bull-baiting and the playing of interludes, as well as bowling.[5]

The detailed descriptions provided by these reports of the circumstances in which accidental deaths occurred shed light on the social range of participants in these activities and those who watched them play. Archery accidents were more frequent than those for any other pastime. They show that men and boys of all social ranks, from gentlemen to labourers, urban and rural, craftsmen and farmers, practised archery in groups of up to a dozen or more.[6] Football was played by boys aged 15 or 16, young men, labourers, husbandmen, brewers' men

---

[2]   The findings here are drawn in part from research conducted for Gunn, 'Archery Practice', and partly from a research project, running from 2011 to 2015, funded by the Economic and Social Research Council and conducted by both authors, from which the figures and examples for 1551–60 and 1590–7 derive.

[3]   Steven Gunn and Tomasz Gromelski, 'Toys and Games that Killed in Tudor England', *BBC History Magazine*, 13/13 (2012): pp. 37–40.

[4]   *Tudor Royal Proclamations*, ed. Paul L. Hughes and James F. Larkin (3 vols, New Haven and London, 1964–9), vol. 1, nos. 108, 183, vol. 2, no. 586.

[5]   *The Constitutional Documents of the Puritan Revolution 1625–1660*, ed. Samuel Rawson Gardiner (London, 1899), pp. 99–103.

[6]   Gunn, 'Archery Practice': pp. 60–61.

and stonemasons.[7] Those who threw the hammer or cast the bar were a similar mix to those pursuing other sports: yeomen, husbandmen, weavers, lightermen.[8] So were those who wrestled or practised fighting with swords, bucklers, staffs and other weapons: labourers, husbandmen, yeomen, servants, a bellows-maker, a cartwright and a furrier.[9]

Some games were even enjoyed in mixed groups. Stoolball, though we have as yet found no accidents involving it, may have been so.[10] More commonly it was less organised pastimes, especially among the young, that brought the sexes together. John Keynesham, husbandman, John Norcott, labourer, four boys who were the sons of named local men and some girls spent the afternoon of St Matthew's Day 1554, 'running ... and playing' in a close next to the churchyard at Chesterton in Oxfordshire. Keynesham ran into Norcott and was wounded by the knives hanging at his belt.[11] Edith Baron, spinster, was gathering barley with a boy called William Hokey at Ashton in Dorset in August 1554 when they began 'fighting in fun'; she playfully pushed him over, fell on top of him and accidentally stabbed herself in the side with his knife.[12] Equally spur-of-the-moment and perhaps flirtatious was the 'joking and playing' that John Beeley and Alice Higgot indulged in at the top of a flight of stairs in the house of Patrick Lowe Esquire at Breadsall in Derbyshire in November 1595, causing them both to fall down the stairs and John to die from his injuries.[13] And it was of course the mixed nature of dancing that sharpened concerns about its effects on public decency and the illegitimacy rate, concerns summed up in the title of Christopher Fetherston's 1582 *Dialogue against Light, Lewd and Lascivious Dauncing*.[14]

Accidents support the view that hunting was the most socially exclusive sport for men, at least when practised with fine horses in large parks to provide venison for exchange as politically charged gifts.[15] Archery was probably the most socially inclusive, for gentlemen are recorded as shooting with groups of other 'honest persons' and took their servants to visit local towns for shooting

---

[7]   The National Archives, PRO, KB9/490/54, 494/47, 578/15, 610/263, 639/135, 688/97, 1004/108.

[8]   *Sussex 1558–1603*, nos. 41, 152, 162; PRO, KB9/1037b/244.

[9]   PRO, KB9/450/28, 474/47, 486/46, 580/141, 985/133, 1004/5, 1040c/288.

[10]   David Underdown, *Start of Play: Cricket and Culture in Eighteenth-Century England* (London, 2000), p. 11.

[11]   PRO, KB9/9/587/192: 'currentes ... & ludentes'.

[12]   PRO, KB9/9/587/41: 'in ioco luctantes'.

[13]   PRO, KB9/690a/115: 'jocantes & ludentes'.

[14]   Underdown, *Revel, Riot and Rebellion*, pp. 46–7; Ronald Hutton, *The Rise and Fall of Merry England: The Ritual Year 1400–1700* (Oxford, 1994), pp. 127–46.

[15]   James Williams, 'Sport and the Elite in Early Modern England', *Sport in History*, 28 (2008): pp. 389–413.

matches against the townsfolk.[16] Football perhaps drew in the widest range of men below the gentry, but even the great seem to have played it on occasion. Henry VIII himself, we learn from his wardrobe accounts, had a pair of special football shoes, but it is not clear whether he played with his courtiers or with men of lower status, perhaps the yeomen of his guard with whom he practised archery.[17] All these activities must have provided sociable interaction, though the wording of the inquests rarely if ever allows us to judge its quality.

Many sports attracted spectators. Archers were often watched by other men and, more rarely, by women.[18] Those who shot apparently took some care not to hit spectators, shouting out a warning when they were about to shoot or if they saw their arrow was likely to hit someone, but accidents would happen, especially to men like Alexander Godbye.[19] He sat on the churchyard wall at Lowick in Northamptonshire on Friday 2 June 1542, watching archers shooting at targets next to the wall. Despite several warnings he would not leave the wall, and John Fryssby's arrow hit him on the left side of the head.[20] Football sometimes had spectators, but the game was inherently less dangerous to them than archery was, so they do not appear in the coroners' reports.[21] It was another matter for those who watched sledge-hammer throwing, who faced nasty injuries if they got in the way. On Monday 18 June 1565, at Ardington in Oxfordshire, Elizabeth Albott was sitting with Robert Phyppes next to the wall of her house watching Phyppes, Francis Robynson and others throw a workman's hammer called 'a sledge'. Robynson threw the hammer, warning those standing by, but Elizabeth got up and ran off and the hammer struck her on the head. She languished until 6 July and then died. The jurors pointed out, just for the sake of completeness, that if she had stayed by the wall with Phyppes she would not have got hurt.[22] Other spectators were caught on the neck or head by sledge hammers or stone quoits, in one case because they trespassed on the target area which all present had been warned three times to vacate at their peril.[23]

[16]   PRO, KB9/442/116, 683b/190; Gunn, 'Archery Practice': p. 64.

[17]   Maria Hayward, *Dress at the Court of King Henry VIII* (Leeds, 2007), pp. 113–14; Anita Hewerdine, *The Yeomen of the Guard and the Early Tudors: The Formation of a Royal Bodyguard* (London, 2012), p. 78.

[18]   Gunn, 'Archery Practice': p. 61; PRO, KB9/689/103; for female spectators see KB9/625/161 and perhaps KB9/469/86 (though the victim in the latter may have been an accidental bystander rather than a spectator).

[19]   PRO, KB9/579/49, 625/161, 683b/190, 9/1037a/127.

[20]   Gunn, 'Archery Practice': p. 61.

[21]   James Sharpe, *The Bewitching of Anne Gunter* (London, 1999), pp. 14–19.

[22]   PRO, KB9/613/109. In quotations from primary documents, capitalisation has been modernised and Latin translated into English.

[23]   PRO, KB9/582/112, 633/191, 1037b/244; *Sussex Coroners' Inquests, 1558–1603*, ed. R.F. Hunnisett (Kew, 1996), nos 152, 162.

The reports also indicate the specific locations within towns and villages where sports took place. Archery, which ideally needed targets set at 200 yards' range or more, was practised almost anywhere large enough spaces were available: in fields, closes, gardens, yards, parks, disused castles, near rivers or by the seashore; sometimes near churches, favoured centres of communal activity, as in 'the church lease' at Appledore in Kent in 1571, or near the old chapel of ease at Fishtoft, Lincolnshire, 1550.[24] Football, likewise, seems to have been played wherever there was room. In East Anglia, above all Suffolk, village or town camping closes were maintained for playing football and other recreations. These were small fields, often close to churches or other nuclei of settlement, sometimes attached to inns or held by community trustees.[25] Some villages in other regions seem to have had such sites, but play is also recorded in churchyards, on village greens, in a close in private ownership in Hertfordshire and a meadow in Essex.[26] Some pitches were rough enough that falls could cause serious injury, as players tripped over molehills, bruised their sides falling onto stones, or stabbed their legs on stubby maple trees.[27] Throwing sports too needed room, whether in gardens or on open ground like the downs to the west of Lewes in Sussex, though they might involve throwing hammers over houses, with obvious risk to passers-by.[28] Churches, churchyards and rectories seem to have been natural centres for other kinds of sociable activity, wrestling, sword-fighting and maypole-dancing.[29] The one place we have found a dedicated 'sporting place' was in Nottingham Gaol in 1593. There John Boothe, a prisoner, broke his neck when he took a few steps backwards to lengthen his run-up when leaping and fell over a low hedge into a pit.[30]

The dates of accidents show the times of year when different activities were most popular. February was the football season, accounting for nearly three-quarters of all accidents, with outliers in March, April and May; none of the games found so far took place on Shrove Tuesday, so it seems to have been the month in general rather than the day in particular that was thought best.[31] April

---

[24] Gunn, 'Archery Practice': pp. 62–4.

[25] David Dymond, 'A Lost Social Institution: The Camping Close', *Rural History*, 1 (1990): pp. 165–92.

[26] Dymond, 'Camping Close', pp. 182–5; PRO, KB9/494/47, 610/263, 639/135, 688/97.

[27] PRO, KB9/578/15, 610/263, 633/135.

[28] *Sussex 1558–1601*, vol. I, nos. 41, 152; PRO, KB9/1037b/244.

[29] PRO, KB9/486/46, 595a/80, 970/78; *Calendar of Nottinghamshire Coroners' Inquests, 1485–1558*, ed. R.F. Hunnisett (Thoroton Soc., Record ser. xxv, Nottingham, 1969), no. 278.

[30] PRO, KB9/683a/100.

[31] PRO, KB9/448/44, 451/11, 490/54, 494/47, 578/15, 610/263, 633/135, 639/135, 688/97, 1004/108; Adrian Harvey, *Football: The First Hundred Years. The Untold Story*

and May were, unsurprisingly, the time for maypoles.[32] Archery took place all year, with peaks in spring, early summer and autumn, the seasons recommended by Roger Ascham in his 1545 guide to archery, *Toxophilus*.[33] Casting the bar and throwing the hammer were concentrated in summer, June and July, and went on into harvest time.[34] Swimming too was a summer recreation: May to August were the best months, thought Everard Digby, author of the first English treatise on swimming, and accidents clustered then.[35] Indoor activities were more appropriate to Christmas, but could still be perilous. John Sanway, husbandman, fell off a bench and broke his neck while performing a 'Cristmas playe' in a gentleman's house at Toller Fratrum in Dorset in 1552.[36] Thomas Bunting wrestled with a neighbour in the hall of Kneesall rectory in Nottinghamshire on New Year's Day 1549, but fell on his opponent's knife.[37] John Hypper crushed his testicles with fatal effects while 'playinge Christenmas games' in the house of Thomas Purdew, husbandman, at about 6 p.m. on 26 December 1563.[38] Whatever the season, Sundays and church holidays were prime times for most forms of recreation. They accounted for over half of all archery, throwing and wrestling accidents and nearly half of football accidents.[39]

Beyond such statistics, accidents give us closer insight into a number of sporting cultures. East Anglia, Yorkshire and perhaps Cumbria seem to have been footballing areas in the sixteenth century as they were in the eighteenth and nineteenth, while Cornwall had its own variant, hurling or 'whurlyng', apparently played differently in the east and west of the county, one in enclosed fields with goals, the other across country.[40] Inquest reports reinforce the view that football could be 'a ritualized expression of communal rivalry'.[41] In Cornwall in 1509

(London, 2005), pp. 1–17.

[32]   PRO, KB9/595a/80, 681b/126, 686b/240; *Sussex 1558–1601*, nos. 96, 281.

[33]   Gunn, 'Archery Practice': p. 60.

[34]   PRO, KB9/582/112, 613/109, 1037b/244; *Sussex 1558–1603*, nos. 41, 152, 162; Underdown, *Revel, Riot and Rebellion*, p. 93.

[35]   PRO, KB9/458/17, 579/179, 587/189, 587/247, 589b/196, 599a/88, 682a/45, 690b/238; 1040c/233; Nicholas Orme, *Early British Swimming, 55BC–AD1719: With the First Swimming Treatise in English, 1595* (Exeter, 1983), p. 120.

[36]   PRO, KB9/985/136.

[37]   *Nottinghamshire 1485–1558*, no. 278.

[38]   PRO, KB9/608/234.

[39]   Gunn, 'Archery Practice': p. 60; PRO, KB9/489/63, 970/78, 1040c/288; *Nottinghamshire 1485–1558*, no. 278; and see references in fn. 31 (football) and 34 (throwing sports).

[40]   Emma Griffin, *England's Revelry: A History of Popular Sports and Pastimes 1660–1830* (Oxford, 2005), pp. 43–7; Harvey, *Football*, pp. 52–67; Dymond, 'Camping Close', pp. 169–73; PRO, KB9/451/11.

[41]   Underdown, *Revel, Riot and Rebellion*, p. 96.

men from Bodieve and Benbole, 60 in all, faced each other at Tregorden, midway between their villages, playing, as the jurors stressed, 'for their recreation or play ... according to the form and usage of the county used for this cause from old times'.[42] In Cambridgeshire Great Shelford men played Cambridge men at Waterbeach.[43] But many other games seem to have involved players from a single village, sometimes indeed described as neighbours.[44] The game was certainly rough, as players violently obstructed one another, knocked one another to the ground, 'contending in the game and struggle' as one report put it, or threw those who grabbed hold of them forcefully away.[45] Simon Hogeson just 'fell to the ground amongst the players', so that no one knew who had knocked him down.[46] It was no accident that the East Anglian name for the game, camping, derived from the Anglo-Saxon *campian*, to fight.[47]

Yet however rough, the game was not merely an excuse for a punch-up. Accidents show that the ball – in one case made from an old shoe – was central.[48] John Langbern and Roger Bridkirk were running after it and both reached it at the same time, Roger falling on top of John and crushing him.[49] John Coulyng was holding the ball in his right hand, running very strongly and rapidly, when Nicholas Jaane tried to tackle him and broke his left leg in the process.[50] And many injuries resulted simply from the speed and vigour of the game, especially when played on hard or even frozen ground in February. John Pyrry tripped over another player's leg as he ran for the ball and hit his chest and stomach so hard on the ground that he felt sick. He ran off to a hedge 40 yards away, vomited up the entire contents of his stomach and immediately died.[51] John Tyler injured his body so badly when he ran after the ball, tripped and fell on his stomach, that he too died instantly.[52] Giles Hull ran fast to intercept the ball that John Waylett had thrown towards the goal with his hands, but crashed to the ground, surviving the injuries he sustained only till the following day.[53] Richard Mulcaster, the schoolmaster who thought a reformed version of football might be useful exercise, recognised that it was not only the 'thronging of a rude multitude, with

[42] PRO, KB KB9/451/11: 'recreacion[is] sive ludendi causa ... s[e]c[un]d[u]m modum & usum com[itatus] p[re]d[ic]ti ex causa p[re]d[ic]ta ab antiquo temp[or]e'.
[43] PRO, KB9/494/47.
[44] PRO, KB9/451/11, 490/54, 610/263, 633/135, 639/135.
[45] PRO, KB9/494/47, 639/135: 'lusu et lucta concerta[ntes]'.
[46] PRO, KB9/633/135: 'int[er] ludentes p[ro]strat[us] fuit ad terram'.
[47] Dymond, 'Camping Close', pp. 165, 181–5.
[48] PRO, KB9/1004/108.
[49] PRO, KB9/490/54.
[50] PRO, KB9/451/11.
[51] PRO, KB9/1004/108.
[52] PRO, KB9/578/15.
[53] PRO, KB9/688/97.

bursting of shinnes, & breaking of legges' but also the 'rash running & to much force' that made it dangerous under normal sixteenth-century conditions.[54]

Mulcaster thought wrestling was 'contemned by the most, and cared for but by the meanest', but worthy of revival, as practised by the ancients and healthful in its effects: 'it makes the breath firme and strong, the bodie sound and brawnie, it tightes the sinews, and backes all the naturall operations'.[55] It was friendly, but challenging and virile, for, as Mulcaster put it, 'the attemptes to get vantage in wrastling be very eager & earnest'.[56] John Thurkyll 'dyd wrestyll' with Ralph Otley at Bocking in Essex in May 1522, we are told, out of familiarity with him and for recreation, without malice or premeditated harm. Two days after John fell heavily on top of him, Ralph died.[57] James Chapplehowe was wrestling with his brother John when John's knife fell out of its scabbard and James fell on it.[58] Three Yorkshiremen, Thomas Tenyson, John Homler and William Lamrose, were wrestling amicably on a Sunday afternoon in October 1518 in the churchyard at Skeckling, near Burstwick in Holderness. A fourth neighbour, Stephen Kayngham, arrived and announced that he was a 'manly man' who could throw all three of them over the churchyard wall. Homler denied it, but had to eat his words when Kayngham put him over the wall. Unfortunately, as he fell, his own knife went into a vein in his arm.[59]

Other combat sports shared the same virile air. John Coksegge and Richard Chelliffeld, labourers of Gillingham, Kent, chose St George's Day as the time to show off their sword-fighting skills, and the 'churcheplayn' as the place to do it – acting '*insolenter*', in an unrestrained manner, carelessly, or proudly, opined the inquest jurors.[60] Walter Churke, servant of William Rugge of Ashford, had some of the same spirit. At 5 p.m. on 24 January 1552, he came out of his master's house and met George Lawner on the road between Great Chart and Ashford. Churke took Lawner's staff in his hands and said 'This ys a good staff, I prey the geve yt me'. Lawner declined, but said that if Churke wished to play with him he would show him some points for his learning; we might say he offered to teach him a thing or two. Lawner equipped Churke with a six-foot staff and they went into Rugge's close for some amicable 'staffpleyeing', giving one another blows. Their

---

[54] Richard Mulcaster, *Positions vwherin those primitiue circumstances be examined, which are necessarie for the training vp of children, either for skill in their booke, or health in their bodie* (London, 1581), pp. 104–5.

[55] Mulcaster, *Positions*, pp. 75–6.

[56] Mulcaster, *Positions*, p. 76.

[57] PRO, KB9/489/63.

[58] PRO, KB9/1040c/288.

[59] PRO, KB9/970/78: 'virilis homo'.

[60] PRO, KB9/486/46.

bantering combat turned sour only when Churke unintentionally hit Lawner on the left side of his head and he fell to the ground, dying the following afternoon.[61]

Bell-ringing, an increasingly popular activity, was collaborative: up to five people are recorded as ringing together in belfries when accidents took place.[62] But when things went wrong and bells broke or ropes malfunctioned, with falling metal, swinging ropes and 'great and terrible noise', it was every man for himself. William Stuard's foot got tangled in the rope of the third bell at Northfleet in Kent on Easter Sunday 1559 as he tried to avoid a broken bell; he was lifted six feet in the air and smashed his head against the edge of a paving slab.[63] Much the same happened to Adam Strutt in August 1568 at Preston, Suffolk, except that he was ringing for evensong and Stuard for matins: his rope pulled him seven feet off the ground and he landed head-first, dying the next day.[64] John Robinson was standing on a bench to ring for the anniversary of Elizabeth's accession on the evening of 17 November 1592 at Cobham in Kent. The rope caught round the bench and lifted it and him six feet into the air, dropping him onto the paved floor. He died from injuries to his head and body just after noon the next day.[65]

It was the bell itself that did for John Brock. He rang a small church bell at Lenton in Nottinghamshire too vigorously on Ash Wednesday 1573 and it fell out of its frame and hit him on the head.[66] Standers-by could be in danger too. On All Hallows' Eve 1570 Thomas Lockley and William Garden were ringing the great bell in the bell-tower of All Saints' church, Northampton, for evening prayer. A piece of the bell-clapper, 33¾ pounds of ironwork, broke off and fell out of the bell-tower, bounced off the wall of the church and then, 'in the sight and presence of many of the queen's subjects', hit John Dambroke, son of John Dambroke, haberdasher, breaking much of the left side of his head and knocking out part of his brain.[67] If his fate was unexpected, that of John Smithe, the jurors seem to have thought, was more predictable. On 21 December 1590, they reported, he went into the parish church of St Mary, Nottingham, pulled on the rope of the middle bell in an incautious manner and, 'playing childishly', climbed up the rope. He fell off, badly bruised, and died three days

---

[61]   PRO, KB9/1004/5: 'si vis ... ludere mecum monstravero tibi puncta erudic[i]o[n]is tue'.

[62]   David Cressy, *Bonfires and Bells: National Memory and the Protestant Calendar in Elizabethan and Stuart England* (London, 1989), pp. 68–80; Diarmaid MacCulloch, *The Later Reformation in England, 1547–1603* (2nd edn, Basingstoke, 2001), p. 116.

[63]   PRO, KB9/597a/75: 'cum maximo & terribili sonitu'.

[64]   PRO, KB9/1014/290.

[65]   PRO, KB9/1038/22.

[66]   PRO, KB9/635/220.

[67]   PRO, KB9/625/342: 'in visu et p[rese]ncia multoru[m] ligio[rum] d[ic]te d[omi]ne regine'.

later.[68] Boyish exuberance might be more excusable in the case of nine-year-old Edward Hurford, who took hold of the bell-rope in the porch of the chapel at Leighland Chapel in Somerset on 24 August 1595 and 'did swinge himselfe w[i]th the said rope from one side of the wall to the other of the said porche'. He knocked himself out when his forehead hit the wall and was hanged when the rope caught under his chin.[69]

Swimming was more solitary and therein lay part of its danger. As Digby's swimming manual pointed out, when entering the water it was best to have a strong companion.[70] Some of those who drowned were in company, but it did them no good. John Kent, 10-year-old son of Thomas Kent of Little Wittenham, husbandman, was with other boys at Nuneham Courtenay, Oxfordshire, in June 1554, but he went into the Thames first and a sudden rush of water dragged him into a whirlpool.[71] Most died alone. James Astrell of Winwick, Northamptonshire, labourer, went to a pond called 'Growton Poole' to learn to swim in July 1559, but entered deep water and drowned due to lack of experience.[72] Robert Romesey of Gloucester, capper, tried to take precautions, swimming in the Severn at Llanthony Quay in July 1553 with bladders attached to his body – as recommend by Digby particularly for learning breast-stroke – but got into trouble when the current swept away his buoyancy aids.[73]

In many activities the everyday wearing of knives or daggers at the belt made falls and collisions dangerous. Footballers, wrestlers, runners and Nicholas More of Staverton, Wiltshire, who was playing tip-cat, a game that involved flicking a tapered stick out of the ground and then hitting it some distance, all fell on their own knives or daggers or those of their companions and bled from their thighs, elbows, stomachs and chests, often because their sheaths were faulty.[74] Martial sports were dangerous by definition, but accidental deaths might come about in freakish ways. John Smyth was wielding a partisan on May Day 1555, playing with his friends at eight in the morning in the fields of Wishford, Wiltshire. He accidentally hit a great gelding belonging to William Herbert, Earl of Pembroke, in the right buttock and the horse turned on him and broke his leg. He died, presumably from infection, four weeks later.[75] Sword-fighters in Derbyshire and Kent stabbed themselves in the leg with their own swords and one in Somerset impaled his leg on his opponent's sword-point as he stamped on

---

68   PRO, KB9/678b/166: 'purilite[r] colludens'.

69   PRO, KB9/690b/183.

70   Orme, *Early British Swimming*, p. 121.

71   PRO, KB9/587/189.

72   PRO, KB9/599a/88.

73   PRO, KB9/587/247; Orme, *Early British Swimming*, p. 132.

74   PRO, KB9/9/448/44, 580/141, 587/192, 588a/97, 639/135, 970/78, 1040c/288; *Nottinghamshire 1485–1558*, no. 278.

75   PRO, KB9/588a/94.

the buckler he had dropped to prevent the other man picking it up.[76] In hunting, too, the danger was part of the attraction, but it sometimes came in unexpected forms.[77] On Wednesday 12 September 1537, just as the buck-hunting season was ending, Ellis ap Euan was out hunting with his buckhounds in Brickhill Park, Buckinghamshire. He shot a buck with a broad-headed arrow, but it suddenly ran back towards him and butted him on the left side of his head with its antlers, so that he died instantly.[78] William Gryffethe, being 'expert in the art of swimming', must have thought the odds were in his favour when he set off across a pond in Wedgnock Park, Warwickshire on a July afternoon in 1555 to retrieve a drowned buck, but he got cramp 15 feet from safety and drowned.[79]

The incidence of accidents suggests the rise and fall of certain activities. Contemporary commentators were sure that archery was in decline, the victim of idleness, moral decay, poor diet, alternative attractions, superior weapons and magisterial negligence. Archery accidents do indeed seem to have peaked in the 1540s and 1550s and declined thereafter.[80] Conversely, the number of swimming accidents seems to have risen over time. This may have been encouraged by the example of the manly Romans, much praised by English Renaissance scholars such as Sir Thomas Elyot and Richard Mulcaster.[81] As we have seen, not all those who tried their hand at swimming were scholars, but many were. An early victim was Walter Elmes, rector of Harpsden in Oxfordshire, drowned in the Thames at Wargrave in 1511.[82] Sampson Butler, scholar of Eton, followed in 1556, trying to swim across the Thames to pick nuts on the far bank.[83] By the late 1560s and 1570s, Cambridge students were regularly drowning while swimming at Grantchester, and this despite Vice-Chancellor John Whitgift's order in 1571 that no scholar should enter any river, pond or water in Cambridgeshire by day or night to swim, on pain of public beating or, for a second offence, expulsion from the university. Digby for one did not toe the party line with his swimming manual of 1587, *De arte natandi*, for he was a fellow of St John's.[84]

---

[76] PRO, KB9/474/47, 486/46, 600b/120.
[77] Roger B. Manning, *Hunters and Poachers: A Social and Cultural History of Unlawful Hunting in England 1485–1640* (Oxford, 1993), pp. 8–9.
[78] PRO, KB9/539/119; Emma Griffin, *Blood Sport: Hunting in Britain since 1066* (New Haven and London, 2007), p. 56.
[79] PRO, KB9/588b/173: 'expers in arte natandi'.
[80] Gunn, 'Archery Practice': pp. 53–4, 57, 66–75.
[81] Orme, *Early British Swimming*, pp. 1–9, 50–54, 62–3.
[82] PRO, KB9/458/17.
[83] PRO, KB9/589b/196.
[84] S.J. Stevenson, 'Social and Economic Contributions to the Pattern of "Suicide" in South–East England, 1530–1590', *Continuity and Change*, 2 (1987): pp. 251, 261; Orme, *Early British Swimming*, pp. 64, 71–88.

Fatal accidents cannot give us a comprehensive picture of sporting culture. Some popular recreations caused mishaps only tangentially. Maypole-dancing was dangerous not to the dancers, but to those who erected the poles and might be struck on the head if they fell; those who delivered them by cart and might have a traffic accident; or unluckier still, passers-by who might be missed by a falling pole but hit by a stone it dislodged from a nearby wall.[85] The one dancing fatality we have found so far brought his trouble on himself, falling inebriatedly into a fire while trying to dance on one leg in a kitchen at Fulstow in Lincolnshire in 1552 and scalding his back and legs with boiling water from a kettle.[86] Dicing, the bane of many local authorities in their efforts to maintain moral order, likewise came to light only when it caused a dispute that led to a fatal scuffle. Between 9 and 10 p.m. on Monday 23 February 1556, half a dozen Bedford men including a tiler, a glover, a shoemaker and an ostler were playing dice on the northern side of the town's great river bridge. John Clapham and Thomas Philips, alias Bowyer, quarrelled over the game and Clapham snatched off Philips's woollen hat. Philips tried to grab it back and Clapham drew a dagger, but succeeded only in cutting himself in the leg, bleeding to death two hours later.[87] Flower-picking was innocuous in itself but took women, boys and, most often, girls too close to water, where they drowned in steady numbers reaching out for corn-marigolds, cowslips and other blooms, or crossing rivers to find better places to pick.[88]

Entertainments watched by the public might be dangerous to performers. Thomas Talior of Scarborough was a minstrel with an attractively risky routine, juggling with two daggers. It went wrong at about 9 p.m. on 2 May 1556 at Malton in Rydale, 20 miles from his home, when one of the daggers hit him in the neck and he died instantly.[89] William Hobson, a Scot, offered to show bystanders at Over in Cambridgeshire in December 1523 a pastime so risky that, when it went wrong, the jurors classed it as suicide. He described it as 'a certain game used in his country' and it seems to have involved his lying on the ground on his back tied to a beam or door-post while six men tried to pull him along; his right leg got broken in the process and he died three weeks later.[90]

Spectators could be in danger when viewing arrangements were perilous. On 28 June 1592, between 6 and 7 p.m., eight-year-old Thomas Johnson, son of Richard Johnson, weaver, was standing with other boys under the 'preaching place or crosse' in the upper part of Gloucester Cathedral churchyard to watch

---

[85]　*Sussex 1558–1603*, no. 281; PRO, KB9/595a/80, 681b/126, 686b/240.

[86]　PRO, KB9/1004/90.

[87]　McIntosh, *Controlling Misbehavior*, pp. 100–101, 199–200; PRO, KB9/1072/169.

[88]　PRO, KB 9/579/170, 579/173, 625/241, 985/20, 1004/167, 1014/85; *Nottinghamshire 1485–1558*, no. 46.

[89]　PRO, KB9/589/101.

[90]　PRO, KB9/494/67: 'quoddam ludu[m] usitat[um] in patria sua'.

a play. John Thomas, labourer, climbed up the cross to get a better view, but the weight of his body put a strain on the upper part of the cross and a loose stone broke off and fell on the back of Thomas's head. He fell to the ground and four days later he was dead.[91] Forty years earlier, at Warslow in Staffordshire, Thomas Dakyns was distracted from watching his neighbours practise archery by an entertainer who arrived at the butts. Dakyns never saw the arrow that hit him in the forehead.[92] In bull-baiting the line between spectators and participants was a fine one. Peter Singleman alias Tucker, a sailor, was watching his mastiff fight a bull at Bridport in Dorset in 1595. He stepped in to pull his dog off the bull's legs and encourage it to attack head-on, but the bull gored his right thigh and he died two hours later.[93]

Gunpowder created spectacular special effects, but its presence made royal pageantry and street theatre dangerous for participants and spectators alike. On 1 May 1559, John Penne, mariner, was on a boat on the Thames by Whitehall Palace, taking part in the entertainments for Queen Elizabeth. He drowned when panic at a burning barrel of gunpowder made his crew-mates capsize the boat.[94] Thomas David was shot in the chest by a handgun that went off prematurely on Good Friday 1555 when it was propped against a wall in Usk, Monmouthshire, ready to be used in a 'stache playe'.[95] Jane Smyth, servant of John Wylkenson of Newcastle upon Tyne, merchant, and Edmund Fenwycke, a boy, died in the same accident in 1552. They were watching the annual Corpus Christi plays on the Clothmarket at Newcastle, she walking in the street, he lying on a scaffold set up for spectators. At 4 p.m. a keelman, who worked on the Tyne coal-ships, and a yeoman set off the charges in three gun chambers, but one exploded and pieces of shrapnel hit Edmund in the head and Jane in the stomach; he died instantly, she at 11 p.m.[96] Similar dangers were present in London in 1590, the only year for which inquest returns for the capital survive. At 8 a.m. on 28 May Richard Hawkesforth, shoemaker, fired off a caliver in a May game but gave himself a burn two feet long by eight inches wide when the spark ignited loose gunpowder that had fallen onto his sleeve.[97]

Some died without even enjoying the show. Part of the attraction of bear-baiting was the power and aggression of the bears, but that made them a threat if they got loose when they were not performing. Agnes Rapte, widow, was killed by Lord Bergavenny's bear when it broke loose at his house at Birling

---

[91]   PRO, KB9/682b/192.
[92]   PRO, KB9/1004/141.
[93]   PRO, KB9/690b/190.
[94]   PRO, KB9/598/21.
[95]   PRO, KB9/588b/167
[96]   PRO, KB9/1004/168, 169.
[97]   Thomas R. Forbes, 'London Coroner's Inquests for 1590', *Journal of the History of Medicine and Allied Sciences*, 28 (1973): p. 380.

in Kent at about 8 a.m. on 3 August 1563. She was in the hall of the house and it attacked her furiously, biting and tearing her head, body and legs. Lord Bergavenny ordered his servant John Washenes to shoot the bear immediately with a handgun, but Agnes died within six hours.[98] Two years later a bear bit and killed a man at the old Austin Friars in Holywell parish, just outside the Oxford city wall, and in 1570 Agnes verch Owen was killed in her bed by a bear that got loose near Hereford.[99] On one occasion it was merely the advertising for an entertainment that proved deadly. On 4 June 1567 the servants of Simon Poulter of Paris Garden in Southwark came past Charing Cross between 10 and 11 in the morning, proclaiming that bears and a bull were to be baited with dogs at Paris Garden on Friday 6 June. To attract attention they had with them a drum, a bull and a bear. Startled by the drum and scared of the bull and bear, the horse drawing a collier's cart bolted and five-year-old George Jeames was run over.[100]

Some recreations were not dangerous enough to show up in records of accidental death at all. Bowls was widely played but generated no fatalities that we have found so far; likewise tennis, though it was popular at court and elsewhere.[101] Other activities were revealed only as the context for accidents. Walking, thought Richard Mulcaster, was a very popular form of exercise. 'I dare saye', he wrote, 'that there is none, whether young or olde, whether man or woman, but accounteth it not onely the most excellent exercise, but almost alone worthy to beare the name of an exercise'.[102] Yet it rarely featured in accidental deaths. Agnes Hemyng, wife of Lewis Hemyng of Coventry, sawyer, took their eight-year-old daughter Elizabeth for an hour-long walk in Cheylesmore Park on the afternoon of 27 May 1556. On the way back to their home in Little Park Street, Elizabeth spotted a ladder propped against a stone wall and climbed it, but slipped, fell, broke her neck and died in her mother's arms.[103] Elizabeth Holecat was ill, perhaps suffering from the fierce influenza epidemic of that year, when she went to Jane Martyn's garden on 6 June 1558. She was going for recreation, the jurors said, but she fell into a pond by the garden and drowned.[104]

---

[98]   PRO, KB9/608/125.

[99]   PRO, KB9/628/175, 1110/unnumbered.

[100]   PRO, KB9/619/11; Simon Poulter and Simon Poulton, recalled by witnesses in 1620 as the probable constructor of stands to watch bear-baiting in Southwark, were presumably one and the same: C.L. Kingsford, 'Paris Garden and the Bearbaiting', *Archaeologia*, 70 (1920): pp. 161–6.

[101]   McIntosh, *Controlling Misbehavior*, pp. 103–7; Underdown, *Revel, Riot and Rebellion*, pp. 86, 88, 90, 93–4, 97, 99; Simon Thurley, *The Royal Palaces of Tudor England* (New Haven and London, 1993), pp. 182–90.

[102]   Mulcaster, *Positions*, p. 81.

[103]   PRO, KB9/589b/225.

[104]   PRO, KB9/595a/21.

Accident inquests, then, cannot tell us everything we would like to know about sport and recreation in early modern England, but they can provide insights that no other source can easily give. Their chronological and geographical coverage is wider than that of most other sources and they provide incidental detail that is invaluable in reconstructing when, where, how and by whom different activities were pursued. They sometimes confirm, sometimes amplify or contradict what legislation, litigation and treatises – the primary sources for previous histories of early modern sport – suggest about sporting cultures and practices. They illuminate much of the spectrum of leisure activities that contemporaries thought of as 'sports' or 'games', a spectrum that crossed the boundaries between our categories of sport, drama and casual play. They tell us less about the moral status, medical functions and cultural resonances of activities than do the treatises and less about their role in local social, political and religious conflict than the records of litigation. But they can reveal more than these other sources about the times, locations and methods of play and the ages and social positions of participants. With careful handling to take into account the relative dangers of different types of activity, they can also reveal something of the changing popularity of different activities over space and time and illustrate the degree to which sporting cultures varied from region to region.[105]

On the larger scale, accidents suggest that sixteenth-century English sports and games were more regular and informal and less tied to the festive calendar of 'rustic merrymaking', less part of the ritual world of 'folk sport' barely emerged from its 'primitive state', than has often been assumed.[106] Yet they show little sign of the rationalisation and quantification of sporting practice attributed to contemporary Italy and France.[107] In the details accident reports provide of activities, times, places and vocabulary, they may provide the means to test sociological or semiotic generalisations about the genealogy and distinctiveness of modern sporting practices.[108] As our project to analyse all those that survive from the sixteenth century continues, we hope to shed more light on the ways that early modern English men, women and children played, lived and died.

[105] Underdown, *Start of Play*, pp. 4–11; Griffin, *England's Revelry*, pp. 43–52, 141–66.

[106] Dennis Brailsford, *Sport and Society: Elizabeth to Anne* (London, 1969), pp. 51–9; Peter Burke, 'The Invention of Leisure in Early Modern Europe', *Past and Present*, 146 (1995): p. 148; Joan-Lluís Marfany, 'Debate: The Invention of Leisure in Early Modern Europe', *Past and Present,* 156 (1997): pp. 187–91.

[107] John McClelland, 'The Numbers of Reason: Luck, Logic and Art in Renaissance Conceptions of Sport', in *Ritual and Record: Sports Records and Quantification in Pre-Modern Societies*, ed. John Marshall Carter and Arnd Krüger (Westport, CT, 1990), pp. 53–64.

[108] Allen Guttmann, *From Ritual to Record: The Nature of Modern Sports* (New York, 2004), pp. 54–5, 172; McClelland, *Body and Mind*, pp. 11–18.

Chapter 3

Putting Sports in Place: Sports Venues in Sixteenth- and Seventeenth-Century England and their Social Significance

Angela Schattner

The history of early modern sports has so far largely been written as macro-histories mainly based on normative sources and discourses, describing long-term developments.[1] When sports practices have been described, these descriptions are normally based on the study of one specific sport or focus on the practises of one social milieu.[2] However, the attempt to contextualise the practice of sport or sportive physical movements more broadly in early modern culture and society poses several methodological difficulties: What should be the parameters to compare the social practice of different sports? How can the sports practices of different social milieus be compared? And how can changes and developments in those practices be captured?

Confronted with similar conceptual difficulties while analysing the culture of celebrations, amusements and pastimes in the long eighteenth century, Emma Griffin and Ulrich Rosseaux decided to use space as an analytical framework to tackle these difficulties. Emma Griffin compares in her study outdoor public places used for popular recreations including sports in provincial and industrial towns as well as rural villages from 1660 to 1830 and asks who had the power to control these public places to explain social changes in pastime behaviour

---

[1] Dennis Brailsford, *Sport and Society, Elizabeth to Anne* (London, 1969); John McClelland, *Body and Mind: Sport in Europe from the Roman Empire to the Renaissance* (London, 2007); Wolfgang Behringer, *Kulturgeschichte des Sports: Vom antiken Olympia bis ins 21. Jahrhundert* (Munich, 2012).

[2] Norbert Elias, 'An Essay on Sport and Violence', in Norbert Elias and Eric Dunning, *Quest for Excitement: Sport and Leisure in the Civilising Process* (Oxford and New York, 1986), pp. 150–74; Michael Flannery and Richard Leech, *Golf through the Ages: Six Hundred Years of Golfing Art* (Fairfield, 2004); Sydney Anglo, *The Martial Arts of Renaissance Europe* (New Haven and London, 2000); James Walvin, *The People's Game: The History of Football Revisited* (Edinburgh, 1994); Heiner Gillmeister, *Tennis: A Cultural History* (Leicester, 1997); Jean-Michel Mehl, *Les jeux au royaume de France du XIIIe au début de XVIe siècle* (Paris, 1990).

from the eighteenth to the nineteenth century.[3] Ulrich Rosseaux concentrates on the leisure spaces in one city, comprising and comparing the interaction of different social milieus in their leisure pursuits and amusements.[4] Although neither Emma Griffin nor Ulrich Rosseaux are really concerned with developing a cultural theory of space, their studies show that using space as an analytical tool has three distinctive methodological advantages that could also prove fruitful for a history of early modern sports as suggested in this anthology:[5]

1. comparing the use of spaces proves sensitive to regional and temporal variations;
2. conflicts over the use of spaces reflect relationships of power and cultural forces that contributed to these changes;[6]
3. when conceptualising space as relative configuration, looking at the process of the constitution of space can reveal the agency of historical actors to include or exclude people in or from specific spaces, reflecting the practices of social milieus and social inequalities in practices.[7]

This chapter tests the benefits of using space as an analytical framework to explore early modern sportive practices and the social significance of sports in early modern society by comparing the constitution of different sportive spaces. Unlike the above mentioned studies of Griffin and Rosseaux, the chapter focuses not on spaces of leisure and popular pastimes in general but exclusively on spaces in which sports, here with a concentration on playful physical contests like ball games, martial arts or athletics, were practised. In the early modern period, these activities often took place not physically separated from other activities (e.g. related to leisure, work or spirituality) as most places provided space for multiple activities and purposes. It is exactly the relationship to and the interaction with these other fields of early modern society that this chapter wants to investigate to explore early modern sports in their social context.

The approach to space applied in this chapter builds on relativist concepts of space, especially on the sociology of space developed by Martina Löw. In contrast to an absolute approach to space, which conceptualises space as divided from bodies and their actions and thus imagining space as a container in which human action takes place, relativist approaches describe space as a relational

---

[3] Emma Griffin, *England's Revelry: A History of Popular Sports and Pastimes, 1660–1830* (Oxford, 2005), pp. 19–20.

[4] Ulrich Rosseaux, *Freiräume. Unterhaltung, Vergnügen und Erholung in Dresden 1694–1830* (Köln, Weimar and Wien, 2007), pp. 12–14.

[5] See Introduction, pp. 1–17.

[6] Griffin, *England's Revelry*, pp. 19–20.

[7] Rosseaux, *Freiräume*, p. 13.

configuration of bodies to each other.[8] Martina Löw defines space as a relational configuration of living beings and social goods that takes shape in places.[9] Spaces are formed by human (inter)action at specific places (e.g. a park, a church) in the simultaneous process of 'spacing' and 'synthesis': Spacing describes the process of building or placing material social goods but also the active and passive positioning of human beings in relation to each other and to the social goods. However, it is only in combination with the process of synthesis, that is the process of recognising, imagining or remembering the specific configuration of living beings and social goods, that these relational configurations of goods and people are connected to spaces. Human beings play a creative role in the constitutional process of space but can also be a placed or interrelated part in the spatial constitution of others.[10] Spaces are institutionalised when their relational configurations are recognisable and their process of spacing and synthesis is standardised for a group of people. The social rules and symbolism inscribed in these spaces reproduced in repetitive routines give this configuration its objective social validity.[11] Institutionalised spatial structures are a form of social structures and as such are also permeated by structural principles like power, status and gender relations. In this, they reflect and (re-)produce social inequalities.[12] Martina Löw's approach has already been successfully applied in the historical study of public spaces like taverns, town-halls and churches in early modern Europe.[13]

Following the above mentioned approaches, the chapter compares the constitution and social context of three sportive spaces in England in the sixteenth and seventeenth century: The churchyards, sports venues in drinking establishments, and purpose-built sports venues at the royal court. The examples have been chosen to compare spaces constituted in different social contexts and with different forms of accessibility.

In historical research, space has primarily been examined in the categories public and private, mostly using Habermas's theory of the private and the public sphere, constructing a duality of the private domestic sphere and the public.[14] In these categories the chosen sample cases have also been discussed: While the

---

[8] Martina Löw, *Raumsoziologie* (Frankfurt/Main, 2001), pp. 17–19.

[9] Löw, *Raumsoziologie*, pp. 154 and 198.

[10] Löw, *Raumsoziologie*, pp. 158–60.

[11] Löw, *Raumsoziologie*, pp. 161–4.

[12] Löw, *Raumsoziologie*, pp. 166–72 and 173–8.

[13] Susanne Rau and Gerd Schwerhoff (eds), *Zwischen Gotteshaus und Taverne: Öffentliche Räume in Spätmittelalter und Früher Neuzeit* (Köln, 2004); Susanne Rau and Gerd Schwerhoff (eds), *Topographien des Sakralen: Religion und Raumordnung in der Vormoderne* (München, 2008); Gerd Schwerhoff (ed.), *Stadt und Öffentlichkeit* (Köln, 2011).

[14] Jürgen Habermas, *The Structural Transformation of the Public Sphere* (Cambridge, MA, 1989), pp. 43–51; Susanne Rau and Gerd Schwerhoff, 'Öffentliche Räume in der

churchyard and drinking venues are usually categorised as public places, venues at the royal court could be described as private institutions. However, newer research on private and public spaces has shown that the boundaries between private and public are not as clear-cut in early modern society and that there are several intermediate stages between public and exclusively private in venues and houses themselves.[15] Thinking about private and public spaces in terms of ownership also seems only partially helpful in early modern society, especially when considering that places like the church or drinking establishments were officially owned by private parties or organisations, for example by the Church of England, the king, or a landlord, nevertheless they were publicly accessible for large parts of specific communities. The privacy and publicity of spaces thus have again to be considered as cultural constructs that are (re-)produced in social codes of behaviour and safeguarded in legal measures but also materially, e.g. through fences, doors or gates to keep the public out. In this respect, it seems more helpful to examine the inclusiveness or exclusiveness of specific places,[16] and to ask who was in power to allow or restrict access, to whom was access allowed or denied and who would voluntarily choose not to use specific places?[17]

Public Spaces: The Churchyard

Churches and churchyards were important public institutions in early modern society. Following Gerd Schwerhoff's and Susanne Rau's definition of public space, church and churchyard were in principle accessible for everyone independent of their gender or social status and at the same time they were centres of communication and social interaction between people of various provenance.[18] In this latter function, they provided various, overlapping spaces

Frühen Neuzeit. Überlegungen zu Leitbegriffen und Themen eines Forschungsfeldes', in Rau and Schwerhoff, *Zwischen Gotteshaus und Taverne*, pp. 11–52, here pp. 13–20.

[15]   For newer research on the notions of public and private see: Rau and Schwerhoff, 'Öffentliche Räume in der Frühen Neuzeit', pp. 11–52; Caroline Emmelius, Fridrun Freise, Rebekka von Mallinckrodt, Petra Paschinger, Claudius Sittig and Regina Töpfer (eds), *Offen und Verborgen: Vorstellungen und Praktiken des Öffentlichen und Privaten in Mittelalter und Früher Neuzeit* (Göttingen, 2004); Amanda Vickery, 'An Englisman's Home is His Castle? Thresholds, Boundaries and Privacies in the Eighteenth-Century London House', *Past and Present*, 199 (2008): pp. 147–73; Benjamin Heller, 'Leisure and the Use of Domestic Space in Georgian London', *The Historical Journal*, 53/3 (2010): pp. 623–45.

[16]   Löw, *Raumsoziologie*, pp. 168–9, 216–17 and 465–6.

[17]   I am following an approach brought forward by Vickery, 'An Englisman's Home is His Castle?', pp. 153–8; and Heller, 'Leisure and the Use of Domestic Space', pp. 626–8 in their research on the gendered use of space.

[18]   Rau and Schwerhoff, 'Öffentliche Räume in der Frühen Neuzeit', p. 48.

for multiple purposes at the same time. Although churches were primarily the space for communal worship and the churchyard for Christian burial, members of the parish constituted church and churchyard as spaces for other activities of the parish community as well.

Church and churchyard formed the geographical core of the parish community;[19] they were centres of parish communication but also centres of parish sociability.[20] In the church, royal proclamations were read, parish meetings took place and in the churchyard parish celebrations such as church ales, plays and pageants were organised.[21] However, the churchyards were not exclusively used for clearly church-related events, they also served as a place for more profane festivities and meetings as well as for a whole range of recreations and sports sometimes linked to these church festivals, more often separated from them.[22] Church court records and churchwarden presentments, in which parishioners were presented for playing during service or for using the churchyards for their activities, provide an impressive list of sportive games played in the churchyard. These range from contemporary popular ball games such as football or hurling, cricket, tennis, fives, bowling and quoits to martial sports such as cudgelling, wrestling or archery.[23] The constitution of this sporting place was clearly led by the parishioners who started to use the churchyard for games and sports already in the thirteenth century.

The choice of the churchyard as place for sports grew probably out of its status as a public place, which was often placed centrally in the town or village, and as a central meeting place on Sunday. Emma Griffin has already pointed out the importance of public places as spaces for recreation and sports for the poor and landless members of society. As these classes had no land of their own where they could constitute sporting spaces, they were either dependent on the

---

[19] For a detailed discussion of the term parish community and its shaping in the late Middle Ages see: Beat Kümin, *The Shaping of a Community: The Rise and Reformation of the English Parish c. 1400–1560* (Aldershot, 1996); Katherine L. French, *The People of the Parish: Community Life in a Late Medieval English Diocese* (Philadelphia, 2001), pp. 22–7.

[20] Peter Clark, *The English Alehouse: A Social History 1200–1830* (London, 1983), pp. 25–8; David Dymond, 'God's Disputed Acre', *Journal of Ecclesiastical History*, 50/3 (1999): pp. 464–97, here pp. 478–9.

[21] Dymond, 'God's Disputed Acre': p. 467.

[22] Clark, English Alehouse, pp. 25–8; Dymond, 'God's Disputed Acre': pp. 478–9.

[23] See for example: Records of Early English Drama (REED): Elizabeth Baldwin, Lawrence M. Clopper and David Mills (eds), *REED Cheshire including Chester* (Toronto, 2007), pp. 713, 735–6; James Stoke (ed.), *REED Somerset*, 2 vols, vol. 1, (Toronto, 1996), pp. 97, 103–4, 207, 390, 396; David N. Klausner (ed.), *REED Wales* (Toronto, 2005), p. 37; Timothy J. McCann and Peter M. Wilkinson, 'The Cricket Match at Boxgrove in 1622', *Sussex Archaeological Collections*, 110 (1972): pp. 118–22.

goodwill of landowners to make space for this purpose available or they had to appropriate publicly accessible space for their recreational activities.[24]

Still the use of the churchyard as place for sport seems rather strange to us nowadays, especially when considering that other publicly accessible places such as commons, moors or village greens could be used to the same end and were widely available at least in the rural areas of England and Wales. Considering that the aforementioned places served in fact in many villages and towns as spaces for sport alongside the churchyards rather than an alternative to them, the choice for the churchyard as a place for sport must have had reasons beyond its centrality and its accessibility. The main difference between churchyard and commons as spaces for sport was less the games played there but rather the times and mode in which they were constituted as such.

Normally, a specific green or part of a common was used by different groups of men, young women and children to play football, cricket or stoolball during the weekdays in the afternoons or evenings. In the small Welsh village of Llwyn-on in the county of Denbighshire, for example, this place was Lloynon Green where the villagers, young and old, regularly assembled at presumably well-known 'times of recreation ... to make matches for triall of their strength and activitie'. This coming together seems to have been organised quite informally as one inhabitant described his habit 'to walke and resorte thyther [at the green] for one houre or two ... to partake in the said excercises yf occasion shoulde be, or e[lse] to behoulde others performe the same'.[25] The commons and greens thus were well-known and institutionalised sports venues constituted by those inhabitants who had the knowledge of the place and time and who came to join in those sports as players or as spectators.

While the sportive encounters on the village green were more variable as presumably their times and participants varied during the week, sports at the churchyard were a bit more predictable as church service brought regularly together a specific community of people, namely the parishioners, at a specific place (the church/churchyard) and time (Sunday).[26] It was probably these three factors that facilitated the constitution of the churchyard as an important space for sports.

As Sunday and other holy days were days when work had to stop, the times before, between, after and even during service offered convenient occasions

[24]   Griffin, *England's Revelry*, pp. 20–21.

[25]   REED Wales, p. 121.

[26]   On the relationship of time, space and socialisation see: Anthony Giddens, *The Constitution of Society* (Berkeley, 1986), pp. 118–19 and 132–3; Allan Pred, 'Place as Historically Contingent Process: Structuration and the Time-Geography of Becoming Places', *Annals of the Association of American Geographers*, 74 (1984): pp. 279–97, 281.

for recreational or sportive activities to pass the time.[27] In this situation, the churchyard offered enough space for the parishioners to meet and mingle but also provided open space for sports and games outside the actual burial grounds. In addition to this open space, which was in this form also available on the greens and commons, the churchyards' distinctive features such as the high walls and roofs of the church building presumably helped to develop churchyard-specific ball games such as tennis and fives. For example, a pre-form of real tennis was played against the walls of churches, probably also using the slopes of the roofs as game features.[28] Likewise the game of fives[29] featured regularly in church court records and churchwarden accounts in south-west England and Wales as a game played in the churchyard against the walls of the church. Considering that the church building was in most country towns and villages the only building with a wall strong and high enough for such a game and with special roof features that could be used in the game, the church-building was a crucial element for these games at least in the countryside.[30]

Studies on the English parish suggest that a parish identity formed in the late Middle Ages based on common parish charitability and common responsibility for the parish church or village chapel.[31] It was presumably this kind of solidarity that favoured bonds between the parish members and formed their identity as a community which facilitated a sociable atmosphere in which sports between the parish members became possible. At the same time, it can be argued that the parish community bonded exactly through these kinds of regular, more or less structured, communal activities in addition to the aforementioned factors.

Through the process of regular repetition on Sundays, parishioners could expect to play or watch sports on Sundays in the churchyard, thus actively reinforcing and institutionalising the churchyard as space for sport.[32] In this light, it does not seem unlikely that informal teams of fives or tennis players,

---

[27] Chapter 2 in this volume; Dymond, 'God's Disputed Acre': p. 191, footnote 125.

[28] This was at least suggested in the accusation of Bishop Lacy against the canons of the Ottery St Mary of 1451, Gordon Reginald Dunstan (ed.), *The Register of Edmund Lacy Bishop of Exeter 1420-1455,* vol. III. (Torquay, 1967), p. 119-20, cited in: Gillmeister, Tennis, pp. 32-33, also pp. 29-30; see also: Dennis Brailsford, *A Taste for Diversions. Sport in Georgian England* (Cambridge, 1999), p. 45–6

[29] Tony Collins and Emma Lile, 'Fives', in Tony Collins, John Martin and Wray Vamplew (eds), *Encyclopedia of Traditional British Rural Sports* (London, 2005), pp. 114–15.

[30] Brailsford, *A Taste for Diversions,* pp. 45–6; Donald Gregory, *Yesterday in Village Church and Churchyard* (Llandysul, 1989), p. 64-5; Dymond, 'God's Disputed Acre': pp. 490–92.

[31] French, *People of the Parish,* pp. 20–31; Kümin, *Shaping of a Community,* pp. 13–64.

[32] For the process of institutionalisation see: Löw, *Raumsoziologie,* pp. 161–4.

cricketers, wrestlers or footballers formed that way and that other parishioners regularly joined these activities as spectators.

This sportive space in the churchyard was structured by the age, class and gender of the sport's participants and spectators. According to Martina Löw, class and gender have to be considered as structural principles in the constitution of space as they influence the habitus of those constituting spaces which in turn influences the way they will act in specific places or spaces. This habitus can either reflect contemporary acknowledged social behaviour or it can form an alternative culture.[33] In the case of sports, games played in the churchyard were divided into sports for young and middle aged men, such as fives, tennis or football, and sports for young women and children such as stoolball.[34] These different games could take place simultaneously with other recreational activities on the churchground, but occupying different spaces on it. Unfortunately, there is no way to reconstruct the organisation of these games nor the exact place where they were played as these games on the churchyard – or the commons for that matter – are not described anywhere in any detail. So we do not know how regularly the same groups played together, if specific spots on the churchground were reserved for specific games or if the space for these games had to be negotiated each time with other activities taking place on the churchground, and if age and gender played a part in these space negotiations. The only thing we can at least sketchily reconstruct is the role gender and age played in constituting the mode of participation in specific games.

Although young women had their own forms of games, more often women took on the role of spectators. Likewise elderly men and women who were no longer capable of participating and for whom physically playing did not seem appropriate anymore would also join the spectators.[35] Thus the parish members joined differently in sports and games according to their age and gender but shared a common experience of sociability. This does not mean, however, that every member of the community had to or did in fact join in these activities as these games were also confessionally and socially encoded. Parishioners, who perceived the churchyard as consecrated ground, most definitely would not use it as a place for sport. Equally, staunch puritans such as the London wood turner Nehemiah Wallington would not agree to, nor do, any sports on Sundays.[36] Similarly, it was the choice of the 'better sort of people' not to use common

---

[33] Löw, *Raumsoziologie*, pp. 183–91.

[34] See for example the description of games in: Roger North, *The Lives of the Right Hon. Francis North, Baron Guildford ... Together with the Autobiography of the Author*, ed. Augustus Jessop (3 vols, London, 1890), vol. 3, pp. 9–10; Paul Griffiths, *Youth and Authority: Formative Experiences in England 1560–1640* (Oxford, 1996), p. 133.

[35] Dymond, 'God's Disputed Acre': p. 488.

[36] British Library Add. Ms 21935, fol. 45–7.

places for their leisure and sportive activities but to segregate their sports in privately owned facilities.

We do not know when exactly the churchyard had become a firmly but unofficially established institution for parish sports in most English parishes. It was certainly widely accepted by large numbers of parishioners all over England and Wales at the end of the sixteenth and in the seventeenth century when this institution was challenged by a growing fraction of local authorities and the local clergy.[37]

Measures against the profanisation of consecrated ground of church and churchyard were formulated in visitation articles by the higher clergy throughout the Middle Ages.[38] However, these measures had not had very much relevance for the practice of Sunday sports during the Middle Ages as most parish members and even parts of the local clergy were prepared to accept the churchyard and Sunday as the appropriate time and space for sports. This changed at the end of the sixteenth and the beginning of the seventeenth century when various local authorities and some parishioners themselves re-evaluated both the churchyard as a communal place for sports and Sunday as a timeframe for sports under the influence of the Reformation. These changes did not take place without conflicts with those parishioners who still perceived, remembered and used the churchyard as traditional space for sports on Sunday. The resulting conflicts are vividly illustrated in churchwarden presentments and church court records. The increasing number of presentments and church court cases at the end of the sixteenth century and the beginning of the seventeenth century was the result of a stricter implementation of already existing rules against playing in the churchyard by local authorities and the often stubborn ignorance of the same by various parish members who felt they had the right to play there.[39] The *Declaration of Sports*[40] published by James I in 1618 and re-published by Charles I in 1633 in its official approval of Sunday sports often even spurred this attitude although both texts never approved of using the churchyard for Sunday sports. John Brooke, parishioner in Dundry in the county of Somerset, obviously felt he was in the right when he angrily told the churchwarden, who had just rebuked him and his friends 'for vsually playing of fiues, and cudgills in the curchyard theare on sabboath daies and holie daies', to leave them alone as 'wee are att

[37] Dymond, 'God's Disputed Acre': p. 480.

[38] Dymond, 'God's Disputed Acre': pp. 476–8.

[39] Kenneth L. Parker, *The English Sabbath: A Study of Doctrine and Discipline from the Reformation to the Civil War* (Cambridge, 1988), pp. 144, 220–21.

[40] 'The King's Majesty's Declaration to His Subjects, Concerning Lawful Sports to be Used', in Neil Rhodes, Jennifer Richards and Joseph Marshall (eds), *King James VI and I: Selected Writings* (Burlington, 2003), pp. 355–7.

an exercise to doe the kinge service' and called the churchwarden a neighbours' 'cut-throat' if he insisted on reporting them to the church court.[41]

Conflicts also arose about the actual borders of consecrated ground and about the power to decide upon the use of the churchyard. For example, in 1634, again in the parish of Dundry, John Fabian, vicar of Chew Magna, and his curate, Simon Cotton, accused several parishioners of setting up a maypole on consecrated ground. The vicar and the curate claimed that the ground where the maypole stood belonged to them as local church officials and sports as well as festivities on this ground posed a profanisation of the same. While some parishioners backed the vicar's claim, others such as the 64-year-old William Brooke and the 65-year-old Thomas Loscomb challenged the perception of this plot as sacred space. They argued that the disputed plot of ground was apportioned by two walls and that the churchground stretched from the walls of the church building to the first wall and that the plot from the inner to the outer wall was already part of the 'churchhay'. The use of the plot between the inner and the outer wall, where the maypole stood, was no profanisation of consecrated ground according to William Brooke as no 'dead Corps of anie christian deceased was euer buried in the said plott of ground'.[42] Moreover, he and Thomas Loscomb argued that this plot was the traditional place for various parish sports and had never been questioned as such before John Fabian became the vicar of Chew Magna:

> that during all the time of this deponents memorie the said plott of grownd hath been a place wherin some sports or other, & recreations haue byn used and noe contradiction therof that euer this deponent hard [*sic*] or knew of untill since the aforementioned Mr ffabian came to be vicar of Chew magna ... and he him self in his youth & since hath severall tymes used & byn actor in some of the recreations and sportes aforementioned and the use of [such] sportes & recreations in the said plott of ground hath byn from tyme to tyme commonlie known in dundrie & other places & parishes thereaboutes.[43]

These developments did not affect every English and Welsh community to the same extent. In some parts of England the churchyard was still used for sports until the end of the seventeenth century.[44] It depended on local authorities if they accepted this use or not and this was very much dependent on the persons in office. In 1603, the parish priest of Donyatt near Taunton in Somerset complained that the churchwardens and sidemen not only organised church-ales

[41]   Cited in: REED Somerset, p. 100.
[42]   REED Somerset, pp. 104 and 900.
[43]   REED Somerset, pp. 103–4.
[44]   Brailsford, *A Taste for Diversions*, pp. 45–6.

on sacred ground but also allowed games like tennis or bowling to be played in the churchyard.[45]

Some sportive games clung more persistently at the churchyard than others. Games such as fives and tennis, that were dependent upon the specific structure of the church and churchyard, could not be transferred easily to alternative places. In rural areas alternative structures were often not available and purpose-built tennis and fives courts in towns and cities had either only restricted access or had to be paid for. Although most parishes had successfully enforced the banishment of festivities and sports from the churchground by the end of the seventeenth century, these games survived illegally for much longer in the churchyard. In some Welsh parishes fives was still played in the churchyards with approval by local church authorities in the nineteenth century and had developed into local Sunday sports events followed by the whole parish community and transients.[46]

Other sports such as football, cricket, running competitions or wrestling could be transplanted more easily to alternative, often newly created, places. This process of creating alternatives to the churchyard was often actively supported, if not initiated, by village communities and local authorities. In the seventeenth century, newly designated sports grounds for the sole purpose of communal sociability developed in different parishes in central places, namely either close to the churchground or in the middle of the village or town. David Dymond has explored this development in detail for East Anglia where the segregation of the churchyard as a sacred space was enforced early on at the end of the sixteenth and beginning of the seventeenth century.[47] In East Anglia so-called *camping closes* developed, presumably as a response to the segregational efforts. Although the name suggests that these were solely used for the sport of *camp-ball*, which can be best described as a mixture of handball and football, these grounds were used in a similar manner as the churchyards and commons. Their often close proximity to the churchyard – many of the closes were immediately adjacent to it – indicates that their establishment was meant to be an alternative to the churchyard as a playing ground and must have involved at least some degree of general consent and to some extent the support of the local gentry and clergy. Those playing fields were often private land which were lent for recreational use at appropriate times, for example when the harvest was over. In other cases sites were bequeathed by individuals to the township for its inhabitants to use or belonged to the local inn.[48] Thus communally or parish organised sports survived even after they were pushed out of the churchyard and show that

---

[45]   REED Somerset, p. 97.

[46]   Dymond, 'God's Disputed Acre': pp. 490–92; Donald Gregory, *Yesterday in Village Church and Churchyard*, pp. 64–5.

[47]   David Dymond, 'A Lost Social Institution: The Camping Close', *Rural History*, 1/2 (1990): pp. 165–92.

[48]   Dymond, 'Camping Close': pp. 166–7, 172–3.

sports obviously played an important role for village and town communities – important enough to purposefully create designated public areas for them. As Emma Griffin has shown in her study, these communal sport institutions even survived the enclosure of common land in the eighteenth and nineteenth century by again being transferred to alternative places.[49]

Semi-Public Spaces: Alehouses, Taverns and Inns

Local drinking establishments such as alehouses, inns and taverns were other important venues that superseded the churchground as centres for communal sociability and sports in the segregational process of the sixteenth and seventeenth century. As Peter Clark and, more currently, Beat Kümin and Susanne Rau demonstrate, these drinking establishments were more closely interconnected with the parish communities and churches than was realised before.[50] Many emerged from former churchhouses built outside the churchgrounds to create alternative venues for church-related festivities such as baptisms, weddings or wakes and other forms of parish sociability.[51] In the towns and cities, the drinking establishments profited also from the urban development in the sixteenth and seventeenth century, which posed a rather different threat to communal places by shifting and reducing open space. In London, for example, public houses gained increasing attraction as they provided necessary space for sociability and sports outside one's own home in the otherwise overcrowded city. This function became particularly important for the middle classes and the gentry, who flocked to London during the parliamentary season beginning in autumn and ending in June.[52]

In the fifteenth century, drinking establishments had become important spaces for leisure and sociability. Like church and churchyard, they were easily accessible and had clear municipal and communicative functions. Various different groups of people would meet there to drink, to share information, to discuss business, to celebrate or just to have fun.[53] Although drinking

---

[49]   Griffin, *England's Revelry*, pp. 211–22.

[50]   Clark, *English Alehouse*, pp. 153–4; Beat Kümin, 'Sacred Church and Worldly Tavern: Reassessing an Early Modern Divide', in Will Coster and Andrew Spicer (eds), *Sacred Space in Early Modern Europe* (Cambridge, 2005), pp. 17–38; Beat Kümin, Drinking Matters: Public Houses and Social Exchange in Early Modern Central Europe (Basingstoke, 2007), pp. 172–8.

[51]   Clark, *English Alehouse*, pp. 27, 152; Dymond, 'God's Disputed Acre': p. 486.

[52]   Michelle O'Callaghan, 'Tavern Societies, the Inns of Court, and the Culture of Conviviality in Early Seventeenth-Century London', in Adam Smyth (ed.), *A Pleasing Sinne: Drink & Conviviality in Seventeenth-Century England* (Cambridge, 2004), pp. 40–41.

[53]   Rau and Schwerhoff, 'Öffentliche Räume', p. 48.

establishments and churchyards were both used for community celebrations and get-togethers, the setting of these get-togethers and access to this space was nevertheless different as alehouses, taverns and inns were first and foremost commercial enterprises and the main purpose for proprietors was to profit from selling drinks and food as well as from providing accommodation.[54] For this reason, proprietors of drinking establishments invested in different forms of pastime activities, including sports, to attract customers. They provided all sorts of games such as cards, dice and table games together with indoor space for play. Most inns, alehouses and taverns additionally held adjacent yards or gardens, which they made available for their customers to use for outdoor sports and provided the respective equipment such as balls, bowls and cudgels.[55] Proprietors also invested in purpose-built sports facilities such as bowling alleys or tennis courts with levelled grounds and purpose-built features, which allowed for a different and more sophisticated playing experience than public places. These sorts of facilities can be found in London from the fifteenth century and even alehouses in smaller villages invested in them.[56]

In contrast to the churchyard where local clergy and parishioners quarrelled over the right to determine the mode of access and the use of the space, the facilities' proprietors were clearly in charge of deciding and enforcing the mode of access to and the use of the space in their facilities. Generally, access to the bar-room and probably also to the gardens was free of charge but the purpose-built sports facilities probably had to be rented. Roger Lowe, a mercer's apprentice living in the small village of Ashton-in-Markerfield in Lancashire, noted several times in his diary that he spent 2d. 'at bowls', which probably meant that he paid for playing there as he noted money spent on ale or lost in bets separately.[57] Tennis courts and equipment would most likely also be rented but for the sixteenth and seventeenth century no prices are handed down to us. From newspaper adverts from the eighteenth century, we know that playing a single match of tennis cost from 6d. and games of fives were even cheaper from 2d.[58] It seems that members of the middle classes could afford to play at these prices. And considering the repeated parliamentary measures in the sixteenth and seventeenth century

---

[54] Kümin, *Drinking Matters*, pp. 87–146.

[55] Clark, *English Alehouse*, pp. 153–4.

[56] For more detail on the commercialisation of these facilities in London and Bath see Angela Schattner, '"For the Recreation of Gentlemen and Other Fit Persons of the Better Sort": Tennis Courts and Bowling Greens as Early Leisure Venues in Sixteenth- to Eighteenth-Century London and Bath', *Sport in History*, 34/2 (2014): pp. 198–222.

[57] William L. Sachse (ed.), *The Diary of Roger Lowe of Ashton-in-Markerfield, Lancashire, 1633–74* (London, 1938), pp. 28, 88–9, 103.

[58] *Daily Advertiser*, 2 December 1742, 18 January 1744.

against servants, apprentices and journeyman playing in these facilities,[59] we can assume that even these groups were able to afford the costs. Nevertheless, it has to be noted that only those with enough money were able to use these facilities, although the percentage of people who probably were able to afford this might have been quite high.

However, access was not only bound to entry charges but often also to status. In towns and cities establishments were frequented by different types of customers and proprietors of 'quality' establishments had to ensure that only people with the right background could gain entry. In London, for example, gentlemen would only frequent facilities where they could meet others of similar rank; so restricting access to these facilities was of crucial importance for the reputation of the facility.[60] At the end of the eighteenth century, similar concerns seem to have troubled Thomas Higginson, proprietor of several tennis courts in London, who repeatedly assured his gentleman customers in his newspaper ads that he was

> determined to preserve the utmost Order and Decorum there, and hath given strict Orders to his Servants not to admit any Journeyman, Labourers, Servants, Apprentices, or any inferior Persons, to play there upon any Terms; therefor 'tis hoped that none such will presume to come there to impede the Entertainment of such Noblemen and Gentlemen as shall honour him with their Company.[61]

So it seems that different establishments existed for different social groups and not everyone who could afford to play at these facilities would also be permitted to enter.

Equally important was the gender aspect when considering the accessibility of drinking establishments. New research has shown that women might have frequented English drinking establishments more regularly than has been assumed so far.[62] Nevertheless, the concern for women's reputation changed

---

[59]   Marjorie Keniston McIntosh, *Controlling Misbehaviour in England, 1370–1600* (Cambridge, 1998), pp. 98–101; Calendar of Patent Rolls (CPR): Ann Morton (ed.), *CPR Elisabeth I* (HMSO, 1891–1986), vol. 2, p. 218, vol. 3, p. 1845, CPR Edward VI, vol. 4, p. 197, vol. 5, p. 47.

[60]   Thomas Brennan, *Public Drinking and Popular Culture in Eighteenth-Century Paris* (Princeton, 1988), pp. 228–68; B. Ann Tlusty, *Bacchus and Civic Order: The Culture of Drink in Early Modern Germany* (Charlottesville, 2001), pp. 147–57; O'Callaghan, 'Tavern Societies', 38–9.

[61]   *Public Advertiser*, 21 April 1760.

[62]   Amanda Flather, *Gender and Space in Early Modern England* (Woodbridge, 2006), pp. 110–21. In contrast Thomas Brennan and Anne Tlusty have characterised taverns in Paris and Augsburg respectively as a 'predominantly male space'. See Brennan, *Public Drinking*, pp. 147–51; and Tlusty, *Bacchus*, pp. 133–45. For a research overview see James R. Brown,

their mode of access and participation in games compared to that of the churchyard where they were more easily included; even if women were restricted to their own games or confined to the role of spectators. Considering these external preconditions of public houses, it might be not too wild a guess that the community of the parish was replaced by other forms of social bonds such as status groups and occupations when sports and sociability found a new home in these facilities.[63] These changes might have developed quite differently in urban spaces in contrast to rural areas, but more research needs to be done here.

Exclusive Places: The Royal Court

While the public and semi-public places described above were easily accessible for large parts of the population, there is a clear trend from the fifteenth century onwards to constitute exclusive and prestigious spaces and purpose-built facilities for sports by urban and aristocratic elites.

In the aristocratic circles building exclusive and prestigious sports facilities formed part of their conspicuous consumption and the representation of their status identity.[64] This became particularly visible at the royal palaces, where the sovereigns installed new purpose-built sports facilities such as tennis courts from the end of the fifteenth century. Although tennis had been popular in France and Spain from the twelfth century and was played in England presumably from the thirteenth century, the first English tennis court at a palace was built by Henry VII in the years 1492 and 1493 in Kenilworth. From 1493 to 1508, several others followed in Richmond, Wycombe, Woodstock, Windsor and Westminster. It was also Henry VII who built the first kind of sports complex[65] at an English royal house, namely in Richmond Palace. He had installed tennis courts, bowling alleys and a designated space with butts for archers in close proximity to each other in the gardens of Richmond at the end of the fifteenth century. This whole complex of sports facilities was complemented by nearby 'housis of pleasure to disporte inn at chesse, tables, dise cardes'[66] and together formed something like a leisure resort for the royal family and their courtiers.

The Landscape of Drink: Inns, Taverns and Alehouses in Early Modern Southampton (PhD thesis, University of Warwick, 2007), pp. 188–9.

[63] Brown, *The Landscape of Drink*, pp. 178–85.

[64] F.J. Fisher, *London and the English Economy, 1500–1700*, P.J. Corfield and N.B. Harte (eds) (London, 1990), pp. 111–15.

[65] Simon Thurley, *The Royal Palaces of Tudor England: Architecture and Court Life 1460–1547* (New Haven and London, 1993), p. 179.

[66] G. Kipling (ed.), *The Receyt of the Ladie Kateryne* (Oxford, 1990), pp. 73–4.

According to Simon Thurley, the whole complex was modelled after those at the Duke of Burgundy's palaces in Princenhof and Ghent.[67]

Permanent sports facilities and these kinds of sports complexes became even more important in Henry VIII's reign. A keen sportsman himself and an enthusiastic jouster in his youth, he installed from 1514 permanent structures for jousting and tilting in Greenwich, Whitehall and Hampton Court.[68] Moreover, new tennis courts were constructed in Westminster, Beaulieu and Bridewell. From 1532 until his death in 1547, Henry VIII equipped all major royal palaces such as Whitehall, Hampton Court Palace and St James's Palace with tennis courts and bowling alleys and even some of the lesser residences as Calais, Eltham, Grafton and Woking were furnished with either of these facilities. In Whitehall and Hampton Court, similar sports complexes as the one in Richmond were created. They all featured a tilting ground, several roofed and unroofed tennis courts and bowling alleys.[69] Jousting, tilting, tennis and bowling had obviously become more than occasional pastimes and the king did not want to do without his sports when changing residence. He and his successors invested quite a lot in maintaining these venues as repairs and alterations were common over the years.[70]

In contrast to the sporting spaces on public grounds, which were constituted by the appropriation through the players and the usage of their specific features, these sports complexes were constituted as spaces for sport through the intentional building of permanent and purpose-built constructions by the monarchs as prestigious facilities to represent group and status identities. However, the constitution of the different sporting spaces varied in terms of access and use depending on the sports and their social function as the examples of the tilting grounds and of the tennis courts and bowling alleys will demonstrate.

It is unclear if the tilting yards were used by sovereigns and courtiers outside of official tournaments but we know for certain that they were used for tournaments quite regularly from Henry VIII to James I and diminished only in Charles I's reign. On average, two tournaments per year took place excluding longer periods without tournaments at the beginning of new reigns. Although the tournament had clearly sportive elements and as such was a sportive spectacle in its own right,[71] it served at the same time as a royal display of power for other royal visitors and diplomats but also for the sovereign's subjects. As such, the tournaments were reserved for special occasions and festivities: Elizabeth I

[67]   Thurley, *Royal Palaces*, p. 179.
[68]   Thurley, *Royal Palaces*, pp. 181–2.
[69]   Thurley, *Royal Palaces*, pp. 185–7, 189.
[70]   David Best, *The Royal Tennis Court: A History of Tennis at Hampton Court Palace* (Oxford, 2002), pp. 271–82.
[71]   Joachim Rühl, 'Sports Quantification in Tudor and Elizabethan Tournaments', in John Marshall Carter and Arnd Krüger (eds), *Ritual and Record: Sports Records and Quantification in Pre-Modern Societies* (New York, 1990), pp. 65–86.

and James I each held a tournament to celebrate their coronation and repeated this almost every year on the anniversary of their accession of the throne. Tournaments were part of the entertainments at royal weddings but also at the celebration of May Day and Shrovetide.[72]

The representative aspect of the tournaments such as the display of royal power and wealth as well as the physical abilities of the courtiers needed publicity and thus made the participation of spectators a crucial element of these sportive events. The importance of spectators is reflected in the construction of the permanent tilting yards of Henry VIII, where viewing stands for the nobility built in brick and stone were the most important structures. The tournaments were never restricted to noble visitors, however, and the tournament grounds, although part of the royal gardens and as such private facilities and normally only accessible for members of the royal household, were opened on these occasions for wider parts of the public.

The representative act was not limited to the physical display in the competition between the courtiers though. Even more important was the spatial arrangement of the spectators on the tournament ground by the royal household. In a tournament in Westminster at the beginning of the sixteenth century, for example, the viewing stand reserved for the royal family and invited guests was positioned at the best point of observation at the tiltyard: with the sun to the back and positioned as close and as near as possible to the centre of the tilt. The stands to the right of the king were reserved for earls, barons and knights and to the left for the ladies of the court.[73] Opposite the king's stands, viewing stands were reserved for the Lord Mayor and his officials. In a similar order as on the king's side, the viewing stands on the north side were descending according to rank. To the right of the mayor's stand was a viewing stand for the gentlemen of the Innes of Court and next to it stands for the members of the London livery companies, to the left were stands for the merchants. The arrangement of these facilities should project an image of the ideal social hierarchy in the kingdom. Considering recent work on the importance of spatial representations of rank in churches, universities, in city and royal festivities,[74] we can assume that conflicts arose about the privileges of entering the different stands as they reflected one's

---

[72]   Alan Young, *Tudor and Jacobean Tournaments* (London, 1987), pp. 196–208.

[73]   Young, *Tudor and Jacobean Tournaments*, pp. 79–80, 85–8.

[74]   See for example: Marian Füssel, 'Rang und Raum: Gesellschaftliche Kartographie und die soziale Logik des Raumes an der vormodernen Universität', in Christoph Dartmann, Marian Füssel and Stefanie Rüther (eds), *Raum und Konflikt: Zur symbolischen Konstituierung gesellschaftlicher Ordnung in Mittelalter und Früher Neuzeit* (Münster, 2004), pp. 175–98; Barbara Stollberg-Rilinger, 'Zeremoniell als politisches Verfahren. Rangordnung und Rangstreit als Strukturmerkmal des frühneuzeitlichen Reichstags', in Johannes Kunisch (ed.), Neue Studien zur frühneuzeitlichen Reichsgeschichte (Berlin, 1997), pp. 91–132; about the 'social logic of space' compare: Peter Burke, 'The Language of Orders in Early

social standing either in court or in the City of London. Attached to either end of the north side's viewing stands for city dignitaries were stands accessible for everyone who could pay a shilling. Separated from the stands, there was designated space for commoners who could watch the spectacle in front of the fences surrounding the tilting ground.[75] So better viewing and social positions were not only constituted by official ranks but also by personal wealth.

While the tournaments were representative competitions which needed publicity and where spectators from all ranks were admitted, access to the royal tennis courts and bowling alleys either as players or spectators was, apart from servants, restricted to members of the royal court. They were places constituted for the private, leisurely play of the sovereign and his courtiers but could also become the venue for royal representation during official visits of other sovereigns, princes and dignitaries.

The tennis courts and bowling alleys were very popular from December to May or June when the hunting and hawking season had not yet started and the court needed to be entertained.[76] Henry VIII made regular use of his own tennis courts as can be seen in the records of his privy expense accounts.[77] In the tennis courts and bowling alleys, Henry VIII played tennis and bowling against his courtiers as we know from betting losses also recorded in the privy purse. He lost, for example, 50 shillings at tennis to Anthony Knyvet or at another time £32 5s. to the Lords Rocheford and Wiltshire at bowling.[78] The matches were presumably informal and played by the courtiers and the king primarily for fun. Nevertheless, it can be assumed that royal court etiquette was still in place and that it was still a privilege and of political significance for courtiers to be asked to play against the king or to attend the royal tennis game. The king also played tennis against hired professionals and even borrowed those of his courtiers as he paid Lord Rochforde in 1530 'for the use of Maister Weston for 4 games of tennis'. Mr Weston and another professional 'Rogers' are again mentioned on several occasions in the accounts of 1531–2.[79]

Courtiers could hire the tennis courts for playing amongst themselves or against tennis professionals,[80] when the king was not at play. For example, Henry Countenay, Earl of Devon, played in the king's court at Richmond and

---

Modern Europe', in Michael L. Bush (ed.), *Social Orders and Social Classes in Europe since 1500: Studies in Social Stratification* (London, 1992), pp. 1–12.

[75]   Young, *Tudor and Jacobean Tournaments*, pp. 79–80, 83–6.

[76]   Thurley, *Royal Palaces*, p. 180.

[77]   L&P: Letters and Papers Foreign and Domestic, Henry VIII, vol. 5 (1880), pp. 754, 757–9.

[78]   L&P, vol. 5, pp. 752, 758.

[79]   L&P, vol. 5, pp. 749, 757.

[80]   L&P, vol. 3, p. 51.

Greenwich for which he paid between 2 shillings 4 pence and 2 shillings 8 pence per day.[81]

Tennis, bowling and archery were sociable activities in the aristocratic circles too, and facilities to cater for spectators were installed. The bowling alleys had waiting areas at either end, one for the players and one for the servants who collected the balls. For the spectators, benches and leaning boards were installed from where they could watch the games. The tennis courts usually had sophisticated galleries for spectators. At the tennis court in Richmond, the spectators could watch matches from galleries above the tennis court, and were protected from stray balls by nets.[82]

While bowling could be played by both sexes, tennis was reserved for the male members of the royal court, leaving female members only the role as spectators. This is also true for the reigning queens Mary I and Elizabeth I who never played tennis themselves. Elizabeth I at least enjoyed watching the game as some anecdotes from letters suggest.[83]

The space for spectators in these facilities was, however, very much restricted. The viewing galleries at the tennis courts, for example, only provided space for a few dozen spectators. We do not know for certain how access was granted for spectators but we can assume that access was restricted to noble spectators and that the mode of access varied on occasion. For example, we can assume that access was more restricted when the king played or when the queen watched games. Likewise on official occasions, probably only selected members of the aristocracy would have been admitted to the tennis courts.[84]

Although games of tennis and bowling were played by the king and courtiers on a leisurely basis, games – especially tennis – could, like the tournaments, gain political significance when staged as part of the entertainments for other sovereigns, princes and dignitaries. On these occasions tennis functioned again as royal display and tennis matches were hosted between select members of different courts.[85] R.J. Lake argues that official invitations to play tennis and officially staged tennis matches formed part of noble conspicuous consumption and representation as tennis courts were a symbol of wealth through the display of craftsmanship and design. Likewise the display of stylish tennis dresses, the accompanying tennis entourage and spectators as well as the tennis play itself should exhibit the refined noble lifestyle.[86]

[81] L&P, vol. 3, p. 51.
[82] Thurley, *Royal Palaces*, pp. 186, 189.
[83] R.J. Lake, 'Real Tennis and the Civilising Process', *Sport in History*, 29/4 (2009): pp. 553–76, pp. 563–4.
[84] Lake, 'Real Tennis', p. 562.
[85] Lake, 'Real Tennis', p. 562.
[86] Lake, 'Real Tennis', pp. 564–7.

Private and prestigious sport facilities were not an exclusive feature of the royal court though. Encouraged by the royal example and as tennis and bowling became fashionable pastimes for courtiers and noblemen in the sixteenth and seventeenth century, tennis courts and bowling alleys or greens became a feature of aristocratic houses such as Somerset House, Essex House and Cecil House.[87] University colleges, for example in Cambridge, built tennis courts for the exclusive use of wealthier students.[88] And most of the London livery companies installed purpose-built bowling alleys in their gardens for the exclusive use of their members and selected friends.[89]

Conclusion

As these admittedly still sketchy sample cases hopefully demonstrate, a relational spatial approach to sports has its own distinctive advantages and disadvantages to contextualise early modern sports practices. On the one hand, this approach is limited by the source materials (e.g. court records, diaries and travel reports, maps and leasing contracts) handed down to us, as in many cases the actual constitution, practices and negotiations of spaces are only partially reconstructable. On the other hand, the analysis of the constitution and use of spaces, as sketchy as they might often be, provide a lens through which the sports practices of historical actors and their agency in these can be revealed and through which sports can be analysed within their specific cultural and social backgrounds. The close examination of spaces and places used for sports also gives us the opportunity to explore the practice and the social significance of sports in connection with other social practices that took place in these spaces and we can examine their interconnectedness. For example, by examining different types of spaces (multi-purpose/purpose-built, public/private/commercial) created for sports in three different places (the churchyard, drinking establishments and the royal court), different practices in sport could be unearthed. Although in all the examined places similar games, especially ball games such as fives, tennis and bowling, were played, the social contexts of these games were quite different and sports could fulfil several functions. Sports consolidated group identities, be it in parish or village communities, the community of the royal court, student or craftsmen communities. This consolidation could be created by the inclusion

---

[87]   Roger Morgan, *Tudor Tennis: A Miscellany* (Oxford, 2001), pp. 30–32.

[88]   John Twigg, 'Student Sports, and their Context, in Seventeenth-Century Cambridge', *International Journal of the History of Sport*, 13/2 (1996): pp. 80–95, see pp. 81–3.

[89]   Brigid Mary Urswick Boardman, 'The Gardens of the London Livery Companies', *Journal of Garden History*, 2/2 (1982): pp. 85–116; Vanessa Harding, 'Gardens and Open Space in Tudor and Early Stuart London', in Mireille Galinou (ed.), *London's Pride: The Glorious History of the Capital's Gardens* (London, 1990), pp. 44–55, here p. 55.

of large parts of communities across status and gender or by social exclusion of large parts of society and were primarily organised over the constitution of space, e.g. the inclusiveness of the churchyard or the exclusiveness of royal tennis courts. Sports and games made up a large portion of recreational activities but with their own distinctive rules and social patterns. However, sports and games were not all fun and play, but could also have representational functions to display social status and a wealthy lifestyle. And sports and games are much more connected to the commercialisation of leisure and luxury goods already in the sixteenth and seventeenth century than has been realised before. Thus the usage and construction of space or places for sports can not only tell us more about the place of sports in society but about recreation, sociability, hierarchies, consumer culture and early modern society more generally.

PART II
Sport for Money and Glory? Commercialization and Professionalization

Chapter 4

The Capital of Tennis: *Jeux de Paume* as Urban Sport Facilities in Fifteenth- and Sixteenth-Century Paris

Christian Jaser

In the eyes of travellers and foreign residents alike, one of the striking features of late sixteenth-century Paris was the sheer quantity and concentration of tennis courts (*jeux de paume*) in the urban landscape. In particular, Italian observers noticed this unique infrastructure: The Venetian ambassador in Paris, Geronimo Lippomano, claimed in 1577 that there existed no less than 1,800 Parisian tennis courts. The author found these noteworthy as they did not only occupy a considerable amount of urban space but, as Lippomano stressed, because of their economic significance as he calculated that more than 1,000 *scudi* were spent daily in these facilities.[1] In 1596, Francesco d'Ierni, accompanying the papal legate Alessandro de' Medici to France, noted in his travel journal that there were 250 'fine and well-equipped tennis courts' in Paris which provided livelihoods for up to 7,000 persons.[2] English visitors like Sir Robert Dallington, travelling through France during his Grand Tour in 1598, also recognised the peculiarities of the French and particularly the Parisian tennis culture:

> As for the exercise of Tennis play, which I aboue remembred, it is more here vsed, then in all Christendome besides; whereof may witnesse the infinite number of Tennis Courts throughout the land, insomuch as yee cannot finde that little Burgade, or towne in France, that hath not one or mo[r]e of them ... and I know

---

[1]   Niccolò Tommaseo (ed.), *Relations des ambassadeurs vénitiens sur les affaires de France au XVIe siècle* (2 vols, Paris, 1838), vol. 2, p. 600; two years after Lippomano's statement, the humanist and Protestant printer, Henri Estienne (1531–1598), tried to prove the superiority of the French over the Italian language. Thereby, he also referred to the *jeu de paume*, in which the French indulged more than any other nation, this being proved by the sheer quantity of *tripots*, i.e. tennis courts, in Paris: Henri Estienne, *Précellence de langage francois*, ed. Edmond Huguet (Paris, 1896), pp. 135–6; see also John McClelland, *Body and Mind: Sport in Europe from the Roman Empire to the Renaissance* (London and New York, 2007), p. 124.

[2]   Gaston Reynaud (ed.), 'Paris en 1596 vu par un italien', *Bulletin de la société de l'histoire de Paris et de l'Ile-de-France*, 12 (1885): p. 166.

not how many hundred there be in Paris: but of this I am sure, that if there were in other places the like proportion, ye should haue two Tennis Courts, for euery one Church through France. Me thinks it also strange, how apt they be here to play well, that ye would thinke they were borne with Rackets in their hands, euen the children themselues manage them so well, and some of their women also.[3]

Likewise impressed was the Swiss-born traveller Thomas Platter the Younger, who visited Paris in the summer of 1599:

> The common play is the tennis court, wherein old and young persons constantly exercise ... Some people say that there are 1,100 tennis courts in Paris. If there exist only half as many, as I believe, in the whole of Paris, it is still an impressive figure. These courts are usually full of people playing tennis, as I have seen it.[4]

Of course, the recurring quantitative references in these diplomatic relations and travel accounts should not be taken at face value. Their significance does not lie so much in statistical evidence but rather in the quite remarkable conformity of quantitative hyperbole. Quite unanimously, the foreign observers reported the omnipresence and density of tennis courts in the Parisian cityscape as being beyond comparison and a typical urbanistic feature of the French capital. The *jeu de paume*, the ball game played with the palm of the hand,[5] is not only presented as the favourite leisure activity of the Parisians but also as a considerable factor in the urban economy. Summing up these aspects, the city of Paris manifests itself as Europe's capital of tennis in the fifteenth and sixteenth centuries, praised for the playing quality and the abundant infrastructure of purpose-built courts within its walls and its suburbs.[6]

From this point of view, the statement of Werner Paravicini that 'the history of medieval sports belongs, in the first instance, to the history of the nobility'[7] has to be reassessed. Whereas the 'tight connection between sport and urbanity'

---

[3]   Robert Dallington, *A method for trauell Shewed by taking the view of France. As it stoode in the yeare of our Lord 1598* (London, 1605), pp. V r–V v.

[4]   Thomas Platter d.J., *Beschreibung der Reisen durch Frankreich, Spanien, England und die Niederlande 1595–1600*, ed. Rut Keiser (2 vols, Basel and Stuttgart, 1968), vol. 2, p. 613: 'Daß gemeinist spil ist daß ballenhauß, darinnen sich iung unndt alts stetigs üebet'; Platter, *Beschreibung*, p. 594: 'Ettliche sagen, daß es bey 1100 ballenheüser zu Paris habe, aber so nur halb so viel, wie ich glaub, in gantz Paris sindt es eine hüpsche zahl. Unndt sindt gemeinlich aller voller leüten, die ballenspilen, wie ichs gesehen' (my translation).

[5]   Heiner Gillmeister, *Kulturgeschichte des Tennis. Sonderausgabe für den Deutschen Tennis-Bund* (Munich, 1990), p. 14.

[6]   Gillmeister, *Kulturgeschichte des Tennis*, pp. 132–3.

[7]   Werner Paravicini, 'Gab es eine einheitliche Adelskultur Europas im späten Mittelalter?', in Rainer C. Schwinges, Christian Hesse and Peter Moraw (eds), *Europa im*

has been studied by some scholars of modern sport, particularly from the United States,[8] the blending of sport and urban history has not yet been systematically analysed with regard to the culturally rich and complex societies of late medieval and early modern cities.[9] This extensively conceptual vacuum is rather strange, given the essential role late medieval and early modern cities played in attracting sport actors and spectators, in employing their established financial and logistical expertise to organise large-scale sport events, in advancing physical competitions of the burghers and, finally, in producing and trading sport equipment.[10] Until recent times, the dominant macrohistorical perspective of premodern sport studies could not have cared less about this agenda, preferring instead vast temporal and spatial scopes like, for example, John McClelland's *Sport in Europe*

---

späten Mittelalter. Politik – Gesellschaft – Kultur (Munich, 2006), pp. 401–34, here p. 409, fn. 29.

   [8]   Christian Koller, 'Einleitung: Stadt und Sport', in Christian Koller (ed.), *Sport als städtisches Ereignis* (Ostfildern, 2008), pp. 7–27, citation on p. 7; Gabriele Klein, 'Urbane Bewegungskulturen. Zum Verhältnis von Sport, Stadt und Kultur', in Jürgen Funk-Wieneke and Gabriele Klein (eds), *Bewegungsraum und Stadtkultur. Sozial- und kulturwissenschaftliche Perspektiven* (Bielefeld, 2008), pp. 13–27; see also Steven A. Riess, *City Games: The Evolution of American Urban Society and the Rise of Sports* (Urbana and Chicago, 1991), esp. pp. 1–48; Stephen Hardy, 'The City and the Rise of American Sport, 1820–1920', *Exercise and Sports Sciences Review*, 9 (1983): pp. 183–219; Melvin L. Adelman, *A Sporting Time: New York City and the Rise of Modern Athletics 1820–1870* (Urbana and Chicago, 1986); for a German perspective, Stefan Nielsen, *Sport und Großstadt 1870–1930. Komparative Studien zur Entstehung bürgerlicher Freizeitkultur* (Frankfurt, 2002).

   [9]   See Erwin Niedermann, 'Die Leibesübungen der Ritter und Bürger', in Horst Ueberhorst (ed.), *Geschichte der Leibesübungen* (6 vols, Berlin, Munich and Frankfurt, 1972–1989), vol. 3/1, pp. 70–96; Roland Renson, 'Leibesübungen der Bürger und Bauern im Mittelalter', in Horst Ueberhorst (ed.), *Geschichte der Leibesübungen* (6 vols, Berlin, Munich and Frankfurt, 1972–1989), vol. 3/1, pp. 97–144; Rudolf Holbach, 'Spiel, Sport und Kurzweil in städtischen Quellen des späten Mittelalters. Bemerkungen zu ihren Bedingungen und Funktionen', in Konstanzer Arbeitskreis für mittelalterliche Geschichte (ed.), *Protokoll der Reichenau-Tagung vom 5.–8. Oktober 1994, nr. 334: Spiel, Sport und Kurzweil in der Gesellschaft des Mittelalters*, Proceedings manuscript, pp. 42–53; Peter Moraw, 'Von Turnieren und anderen Lustbarkeiten. Sport im Mittelalter', in Hans Sarkowicz (ed.), *Schneller, Höher, Weiter: Eine Geschichte des Sports* (Frankfurt, 1996), pp. 68–81, here pp. 79–81; Michael Thomas, 'Leibesübungen, Spiel und "Sport" im europäischen Mittelalter', in Michael Krüger and Hans Langenfeld (eds), *Handbuch Sportgeschichte* (Schorndorf, 2010), pp. 153–66, here pp. 157–8, 160–61.

   [10]   See Rudolf Holbach, 'Feste in spätmittelalterlichen Städten des Hanseraums', in Simonetta Cavaciocchi (ed.), *Il tempo libero: economia e società (loisirs, leisure, tiempo libre, Freizeit), secc. XIII–XVIII* (Prato and Florence, 1995), pp. 213–32, here p. 215.

from the Roman Empire to the Renaissance,[11] or genealogies of specific forms of sport from their beginnings until the present day.[12]

In contrast, I advocate a microhistorical approach to premodern sport history, narrowing the analytical task to focus on a small spatial unit.[13] This approach permits a detailed analysis of the sporting habits in different social milieus of urban society, including reciprocal imitations, adaptations and differentiations beyond the mere confrontation of elite and popular cultures. In addition, the results of such a survey of urban sport practices could and should be contextualised within urban history as a whole and understood against the background of contemporary social, economic, political and urbanistic developments. In this chapter, the Parisian tennis courts from the Middle Ages to the Early Modern Period are interpreted – in the words of Michel de Certeau – as specific 'practised places' of the city's everyday life which were constituted through ludic motions and related social and economic interactions between protagonists of different sociocultural milieus.[14] In this respect, they fulfilled various functions at the same time: For players, they were places of leisure, ludic competition and betting; for the spectators, they were places of sociability and consumption; for proprietors, they were places of economic profit with regard to the renting of playing areas and equipment.

In order to highlight and contextualise these distinctive threads of the Parisian 'tennis cultures', the chapter is divided in three sections: First of all, it will discuss the urbanistic and sociocultural prerequisites for the formation of this peculiar sport culture in the French capital. Based on these findings, the economics of the Parisian *jeux de paume* will be examined. Finally, the chapter

---

[11]　McClelland, *Body*; see also the recent macrohistory of sport by Wolfgang Behringer, *Kulturgeschichte des Sports. Vom antiken Olympia bis ins 21. Jahrhundert* (Munich, 2012).

[12]　See on this genealogical 'obsession des origines' Jean-Michel Mehl, 'Jeux, sports et divertissements au moyen âge et à la Renaissance: rapport introductif', in Jean-Michel Mehl (ed.), *Jeux, sports et divertissements au Moyen Age et à l'age classique. Actes du 116e congrès national des sociétés savantes* (Paris, 1993), pp. 5–22, here p. 12; Norbert Elias, 'An Essay on Sport and Violence', in Norbert Elias and Eric Dunning, *Quest for Excitement: Sport and Leisure in the Civilising Process* (Oxford and New York, 1986), pp. 150–74, here p. 152.

[13]　Moraw, 'Sport', p. 72.

[14]　Michel de Certeau, *The Practice of Everyday Life* (Berkeley, 1984), p. 117. Generally, de Certeau emphasises the impact of experience and motion on the transformation of a rather fixed 'place' into a dynamic 'space' as a socially produced 'practised place'. In this respect, the Parisian tennis courts could be seen as a specific spatial arrangement that implied the practice of bodily movements and ludic dynamics and invoked multi-layered social and economic interactions. For the application of de Certeau's notion to sport history see Patricia Vertinsky, 'Locating a "Sense of Place": Space, Place and Gender in the Gymnasium', in Patricia Vertinsky and John Bale (eds), *Sites of Sport: Space, Place, Experience* (London and New York, 2004), pp. 8–24.

will argue that these commercial units raised rather ambivalent perceptions on the part of city magistrates and contemporary observers, particularly in the context of the contested leisure culture of premodern cities in general.

Urban Spaces and Tennis Cultures

Jeu de paume[15] was bound to a specific kind of spatial arrangement: A flat playing field was necessary that provided enough space for an acceptable hitting-range, a hatch or window as target for the attacking team and a sloping penthouse whereon the service had to be delivered.[16] In late medieval Paris, tennis was mostly played in the courtyards and forecourts of churches and cloisters using their walls as Jean-Michel Mehl's survey of the letters of remission[17] issued by the royal chancellery with regard to ludic activities indicates.[18] Moreover, the Parisians also used public crossroads, squares and streets as temporary tennis

---

[15] For the origins, development and rules of the *jeu de paume* see Yves Carlier and Thierry Bernard-Tambour, *Jeu des rois, roi des jeux. Le jeu de paume en France. Musée national du château de Fontainebleau, 2 octobre 2001–7 janvier 2002* (Paris, 2001); Gillmeister, *Kulturgeschichte*; Roger Morgan, *Tennis: The Development of the European Ball Game* (Oxford, 1995).

[16] Jean-Michel Mehl, *Les jeux au royaume de France du XIIIe au début du XVI siècle* (Paris, 1990), p. 259.

[17] According to Claude Gauvard, *'De grace especial'. Crime, État et société en France à la fin du Moyen Âge* (Paris, 1991), p. 63, a letter of remission could be defined as 'un acte de la Chancellerie par lequel le roi octroie son pardon à la suite d'un crime ou d'un délit, arrêtant ainsi le cours ordinaire de la justice, qu'elle soit royale, seigneuriale, urbaine ou ecclésiastique'. Generally, homicides and physical injuries during a tennis game appear rather frequently in letters of remission of the fifteenth and sixteenth centuries. Consequently, Jean Papon, *Trias Iudiciel du Second Notaire* (Lyon, 1580), p. 470, listed this case under the heading of pardonable homicides; 'Le dixieme cas, est si de plusieurs iouans à la bale, ou paume, l'un par vehemence vient à choquer l'autre, qu'il fait choir, & mourir, poureu que tel choc ne soit faict expres & hors du ieu, mais visiblement selon le ieu, sera tel homicide impuni'; see also Natalie Zemon Davis, *Fiction in the Archives: Pardon Tales and their Tellers in Sixteenth-Century France* (Stanford, 1987), p. 12.

[18] Mehl, *Les jeux*, pp. 260–61. For example, there is evidence dating from April 1383 that the pilgrims' hospice named Saint-Jacques-aux-Pèlerins on the right bank of the river Seine was abused by some vagrant clerics as a temporary tennis court. In 1403, a carpenter was charged with building wooden barriers in front of the entrance to the hospice's fraternity in order to ban the access of 'people playing dice, cards, sticks, hopscotch, tennis and other bad games'. Obviously to no avail because one year later sergeant Jacquet d'Orme was ordered 'to clear the cloister of some players and other impertinent persons'. Henri Bordier and Léon Brièle (eds), *Les archives hospitalières de Paris* (Paris, 1877), pp. 45, 109, 153; see Mehl, *Lex jeux*, pp. 253, 369.

courts.[19] These provisional redefinitions of ecclesiastical and urban spaces posed a continuous challenge to public order.

At the same time, the demand for tennis in Paris gave rise to a steadily growing supply of purpose-built tennis courts both within the city walls and in the suburbs during the fourteenth and fifteenth centuries. Thus, the ludic dynamic of the *jeu de paume* was enclosed in a consolidated spatial arrangement that permitted its serial use and commercialisation in terms of an economically 'practised place'. Of particular importance in this respect were the Parisian taverns that provided tennis as an additional attraction and crowd-puller.[20] Frequently, tavern-keepers assigned an interior space, courtyard or an adjacent parcel of land to this sport activity, or they erected their own tennis court in the form of an outbuilding.[21] Such facilities were mostly open-air courts that could be rented for a certain time-span and supplied the players with spatial accessories for proper rallies and some other services like drinks and equipment.[22]

Together with the large and well-equipped ballhouses situated in the urban residences of the French king, the diversified infrastructure[23] of the Parisian tennis courts was impressive, especially in quantitative terms. About 70 tennis courts could be localised between 1300 and 1600 by gathering data from Parisian notary registers, letters of remission, diaries, travel accounts and chronicles.[24] Their accumulation in certain parts of the city allows us to draw conclusions on the social profiles of tennis players based on socio-topographic data.

The city-space of Paris is characterised by a relatively symmetrical tri-partition.[25] The so-called *Plan de Bâle*[26] from about 1553 by Germain Hoyau

---

[19]   See Jean Favier, *Nouvelle Histoire de Paris: Paris au XVe siècle, 1380–1500* (Paris, 1997), p. 22; Philippe Lorentz and Dany Sandron, *Atlas de Paris au moyen âge. Espace urbain, habitat, société, religion, lieux de pouvoir* (Paris, 2006), pp. 213–14; see also Mehl, *Les jeux*, pp. 260, 353.

[20]   Carlier and Bernard-Tambour, *Jeu des rois*, pp. 92–3.

[21]   Cf. Mehl, *Les jeux*, p. 259; Jean-Michel Mehl, 'Du jeu au sport: l'itinéraire cahoteux du jeu de paume', in Jean-Michel Mehl (ed.), *Des jeux et des hommes dans la société médiévale* (Paris, 2010), pp. 215–26, here p. 219.

[22]   John McClelland, 'Introduction: "Sport" in Early Modern Europe?', in John McClelland and Brian Merrilees (eds), *Sport and Culture in Early Modern Europe / Le Sport dans la Civilisation de l'Europe Pré-Moderne* (Toronto, 2009), pp. 23–40, here p. 29; Carlier and Bernard-Tambour, *Jeu des rois*, pp. 91–2.

[23]   Mehl, *Les jeux*, p. 40.

[24]   Albert de Luze, *La magnifique histoire du jeu de paume* (Bordeaux and Paris, 1933), pp. 118–29.

[25]   Lorentz and Sandron, *Atlas*, pp. 68–9; Favier, *Nouvelle Histoire*, pp. 53–61. See Andreas Sohn, *Von der Residenz zur Hauptstadt. Paris im hohen Mittelalter* (Ostfildern, 2012), pp. 119–22.

[26]   For the *Plan de Bâle* see Jean Boutier, Jean-Yves Sarazin and Marine Sibille (eds), *Les plans de Paris des origines (1493) à la fin du XVIIIe siècle. Étude, carto-bibliographie et*

and Olivier Truschet clearly shows this tripartite structure and their associated affiliation: Firstly, the *Cité* on the Seine island is mainly characterised by political, administrative and religious institutions; secondly, the right bank of the Seine housed the royal residences and the economic and commercial centre around the place de Grève and Les Halles. This district was known as the actual *Ville*. Thirdly, the university quarter was situated on the left bank of the Seine.[27]

While no tennis courts are traceable in the densely built-up *Cité* between 1300 and 1600, 21 tennis courts can be localised, mostly by name, in the urban road network on the right bank of the Seine, with nine records from the fifteenth and 10 records from the sixteenth century.[28] Most of these courts were concentrated in the districts around the royal residences, namely the Louvre in the west and the Hôtel Saint-Pol in the east of the right bank.[29] In the 1360s, King Charles V provided a basis for this development, since he maintained two tennis courts in both residences.[30] In general, Jean-Michel Mehl rightly interpreted tennis as 'jeu par excellence de la noblesse' with regard to the fourteenth and fifteenth centuries.[31] During this time, tennis emerged as a standard element

---

catalogue collectif (Paris, 2002), pp. 86–8.

[27]   Katharina Simon-Muscheid, 'Ordnung, Aufruhr und städtische Plätze. Das Beispiel der Place de Grève in Paris', in Susanne Rau and Gerd Schwerhoff (eds), *Zwischen Gotteshaus und Taverne. Öffentliche Räume in Spätmittelalter und Früher Neuzeit* (Köln, Weimar and Wien, 2004), pp. 273–302, here p. 273; Favier, *Nouvelle Histoire*, p. 13.

[28]   The following figures are based on the inquiry by de Luze, *La magnifique histoire*, pp. 118–29, drawing his information mainly from the Parisian notary registers: Ernest Coyecque (ed.), *Recueil d'actes notariés relatifs à l'histoire de Paris et de ses environs au XVIe siècle* (2 vols, Paris, 1905–1923), vol. 1: 1498–1545, nrs 158, 560, 562, 583, 1152, 1160, 1583, 1608, 1671, 1788, 1882, 1884, 1972, 2145, 2188, 2234, 2252, 2372, 2376, 2506, 2551, 2555, 2556, 2689, 3302, 3418, 3458; vol. 2: 1532–1555, nrs 3955, 4023, 4081, 4102, 4146, 4171, 4256, 4365, 4382, 4486, 4487, 4844, 4894, 5002, 5147, 5210, 5224, 5239, 5260, 5263, 5415, 5651, 5915, 5937, 5945, 5955, 6000, 6027, 6075, 6092, 6153, 6156, 6204.

[29]   See Lorentz and Sandron, *Atlas*, pp. 80–91.

[30]   De Luze, *La magnifique histoire*, pp. 33–4; Adolphe Berty, *Topographie historique du vieux Paris* (6 vols, Paris, 1868–1897), vol. 1: Région du Louvre et des Tuileries, p. 161; Alfred Franklin, *Dictionnaire historique des arts, métiers et professions exercés dans Paris depuis le treizième siècle* (2 vols, Paris and Leipzig, 1905–1906), vol. 2, p. 552; Carlier and Bernard-Tambour, *Jeu des rois*, pp. 130–32. See Alain Salamagne, 'Le Louvre de Charles V', in Alain Salamagne (ed.), *Le Palais et son décor au temps de Jean de Berry* (Tours, 2010), pp. 74–138.

[31]   Jean-Michel Mehl, 'Le jeu de paume: un élément de la sociabilité aristocratique à la fin du moyen âge et au début de la Renaissance', in Mehl, *Des jeux et des hommes*, pp. 227–42, here p. 241. See Cees de Bondt, 'Ballhaus', in Werner Paravicini (ed.), *Höfe und Residenzen im spätmittelalterlichen Reich. Bilder und Begriffe* (4 vols, Sigmaringen, 2003–2012), vol. 2/1, pp. 205–7. Bondt states that in the sixteenth century tennis was the 'most popular physical exercise practised at the princely courts of Europe', p. 205.

of courtly sociability and aristocratic 'conspicuous leisure'.[32] Inevitably, Paris as the capital and residence of the kings of France developed into the epicentre of the aristocratic enthusiasm for tennis. Consequently, the presence of numerous princely and episcopal residences[33] involved a steady demand for leisure and consumption facilities in general and tennis courts in particular. Since the noble residences were centred in the districts of the Louvre and the Hôtel Saint-Pol, the significant density of tennis courts in this part of the right bank area seems not surprising.

A second core area featuring six tennis courts was situated between the central market of Les Halles and the place de Grève together with the harbour of the same name.[34] This area constituted the living and working place of merchants and artisans and the centre of the economic and commercial activities of the capital. Moreover, it was also the seat of the so-called 'guild of the water merchants'. Their head – the *prévôt des marchands* – represented the self-confidence of the rich merchant elite vis-à-vis the city rule of the French king.[35] The statistical analysis of professional backgrounds of tennis players, mentioned in the letters of remission between 1350 and 1550, suggests that Parisian merchants were not regular customers of the commercial tennis courts.[36] Instead, the tennis courts around Les Halles were presumably frequented mainly by artisans, as they accounted for one third of all persons seeking remission.[37] This evidence is

---

[32]   Thorstein Veblen, *The Theory of the Leisure Class* (New York, 1994), pp. 23–62. See Mehl, 'Le jeu de paume', pp. 238–242; Mehl, *Les jeux*, pp. 205–9; Bernard Merdrignac, *Le sport au moyen âge* (Rennes, 2002), pp. 210–13.

[33]   For the noble residences in Paris see Favier, *Nouvelle Histoire*, pp. 93–118; Lorentz and Sandron, *Atlas*, pp. 106–9, 209–11; David Thomson, *Renaissance Paris: Architecture and Growth 1475–1600* (Berkeley, Los Angeles and Oxford, 1985). For the close connection between city and court in general, see Andreas Ranft, 'Residenz und Stadt', in Paravicini, *Höfe*, vol. 2/1, pp. 27–32; Jan Hirschbiegel and Gabriel Zeilinger, 'Urban Space Divided? The Encounter of Civic and Courtly Spheres in Late-Medieval Towns', in Albrecht Classen (ed.), *Urban Space in the Middle Ages and the Early Modern Age* (Berlin and New York, 2009), pp. 481–502.

[34]   Mehl, *Les jeux*, p. 262.

[35]   See Simon-Muscheid, 'Ordnung', pp. 281–86; Favier, *Nouvelle Histoire*, pp. 34, 112; Lorentz and Sandron, *Atlas*, pp. 196–8, 201–3; for Les Halles see also Anna Jourdan, 'La ville étudiée dans ses quartiers: autour des Halles de Paris au moyen âge', *Annales d'histoire économique et sociale*, 7 (1953): pp. 285–301; Jean Martineau, *Les Halles de Paris, des origines au 1789* (Paris, 1960); Léon Biolay, 'Les anciennes Halles de Paris', *Mémoire de la société de l'histoire de Paris et de l'Ile-de-France*, 3 (1876): pp. 293–355.

[36]   Mehl, *Les jeux*, p. 193. Only 0.8 per cent of the tennis players mentioned in the letters of remission were registered as *marchands*.

[37]   Mehl, *Les jeux*, p. 193, this result is based on the following professional groups: *construction* (9.8 per cent), *alimentation* (5.3 per cent), *artisans divers* (8.8 per cent), *transports* (3.5 per cent), *valets* (5.3 per cent).

supported by an ordinance from 1398 by the provost of Paris, the royal official, in which 'artisans and other small people' are explicitly addressed as ardent tennis players preferring this leisure activity to their daily workload.[38] Still around 1550, according to the *Plan de Bâle*, there existed a tennis court at the south end of Les Halles which was dominated by the textile industry. Already in October 1482, King Louis XI bestowed two tennis courts in this area together with the respective proceeds on six new chaplains and six new cantors of the Parisian Sainte-Chapelle, in order to thank John the Baptist for the healing of diverse grave illnesses.[39] And as early as 1427, there existed a tennis court called the 'Little Temple' (Petit Temple) to the north-east of Les Halles, in a side-road (rue Garnier-Saint-Ladre) of the important north-south-axis rue Saint-Martin. According to the *Journal d'un bourgeois de Paris*, it was exactly this 'best tennis court in Paris' which was the place to go for a certain 'young woman of 28 or 30 years' called Margot, who played tennis better than anyone had it seen it played before and outperformed even male opponents, save the most powerful players.[40] This supposed hierarchy of Parisian tennis courts suggests that already in 1427 there were a significant number of such leisure facilities within the city walls.[41] Given the fact that Margot had migrated from Hainaut to Paris only shortly before and without a considerable amount of social capital, it becomes also clear that Parisian tennis courts were far from being frozen in social exclusiveness.

This infrastructure of tennis courts on the right bank of the Seine was a substantial part of an expanding urban sport culture, fed and borne by aristocratic, courtly and civic, artisan milieus. It is not sufficiently clarified if Jean-Michel Mehl is right to postulate that the Parisian burghers simply imitated and adopted noble leisure and consumption habits.[42] It is quite likely that the development of the Parisian tennis culture was more complex; and the district of Les Halles might have served as a space of contact and interaction between aristocratic and civic sport activities. For the period between 1364 and

---

[38]   Ordinance of the provost of Paris (22 January 1398), in: Nicolas Delamare (ed.), *Traité de la police, où l'on trouvera les fonctions et les prérogatives de ses magistrats* (4 vols, Amsterdam, 1729), vol. 1, p. 417; see Alexandre Tuetey (ed.), *Inventaire analytique des livres de couleur et bannières du Châtelet de Paris* (Paris, 1899), no. 301, p. 19, and Mehl, *Les jeux*, p. 228.

[39]   Tuetey, *Inventaire*, no. 2144, p. 6.

[40]   Colette Beaune (ed.), *Journal d'un bourgeois de Paris de 1405 à 1449* (Paris, 2009), p. 239. According to Alexandre Tuetey (ed.), *Journal d'un bourgeois de Paris 1405–1449* (Paris, 1881), p. 222, n. 1, this tennis court belonged at the beginning of the sixteenth century to the Parisian charterhouse, citing a 'sentence des requêtes du Palais' from 21 April 1502 which mentions the payment of rent of 'locateurs de certaines maisons asaises en la rue Garnier-Saint-Ladre, où pend pour enseigne Melusine et la jeu de Paulme'.

[41]   McClelland, *Body*, pp. 123–4; Gillmeister, *Kulturgeschichte*, p. 98.

[42]   Mehl, *Les jeux*, pp. 196, 418–19.

1419, when Paris mutated into the *capitale des ducs de Bourgogne*, it seems at least striking that there developed something like a 'Burgundian quarter' in close proximity to Les Halles.[43] Given the fact that the Burgundian dukes and their entourage had a special passion for the *jeu de paume*, from Philip the Bold to the siege of Neuss 1474,[44] it seems likely that this 'Burgundian connection' involved the heightened presence of noble players and, respectively, contributed to the density of tennis courts in this district.

Of the three parts of the city, the university quarter on the left bank of the Seine was undoubtedly the part with the highest density of ballhouses, at least in the sixteenth century when 41 of its overall 47 tennis courts were built.[45] On this side of the river, only few tennis courts are traceable within the city walls, among them the *Jeu du Château de Nesle* which ranks as the oldest tennis court in Paris with its first mentioning in 1308.[46] Evidently, the building boom of tennis courts in the sixteenth century basically took place in front of the city gates, in the suburbs. In the *faubourgs* Saint-Marcel, Saint-Jacques and Saint-Michel, eight tennis courts can be found, while the majority of ballhouses – 36 out of 47 – were situated in a suburb called Bourg Saint-Germain, just outside the city walls close to the abbey Saint-Germain-des-Prés.[47] This area had developed into the preferred residential area of aristocrats and rich burghers, similarly to the princely residences on the right bank of the Seine, from the end of the fourteenth century.[48] This applies particularly to the Bourg Saint-Germain, with its splendid *hôtels* and residences of nobles, royal officials, Parisian burghers and, particularly, prelates.[49] Moreover, the spacious and undeveloped area between the *bourg* and the Seine happened to be the playground of the about 4,000 Parisian masters

---

[43]   Werner Paravicini and Betrand Schnerb (eds), *Paris, capitale des ducs de Bourgogne* (Ostfildern, 2007); for Les Halles as 'véritable quartier bourguignon', see Werner Paravicini, 'Paris, capitale des ducs de Bourgogne?', in Werner Paravicini and Betrand Schnerb (eds), *Paris, capitale des ducs de Bourgogne* (Ostfildern, 2007), pp. 471–7, here p. 473.

[44]   For the significance of the *jeu de paume* at the Burgundian court see Jean-Michel Mehl, 'Les jeux sportifs de Philippe de Hardi, duc de Bourgogne', in Mehl, *Des jeux et des hommes*, pp. 243–252; Mehl, 'Le jeu de paume', pp. 234–5; Mehl, *Les jeux*, p. 202. For the construction of tennis courts during the siege of Neuss 1474 see Mehl, *Les jeux*, p. 251.

[45]   See de Luze, *La magnifique histoire*, pp. 123–9.

[46]   De Luze, *La magnifique histoire*, p. 128. This tennis court already existed in 1308 when Amaury de Clermont sold the whole complex to King Philip the Fair.

[47]   For the Bourg Saint-Germain see Lorentz and Sandron, *Atlas*, pp. 36–7, 44–5; see also Mehl, *Les jeux*, p. 262, who argues that the local quantity of tennis courts was not only based on the demand of the nearby university quarter, but also on the – compared to the city centre – more loosely-built area of the *rive gauche* and the existence of numerous religious institutions.

[48]   Lorentz and Sandron, *Atlas*, p. 48.

[49]   Lorentz and Sandron, *Atlas*, p. 45.

and students, living in the numerous colleges of the university quarter and in the Bourg Saint-Germain, as a contract between the University of Paris and the abbot of Saint-Germain-des-Prés from 1368 shows.[50] Still in the middle of the sixteenth century, this so-called *Pré aux Clercs* was obviously good for a tennis game in its open air variant as the *Plan de Bâle* demonstrates. The academic milieu distinguished itself by an intensive leisure and consumption culture, like visiting taverns, gambling and enjoying sports contests.[51] The response of the schoolmaster in the *Colloquia* of Erasmus of Rotterdam from 1518 to the question of a scholar if he would allow a game of tennis – 'You are doing nothing else than playing anyway, with or without permission'[52] – could also have been given in the colleges and hostels of the biggest European university. This is attested by numerous prohibitions and, all literary stylisation aside, the lifetime confession of François Villon.[53] In any case, the *jeu de paume* was deeply rooted in the leisure habits of Parisian students[54] as can be seen in a quote by the Spanish humanist Juan Luis Vives in his *Linguae Latinae exercitatio* from 1538. In this text Scintilla responds to the question of Borgia if the Parisians played also other games apart from tennis: 'In Paris there are as many or even more games than here in Valencia, but the scholars are not allowed to play anything else than tennis.'[55] In the same text, Vives suggests that the most famous tennis court of Paris was a place called Brachae.[56] This court represented something like the anchor of student enthusiasm for tennis, known also from a passage in François Rabelais' *Gargantua*: 'This done they went forth, still conferring of the substance of the lecture, either to the Braque or unto the meadows, where they played at the ball, the *jeu de paume* and the triangle ball games, most gallantly exercising their bodies, as formerly they had done their minds.'[57] Brachae and Braque both allude to the tennis court of the tavern called Grand Braque Latin

[50] Lorentz and Sandron, *Atlas*, pp. 44–5. For the quantity of Parisian masters and students see Jacques Verger, 'Paris. D. Die Schulen und Universitäten', *Lexikon des Mittelalters* (10 vols, Munich et al., 1980–1999), vol. 6, cols. 1720–1; Favier, *Nouvelle Histoire*, pp. 68–79, 94; for the student milieu in late medieval Paris in general see Bronislaw Geremek, *Les marginaux parisiens au XIVe et XVe siècles* (Paris, 1976), pp. 165–84.

[51] Mehl, *Les jeux*, pp. 211–12.

[52] Erasmus von Rotterdam, *Colloquia*, ed. Adriano Prosperi and Cecilia Asso (Torino, 2002), p. 94: 'Nihil aliud quam luditis, etiam absque venia' (my translation).

[53] Mehl, *Les jeux*, pp. 221, 366–70 ; see also Jean Favier, *François Villon* (Paris, 1982), pp. 189–91.

[54] Carlier and Bernard-Tambour, *Jeu des rois*, p. 99.

[55] Luis Vives, *Los Diálogos (Linguae Latinae Exercitatio). XXII. Leges ludi. Varius Dialogus de Vrbe Valentia*, ed. M. Pilar García Ruiz (Pamplona, 2005), p. 354.

[56] Luis Vives, *Los Diálogos*, p. 352.

[57] François Rabelais, *Gargantua*, book 1, c. 23, in François Rabelais, *Oeuvres complètes*, ed. Mireille Huchon and François Moreau (Paris, 1994), p. 65. I have slightly changed the

that was situated close to the university quarter and according to the *Plan de Bâle*.[58] Likewise, Thomas Platter accentuated the Bourg Saint-Germain as a preferred location of tennis courts: 'The first suburb, Saint-Germain, is rather huge and populous like a big city. Saint-Germain has its own annual fairs, churches, many alleys, beautiful courtyards and ball houses. Also, many German lords, aristocrats and students live there in the houses of noble people.'[59] Even in the eyes of contemporaries, the correlation between a student customer base and the density of ballhouses was a rather obvious fact.

The Economics of *Jeu de Paume*

Royal residences, princely *hôtels* scattered over the Parisian cityscape, the artisan quarter on the right bank of the Seine, the university quarter on the left – this metropolitan coexistence of different sociocultural milieus entailed a steady clientele of tennis players and spectators. On the basis of this sustained demand, *jeu de paume* established itself as a definite element of the Parisian sport culture. In quantitative terms, this impressive infrastructure of tennis courts in the French capital was largely borne by the initiative of private parties pursuing their commercial interests. These commercial venues opened their doors to every customer able to pay a certain rental charge, whereas the princely ballhouses were reserved from the outset for court members and invited guests.[60] Juan Luis Vives, comparing the Parisian tennis courts to those of the city of Valencia, claimed that in Paris there existed no public, but many private, tennis courts in the suburbs of Saint-Jacques, Saint-Marcel and Saint-Germain on the left bank of the Seine.[61] The Parisian notary records of the sixteenth century, which contain multiple contracts of sales and leases of tennis courts between private parties, support this observation.[62] This development was promoted by demographic and political changes in the fifteenth and sixteenth centuries. According to Alexandre Tuetey, the majority of fifteenth-century Parisian tennis courts had

---

translation in: François Rabelais, *Gargantua and Pantagruel*, trans. by Thomas Urquhart and Peter Anthony Motteux, with an introduction by Michael Randall (New York, 2005), p. 54.

[58]   See de Luze, *La magnifique histoire*, p. 123; Vives, *Los Diálogos*, p. 519; for the inn-signs of the Parisian *jeux de paume*, see Carlier and Bernard-Tambour, *Jeu des rois*, p. 100.

[59]   Platter, *Beschreibung*, vol. 2, pp. 600–601: 'Die erste vorstatt, Saint Germain, ist mechtig groß unndt volckreich wie ein große statt, hatt ihren besonderen jahrmärckt, kirchen, viel gaßen, schöne höf unndt ballen heüser, wie auch viel teütsche herren, edelleüt unndt studenten in der vorstatt bey fürnemmen leüten an der kost sindt.'

[60]   Carlier and Bernard-Tambour, *Jeu des rois*, p. 99.

[61]   Vives, *Los Diálogos*, p. 352.

[62]   See the entries in Coyecque, *Recueil*; see also Mehl, *Les jeux*, p. 379; Carlier and Bernard-Tambour, *Jeu des rois*, pp. 91–3.

been erected on the site of abandoned gypsum mills, for example the playing fields *en la plasterie* and in *rue de la Plaistriere* close to the city gate of Saint-Honoré.[63] Even though Tuetey's statement cannot be verified by contemporary sources,[64] it can certainly be argued that the massive demographic crisis Paris endured in the course of political turmoils, famines and epidemics during the years between 1410 and 1440 led to a significant vacancy of real estate in the Parisian cityscape and indirectly to the deterioration of the building fabric. These developments accompanied and benefited the construction of tennis courts. In the course of the subsequent reconstruction, properties were gutted and courtyards were conveyed to new functions. This spatial redevelopment did not only lay the groundwork for the Parisian garden culture, but also provided the necessary space for tennis facilities.[65] After 1450, a new, well-financed elite consisting of royal officials, administrative and legal experts, intellectuals, rich shop-owners and merchants transformed the Parisian cityscape into an *urbanisme des notables*, as Jean Favier has put it. Moreover, the real estate investments of this group of people shaped the architectonic appearance of the suburbs and the urban surroundings.[66] Altogether, both aspects – on the one hand the availability of fallow land and abandoned constructions in the intramural area and urban periphery, on the other hand the tendency to invest in real property – are the crucial factors for the unique quantity of Parisian tennis courts, apart from the favourable demand situation. Still at the end of the sixteenth century, Thomas Platter regarded such investments in the increased market value of tennis courts as downright plausible:

> A lot of ballhouses are in the city of Paris, but particularly in the suburbs, since ballhouses were erected on the spot of destroyed, dismantled houses. They profit from these tennis courts more than they would from whole houses, and it is easier to borrow money for the courts than for fully developed houses.[67]

Alongside their considerable profitability in the housing market, the Parisian tennis courts can be interpreted, according to Roger Morgan, as 'commercial

---

[63] Tuetey, *Journal*, p. 222, n. 1.

[64] See Mehl, *Les jeux*, p. 262.

[65] Jean Favier, 'Paris', in *Lexikon des Mittelalters*, vol. 6, cols. 1710–11.

[66] Favier, 'Paris', vol. 6, cols. 1710–11; Favier, *Nouvelle Histoire*, pp. 116–18.

[67] Platter, *Beschreibung*, vol. 2, p. 594: 'Mechtig viel ballenheüser sindt auch in der statt Paris, sonderlich aber in den vorstetten, da man auß den zerstörten, abgebrochenen heüsseren ballenheüser aufgebauwen, auß welchen sie mehr nutz ziehen, dann wan sie gantze heüser hetten, unnd leihet man ihnen ehe gelt darauf dann auf außgebauwene heüser' (my translation).

unit[s]'[68] that consisted of a spatially defined range of services offered and, at the same time, covered the demand for specialised sport equipment.[69] Here as elsewhere, for example in London, it formed part of the business plan of owners and tenants to hold available balls, rackets, other pieces of equipment and refreshments, in order to lend or sell them to players if required.[70] These spaces of sociability and sport contests ensured a high level of consumption of easily worn-out tennis balls[71] produced by urban manufacturers of sporting goods.

The commercial character of the Parisian tennis courts becomes all the more evident if the owners or tenants of such facilities acted at the same time as tennis ball manufacturers. Such a double function is sometimes mentioned in the Parisian notary records. For example, the ball manufacturer Claude Dupré assigned the leasehold interest in the tennis court at the rue de Paradis to his colleague Thibault Trichardot in 1545, or the two ball manufacturers David Houllet and Audrien Berthault jointly leased a tennis court called Passe-Temps in the suburb Saint-Marcel in 1547.[72] The Parisian tennis courts served also as locations for the 'direct sale' of tennis balls manufactured by the owner or tenant himself.[73]

In Paris, the manufacturing of tennis balls had a long tradition reaching back to the thirteenth century as the presence of 13 *paumiers* in the tax list of 1292 shows. They were traceable in different parishes of the *rive droite* and the *Cité*, but their core area was the surroundings of the Louvre and the enclos du Temple in the northern part of the city.[74] As chronicles and account books clearly show, Parisian ball producers supplied the demand of the Castilian and Burgundian courts in the fourteenth century.[75] Consequently, the quality of this export commodity became increasingly regulated and standardised, so for example in a

---

[68]   Roger Morgan, 'A Fifteenth-Century Tennis Court in London', *The International Journal of the History of Sport*, 13/3 (1996): pp. 418–31, here p. 422.

[69]   See Carlier and Bernard-Tambour, *Jeu des rois*, p. 91.

[70]   For London see Morgan, 'A Fifteenth-Century Tennis Court in London', p. 422.

[71]   In general, balls for the *jeu de paume* were produced in rather large quantities, since they were usually delivered *par grosse*, that is, in a quantity of 12 dozen. This was due to the fact that, according to Jean A. Gay, normally nine dozen balls were worn out during one game of *jeu de paume*: Jean A. Gay, *Sports et jeux d'exercice en Anjou* (Angers, 1947), p. 127.

[72]   Élisabeth Belmas, *Jouer Autrefois. Essai sur le jeu dans la France moderne (XVIe–XVIIIe siècle)* (Seyssel, 2006), p. 230; de Luze, *La magnifique histoire*, p. 123.

[73]   See Carlier and Bernard-Tambour, *Jeu des rois*, p. 84.

[74]   Hercule Géraud, *Paris sous Philippe-le-Bel. D'après des documents originaux et notamment d'après un manuscrit contenant 'Le Rôle de la Taille' imposée sur les habitants de Paris en 1292 [1837]*, newly ed. by Caroline Bourlet and Lucie Fossier (Tübingen, 1991), pp. xi, 29, 30, 46, 79, 34, 103, 139, 143, 177; for the *paumiers* see also Franklin, *Dictionnaire*, vol. 2, pp. 552–3.

[75]   See Mehl, *Les jeux*, p. 34; Merdrignac, *Sport*, p. 202.

decree of the provost of Paris, Jacques d'Estouteville, from 18 November 1508: 'Nobody is allowed to produce balls in this city or the suburbs, unless from good leather and good filling material, and every ball should weigh 17 *estelins* [approx. 26 g].'[76] In 1538, Juan Luis Vives characterised French in contrast to Spanish tennis balls as smaller, harder, made out of white leather and filled not with cut wool cloth but with dog hairs.[77] Even though tennis balls manufactured *façon de Paris*[78] had become something like an international trademark, the profit margins of this craft were presumably rather modest. In reaction to complaints of the Parisian *confrairie* of ball manufacturers founded in the fifteenth century, an ordinance of King Louis XI from 24 June 1467 sought to readjust this craft 'which creates much hardship and low profit', due to the fact that 'in the past anybody willing to do so could practise it because of missing regulations and visitations'.[79] Closely linked to the building boom of *jeux de paume*, a specialised profession of ball producers unfolded which struggled to control access to the craft and to control quality standards.[80] As Wolfgang Behringer has recently shown, the international trade of tennis equipment gained further momentum when from the end of the fifteenth century the use of rackets came into vogue mainly in aristocratic circles.[81] At the death of the Parisian burgher and merchant Jean Périer in the tennis court of Saint-Jean-de-Latran on the *rive gauche*, his belongings comprised altogether 75 rackets of different quality, 10 bats, 22 differently priced pairs of shoes and 15 pairs of double gloves for

---

[76]   Cited in: René de Lespinasse (ed.), *Les métiers et corporations de la ville de Paris* (3 vols, Paris, 1886–1897), vol. 3, p. 528; see also the similar ordinance of King Louis XI for the ball manufactureres of Rouen from 24 June 1480 in *Ordonnances des roys de France de la troisième race* (21 vols, Paris, 1723–1849), vol. 18, Paris 1828, pp. 544–5, banning the use of 'sand, chalk, bran, fur waste, sawdust, moss, powder or soil' as filling materials, in order to prevent 'injuries of arms and hands'; see also Carlier and Bernard-Tambour, *Jeu des rois*, p. 34.

[77]   Vives, *Los Diálogos*, p. 352.

[78]   Mehl, *Les jeux*, p. 34.

[79]   *Ordonnances des roys de France*, vol. 16, p. 607. Already in 1396, King Charles VI had granted the 'poor' Parisian ball manufacturers a tax exemption, see Mehl, *Les jeux*, p. 501, n. 43. Still, the already mentioned decree of the provost of Paris from 1508 noted the existence of ball producers located in the Parisian suburbs, being regarded by their city centre colleagues as cheap competitors manufacturing low quality products.

[80]   Belmas, *Jouer Autrefois*, p. 230, has identified 40 *paumiers, faiseurs d'esteufs, raquetiers* by name in sixteenth-century Paris.

[81]   Wolfgang Behringer, 'Fugger als Sportartikelhändler. Auf dem Weg zu einer Sportgeschichte der Frühen Neuzeit', in Wolfgang E.J. Weber and Regina Dauser (eds), *Faszinierende Frühneuzeit. Reich, Frieden, Kultur und Kommunikation 1500–1800. Festschrift für Johannes Burkhardt zum 65. Geburtstag* (Berlin, 2008), pp. 115–34; Wolfgang Behringer, 'Arena and Pall Mall: Sport in the Early Modern Period', *German History*, 27/3 (2009): pp. 331–57.

tennis.[82] All this evidence indicates a considerable local market for all sorts of tennis equipment at prices to suit all pockets and based on the steady demand of the urban tennis court agglomeration.

The provision of balls was at times directly linked to another basic process of 'tennis economics': betting. According to a letter of remission of King Charles VI to Philippot Gilles from 3 October 1422, the 'povre homme laboureur' lent balls on pawn from the proprietor of the tennis court in the rue de la Platrière before the game and the losing team was committed to paying for them.[83] Generally, most contemporary tennis players would have approved of Erasmus' statement in his *Colloquia* that 'games tend to cool down without the risk to lose something'.[84] By the beginning of the fourteenth century, the betting of considerable, sometimes even excessive, sums on the results of tennis matches is well-documented for the French and Burgundian courts: On particular occasions, a sum amounting to a year's pension of a Burgundian officer could be at stake, and Duke Louis of Orléans evidentially lost in the 1390s huge amounts of money, up to 2,000 and 3,000 *francs*.[85] Such aristocratic practices of 'conspicuous consumption'[86] were rather unusual in civic circles. Thus the case of the Parisian burgher Symmonet Huppin in September 1398 who lost a wager of 40 francs at the tennis court is a rather atypical example.[87] For the most part, in urban *jeux de paume* only minor wagers between 10 *sous* and 2 *deniers*, or material prizes such as playing equipment or, in the case of a butcher, a leg of mutton were at stake.[88]

Betting practices are also closely linked to processes of ludic quantifications that are clearly visible in the emerging sport cultures in the fifteenth and sixteenth centuries.[89] With regard to tennis, this correlation is particularly reflected in its quindecimal way of counting – 15, 30, 45, 60 – which presumably derived

---

[82]   Inventory of the deceased Jean Périer, August 1525, edited in: Coyecque, *Recueil*, vol. 1, no. 583, p. 113. For the constituent parts of tennis equipment see Mehl, *Les jeux*, pp. 37–8; Gillmeister, *Kulturgeschichte*, pp. 100, 126.

[83]   Ed. in Auguste Longnon (ed.), *Paris pendant la domination anglaise (1420–1436). Documents extraits des registres de la chancellerie de France* (Paris, 1878), no. XXIX, p. 56.

[84]   Erasmus of Rotterdam, *Colloquia*, p. 96.

[85]   See Mehl, *Les jeux*, p. 270, and Mehl, 'Le jeu de paume', p. 235.

[86]   Veblen, *Theory*. For some Italian examples of betting practices in the context of tennis matches, see Cees de Bondt, *Royal Tennis in Renaissance Italy* (Turnhout, 2006), pp. 41–3, 73. On aristocratic betting practices in early modern Venice, see Jonathan Walker, 'Gambling and Venetian Noblemen, c. 1500–1700', *Past and Present*, 162 (1999): pp. 28–69.

[87]   Mehl, *Les jeux*, p. 279.

[88]   See Mehl, *Les jeux*, pp. 279, 281.

[89]   For a general overview over processes of quantification in early modern sport practices, see Henning Eichberg, '"Auf Zoll und Quintlein". Sport und Quantifizierungsprozeß der frühen Neuzeit', *Archiv für Kulturgeschichte*, 56 (1974): pp. 141–76.

from the coin value of the wagers.[90] Through betting, physical performances could be immediately converted into monetary gains and losses. Thus a form of 'second order-competition' was created that caught the attention of both players and spectators in terms of risk and agonistic tension.[91] At the same time, the graduation of wagers according to the respective material resources reflected different circles of sociability and milieus and corresponded to the spatial diversification of Parisian *jeux de paume*.

Contested Leisure and Ambivalent Perceptions

As Peter Burke argued nearly 20 years ago against the mainstream of specialised scholarship, the Later Middle Ages saw virtually the 'invention of leisure' in European history.[92] Indeed, the general trend of an emerging leisure culture could be rightly regarded as a striking feature of urban history in the fifteenth and sixteenth centuries, given the statistical fact of 265 working days on average and, consequently, a considerable amount of potentially free time for the city burghers.[93] Moreover, at the end of the Middle Ages, there emerged the growing tendency to define and differentiate 'work' and 'leisure' in a more precise way.[94] For example, this becomes evident in the regulations of urban craft guilds containing the working hours of masters and journeymen in terms of self-sufficiency.[95] In this light, the city authorities of the Later Middle Ages struggled to manage and control the considerable quantity of civic leisure by a two-step strategy that involved measures of repression as well as public sponsorship.

[90]   Mehl, 'Du jeu', p. 223; Gillmeister, *Kulturgeschichte*, pp. 156–64.

[91]   See Jonathan Crary, *Suspension of Perception: Attention, Spectacle, and Modern Culture* (Cambridge, MA and London, 2001). The quotidianity of spectators' betting practices at *jeux de paume* is for example attested by a woodcut included in the book of hours of the Parisian printer Philippe Pigouchet from about 1510: There, a spectator swinging his purse over the balustrade stands on the left-hand side of a wooden side gallery, see Gillmeister, *Kulturgeschichte*, pp. 27, 157.

[92]   Peter Burke, 'The Invention of Leisure in Early Modern Europe', *Past and Present*, 146 (1995): pp. 136–50, esp. pp. 137–9. See also the debate following Burke's assumption: Joan-Lluís Marfany, 'The Invention of Leisure in Early Modern Europe', *Past and Present*, 156 (1997): pp. 174–91; Peter Burke, 'The Invention of Leisure in Early Modern Europe: Reply', *Past and Present*, 156 (1997): pp. 192–7. For a discussion of the notion of medieval leisure see Gherardo Ortalli, 'Tempo libero e medio evo: tra pulsioni ludiche e schemi culturali', in Cavaciocchi, *Il tempo libero*, pp. 31–54, and Rolf Sprandel, 'Temps libre. Reflet d'un terme moderne dans la vie urbaine du Bas Moyen Age', in Cavaciocchi, *Il tempo libero*, pp. 111–25.

[93]   Holbach, 'Feste', p. 215; Gerhard Fouquet, 'Das Festmahl in den oberdeutschen Städten des Spätmittelalters', *Archiv für Kulturgeschichte*, 74 (1992): pp. 83–124.

[94]   Burke, 'Invention', p. 148.

[95]   Sprandel, 'Temps libre', p. 118.

In Paris, the city authorities had to cope with a unique density of privately operated and financed leisure time facilities in the form of the *jeux de paume*. The expanding network of commercial tennis courts as 'semi-public places'[96] was open for a fee to a wide range of the urban population. Even though admission to specific facilities was certainly governed by social and financial hierarchies, the overall accessibility of the Parisian tennis courts implied a subversive potential appropriate to de Certeau's reading of 'practised places',[97] undercutting the effort of the city authorities to restrict physical exercises during leisure time to military purposes. Insofar, it is not surprising that they disapproved of this urban tennis mania as being contrary to the public good. Following the pattern of royal ordinances from 1319 and 1369 that prohibited the *jeu de paume* in order to urge the population to practice archery and crossbow-shooting 'for the defense of our kingdom',[98] the provost of Paris decreed resolutely in 1394: 'It is forbidden to play any kind of game except archery and crossbow-shooting.'[99] Concomitantly, the city authority sponsored Parisian guilds of crossbowmen and archers, mentioned for the first time in 1359 and 1411 respectively, by providing and maintaining shooting ranges for training purposes.[100] The Parisian magistrate even sought to disqualify tennis by comparing the widespread betting practices to gambling. An ordinance of the provost of Paris from 1398 stated apodictically: 'Many people have lost their whole fortune [by playing tennis], so that they begin to indulge in theft, to kill other people and to lead a very mean life.'[101] Whereas city magistrates and canon and civil lawyers normally showed a rather tolerant attitude towards physical exercises and betting,[102] the Parisian authorities applied in the case of tennis a standard repressive argument

[96]   Riess, *City Games*, p. 38.

[97]   De Certeau, *Practice*, p. 96.

[98]   '*pro nostri defensione regni*', Edict of King Philip V (1319), in Antoine Fontanon and Gabriel Michel (eds), *Les edicts et ordonnances des rois de France depuis Louys VI. dit Le Gros, jusques à present* (4 vols, Paris, 1611), vol. 1, p. 673. Ordinance of Charles V (3 April, 23 May 1369), in: *Ordonnances des roys de France*, vol. 5 (ed. Denis-François Secousse), p. 172 ; see also Mehl, *Les jeux*, p. 361.

[99]   Ordinance of the provost of Paris (23 July 1394), in Delamare, *Traité de la police*, vol. 1, p. 417; see also Mehl, *Les jeux*, p. 361.

[100]   See L.-A. Delaunay, Étude sur les anciennes compagnies d'archers, d'arbalétiers et d'arquebusiers (Paris, 1879), pp. 4, 9.

[101]   Ordinance of the Prévôt de Paris (22 January 1398), in Delamare, *Traité de la police*, p. 417.

[102]   Alessandro Arcangeli, *Recreation in the Renaissance. Attitudes towards Leisure and Pastimes in European Culture, c. 1425–1675* (Basingstoke, 2003), pp. 74–5; see also Giovanni Ceccarelli, 'Gioco tra economia e teologia', *Ludica. Annali di storia e civiltà del gioco*, 7 (2001): pp. 46–60; Giovanni Ceccarelli, 'Risky Business: Theological and Canonical Thought on Insurance from the Thirteenth to the Seventeenth Century', *Journal of Medieval and Early Modern Studies*, 31/3 (2001): pp. 607–58; Renato Ferroglio, 'Ricerche sul gioco

against gambling, claiming that it led quasi-automatically to economic disorder. There is no doubt that this quite extraordinary statement was somehow forced by the uniqueness of the Parisian situation where private facilities competed and collided with the attempt to exploit at least part of the burgher's leisure for military ends.

Nevertheless, the triumphal procession of tennis through the French capital during the fifteenth and sixteenth centuries was unstoppable. In the end, the repudiation of certain aspects of 'tennis economics' by the provost of Paris remained an episode. On the contrary, Christine de Pizan, who had lived most of her life in Paris, recommended at the beginning of the fifteenth century the *jeu de paume* as a recreative physical work and profitable leisure pursuit.[103] Here the above-mentioned devaluating argument was reversed by highlighting its benefits to the body. Similar praise of tennis can be found, for example, in the *Jardin des nobles* of the Franciscan friar Pierre des Gros from 1463: 'It would be fine if lords would forbid playing in their lands, with the exception of archery and crossbow-shooting, tennis, bar- and stone-throwing and other activities that result in bodily effort and work, exercise the members of the body and could be beneficial to the public good.'[104] Against the background of this supposed coincidence of individual body and body politic, the Parisian 'tennis economics' took an unprecedented course of expansion and turned the French metropolis into Europe's uncontested capital of tennis.

---

e sulla scommessa fino al secolo XIII', *Rivista di Storia del Diritto Italiano*, 71 (1998): pp. 273–387.

[103] Christine de Pizan, *Le livre de corps de policie*, ed. Robert H. Lucas (Geneva and Paris, 1967), pp. 181–2; see also Mehl, *Les jeux*, p. 335.

[104] Cited in Mehl, *Les jeux*, p. 362.

Chapter 5

The Bruising Business: Pugilism, Commercial Culture and Celebrity, 1700–1750

Benjamin Litherland

Of all the early modern sports prize-fighting has likely received the most attention from historians. Numerous writers have explored boxing's roots, and the sport's most successful performers during the eighteenth century – James Figg, Jack Broughton, Daniel Mendoza, amongst others – are names that consistently reappear throughout these texts. [1] The reason for this attention might be found in the richness of the sources surrounding this particular sport: prize-fighting is one of the earliest examples of a fully commercialised sport with professionalised performers. These performers used newspapers to spread their names to a growing audience, wittingly and unwittingly helping future historians to spread their name further. In fact, the archives surrounding eighteenth-century prize-fighting can seem deceptively abundant. Newspaper advertisements and reports, which constitute the core of most of the studies available, are complemented by scattered diary accounts, pamphlets, poems and trading cards. By the end of the century new printed material – such as training manuals,[2] a dedicated sporting

---

[1]   See Kasia Boddy, *Boxing: A Cultural History* (London, 2008); Dennis Brailsford, 'Morals and Maulers: The Ethics of Early Pugilism', *Journal of Sport History*, 12/2 (1985): pp. 126–42; Dennis Brailsford, *Bareknuckles: A Social History of Prize-Fighting* (Cambridge, 1988); Peter M. Briggs, 'Daniel Mendoza and Sporting Celebrity: A Case Study', in Tom Mole (ed.), *Romanticism and Celebrity Culture 1750–1850* (Cambridge, 2009); John Ford, *Prizefighting: The Age of Regency Boximania* (Devon, 1971); Kenneth Gordon Sheard, *Boxing in the Civilizing Process* (Cambridge, 1992); Vanessa Toulmin, *A Fair Fight: An Illustrated Review of Boxing on British Fairgrounds* (Oldham, 1999); John Whale, 'Daniel Mendoza's Contests of Identity: Masculinity, Ethnicity and Nation in Georgian Prize-Fighting', *Romanticism*, 14/3 (2008): pp. 259–71.

[2]   See Dave Day, '"Science", "Wind" and "Bottom": Eighteenth-Century Boxing Manuals', *The International Journal of the History of Sport*, 29/10 (2012): pp. 1446–65; and Chapter 6, this volume.

press and autobiographies – further aid our knowledge of the sport's contexts and evolution.[3]

The impressive and painstaking archive work undertaken by these studies has allowed us to build an understanding of the matches fought and the socio-economic backgrounds of the pugilists involved; we are able to trace the changing nature of the fights, seeing weapons replaced by fists; and we can describe the price of entry and speculate on the class and gender of audiences. Yet for all the details we have about the fighters one cannot escape the feeling that these stories are predominantly constructed from sources that were part of the promotional culture that surrounded the sport. The purpose of this chapter, then, is not to speculate on a fighter's heroism, skill or the manner of their victories and losses. What is of concern is the promotional culture itself. Just as a history of advertising's role is not to test the truthfulness of a brand's claims but instead to reflect on the social and cultural milieu that produces these texts, the purpose of this chapter is not to dispel myths but rather to explore the manner in which they were constructed, distributed and disseminated. How did fighting shown alongside animal baiting develop into a popular, professionalised and commercialised sport? What changes were taking place at the turn of the century to allow prize-fighters to become the sporting *celebrities* of their day?

Peter Burke, in his classic study of early modern popular culture, has argued that 'a new type of popular hero made his appearance in the eighteenth century: the sports idol'.[4] He is right, but I would make a more specific claim: in London at the beginning of the eighteenth century a new popular hero emerged: the sports celebrity. A growing body of literature places celebrity culture's roots in the eighteenth century.[5] Tracking the shift from the bear gardens of London to the dedicated boxing amphitheatres offers an illuminating case study in celebrity's history. Advertising and newspapers spread the name of individuals across the country. Similarly, there were changes in the manner in which individuals were sold, turning sporting agents into marketable products in the growing consumer culture. The aim of this chapter is to place pugilism and its promotion into the wider social, cultural and economic context of the early eighteenth century. In this context we see the development of prize-fighters as celebrities.

---

[3]   See Matthew Taylor, 'From Source to Subject: Sport, History and Autobiography', *Journal of Sport History*, 35/3 (2008): pp. 469–91.

[4]   Peter Burke, *Popular Culture in Early Modern Europe* (Burlington, 2006), p. 249.

[5]   Elizabeth Barry, 'From Epitaph to Obituary: Death and Celebrity in Eighteenth-Century British Culture', *International Journal of Cultural Studies*, 11/3 (2008): pp. 259–75; Fred Inglis, *A Short History of Celebrity* (Princeton, 2010); Tom Mole, *Romanticism and Celebrity Culture* (Cambridge, 2009); Simon Morgan, 'Celebrity: Academic "Pseudo-Event" or a Useful Concept for Historians?', *Cultural and Social History*, 8/1 (2011): pp. 95–114; Stella Tillyard, 'Celebrity in 18th-Century London', *History Today*, 55/6 (2005): available at www.historytoday.com/stella-tillyard/celebrity-18th-century-london.

Bear Gardens

The bear gardens of London were an important feature of London's entertainment landscape. They remained – like animal baiting in the towns and at the country fairs – an immensely popular diversion for the public throughout the early modern period. Outside of London animal baiting often took place at local festivals, stressing its communal and rural nature. In London animal baiting was also popular, but its display became increasingly commercialised throughout the seventeenth century and adapted to urban quotidian life.[6] In the city baiting retained some of its original appeal and meanings, particularly regarding the relationship between humans and animal, but was also separated from the festival and agricultural culture of other regions. Rather, events were held frequently and admissions were charged. Audiences at the bear gardens were drawn from all the classes[7] with pricing structures to reflect social standing.[8] At the venues, as the name suggests, one would encounter bear baiting, as well as other animal baiting, including monkeys, bulls, leopards and lions.

In addition to animals, men would also perform, sometimes as supplementary entertainment and at other times as the main attraction. It is difficult to ascertain who owned and directly profited from the venues. Considering audiences would likely have been well-provided with alcohol and that the immediate local publicans would have enjoyed rampant trade on the days of performances, it might not be too wild to speculate that the 'theatre' was owned and operated by one (or more) closely linked to the alcohol trade.

How much the pugilists were likely to earn also remains questionable. Prizes were rewarded to winning competitors but such rewards were often small and infrequent. Many competitors seemed to have retained jobs in 'everyday' employment. While far from a definitive list, advertisements give a sense of the trades occupied by those fighting: 'Felt maker',[9] 'Butcher',[10] 'Carpenter'[11] and former members of the 'troop of horse guards'.[12] Fighters likely earned much

---

[6]   Tobias Hug, '"You Should go to Hockley in the Hole, and to Marybone, Child, to Learn Valour": On the Social Logic of Animal Baiting in Early Modern London', *Renaissance Journal*, 2/1 (2004): pp. 17–26.

[7]   Hug, 'You Should go to Hockley in the Hole'; Allen Guttmann, 'English Sports Spectators: The Restoration to the Early Nineteenth Century', *Journal of Sport History*, 12/2 (1985): pp. 103–25, at p. 115.

[8]   George A. Aitken, *The Tatler, Volume 1: London: Duckworth and Company* (London, 1899), p. 132; Thomas S. Henricks, 'The Democratization of Sport in Eighteenth-Century England', *The Journal of Popular Culture*, 18/3 (1984): pp. 3–20, at p. 14.

[9]   *Post Boy*, 6 April 1700.

[10]   *Post Boy*, 5 April 1701.

[11]   *Flying Post or The Post Master*, 20 September 1701.

[12]   *Daily Courant*, 1 February 1710.

of their wages from aristocratic stake money[13] or, in a similar manner to the travelling showmen of the period, from collections made by the audience at the end of the fight.[14] Because they were reliant on the collection, pugilists were inclined to provide as much of an entertainment as possible. *The London Post's* report of a fight at the turn of the century describes in great detail the drama of the event:

> Terrewest received only one wound, but Hesgate 5 or 6, so that he lost the day. Whilst they were a fighting, Davis, commonly known by the name of the Champion of the west, got upon the stage, and refused to go off again, challenging Terrewest, to fight him for offering to put him off, and afterwards challenged to fight any man there, whereupon one Gorman ... Jumped upon the Stage, and proffered to take up this bold challenger, and accordingly they both stript, and went to it, and at first bout Gorman wounded the Champion in the throat, and at second bout received a wound himself, in the side, but gave the Champion so great a wound on his forehead, that he swooned away; and many thought he had been killed, however he was so far disabled, that he could not try the third bout.[15]

What is most striking about this description is the brutality and bloodiness of the fight. The combatants fought with a range of weapons that had the potential to cause death or serious injury. An advertisement taken from a newspaper in 1699 lists the tools with which the fighters would duel: 'Back-Sword, Sword and Dagger, Sword and Buckler, Single Falchon ... Quarter-Staff'.[16]

As well as the thrill of the blood, violence and competition, the fights between men offered a taste of the theatrical. Colour, costume, music and drama would all be used to present an exciting performance to the crowds. The more interesting and engaging the performance, the more profitable it was for those involved. Richard Steele, a playwright tasked in 1714 with reforming the London stage, was particularly qualified to comment on the theatrical. His 1712 *Spectator* description of a visit to the Bear Garden at Hockley is permeated with theatrical codes and conventions:

> James Miller came on first, preceded by two disabled Drummers, to shew, I suppose, that the prospect of maimed Bodies did not in the least deter him ... Miller had a blue Ribband ty'd round the Sword Arm; which Ornament I conceive

---

13   Ford, *Prizefighting*, p. 90; Guttmann, 'English Sports Spectators': p. 117.
14   *The Spectator*, 21 July 1712.
15   *London Post*, 17 July 1700.
16   *Post Boy*, 21 October 1699.

to be the Remain of that Custom of wearing a Mistrel's Favour on such Occasions of old.[17]

The drama of the fight itself is captured with equally breathless prose.

> It is not easy to describe the many Escapes and imperceptible Defences between the two men of quick Eyes and ready Limbs; but Millar's Heat laid him open to the Rebuke of the calm Buck, by a large cut on the forehead. Much Effusion of Blood covered his eyes in a moment, and the Huzzahs of the crowd undoubtedly quickened the anguish ... The Wound was exposed to the View of all who could delight in it, and sowed up on the stage. The surly Second of Millar declared at this time, that he would that Day Fornight fight Mr. Buck at the same Weapons.[18]

Millar's confrontation and the promise of a fight in the future indicate a form of promotion that boxers and professional wrestlers would draw on for the coming centuries. Other forms of promotion were used, too: on the day of performances there would be a procession through the surrounding area, much to the annoyance of some local residents. Their irritation has left us with a vivid description. In 1701 presentment of the grand jury in Middlesex described what preceded these performances:

> We having observed the late boldness of a sort of men that stile themselves masters of the noble science of defence, passing through this city with beat of drums, colours displayed, swords drawn, with a numerous company of people following them, dispersing their printed bills, thereby inviting persons to be spectators of those inhuman sights which are directly contrary to the practice and profession of the Christian religion ... we think ourselves obliged to represent this matter, that some method may be speedily taken to prevent their passage through the city in such a tumultuous manner, on so unwarrantable a design.[19]

Such processions were clearly designed to garner attention and attract audiences, but their reach was limited. Processions, after all, could only attract those within the immediate vicinity. The blossoming newspaper business, however, had influence across the whole city, and in some cases country, and it was this business that would transform how pugilism presented and promoted itself.

---

[17] Richard Steele, *The Spectator*, 21 July 1712.
[18] Steele, *The Spectator*.
[19] Quoted in James Pellar Malcolm, *Anecdotes of the Manners and Customs of London During the Eighteenth Century* (London, 1810), p. 112.

Commerce

Before analysing the relationship between pugilism and advertising in greater detail, I want to sketch the social and economic changes that were taking place in London and England in the first half of the eighteenth century. In short, this is the beginning of a consumer, commodity and commercial society.[20] It is in this context that we should understand changes in pugilism, sport and popular culture.

For the latter half of the seventeenth century, London was witnessing intense social, economic and political change. London had undergone unprecedented population growth, swelling from 400,000 in 1650 to around 575,000 by 1700.[21] Those moving from rural to urban settings often brought forms of their recreation with them, albeit adapting to the specificities of London life.[22] More importantly, both imported sports and pre-existing amusements in the city benefited from the swelling number of potential audiences. As the city grew so too did consumer habits. The vast majority of skilled labourers and apprentices and an increasing number of unskilled workers in London and the south of England enjoyed higher living standards than their contemporaries in the rest of the country and existed in a 'high wage economy'.[23] Improvements in wages allowed for an increasing number of commodities to be bought with surplus money after basic needs had been met.[24] Inventories of the poor find an ever-growing number of commercial products,[25] and 'cloth, ceramics, glassware, paper, cutlery', T.H. Breen argues, 'transformed the character of everyday

---

[20]   The most influential of these studies remains Neil McKendrick, John Brewer and J.H. Plumb, *The Birth of a Consumer Society: The Commercialization of Eighteenth Century England* (London, 1982). See also Maxine Berg, *Luxury and Pleasure in Eighteenth-Century Britain* (Oxford, 2005); Cissie Fairchilds, 'Consumption in Early Modern Europe: A Review Article', *Comparative Studies in Society and History*, 35/4 (1993): pp. 850–53; Hoh-Cheung Mui and Lorna H. Mui, *Shops and Shopkeeping in Eighteenth Century England* (London, 1989).

[21]   E. Anthony Wrigley, 'A Simple Model of London's Importance in Changing English Society and Economy', *Past and Present*, 37 (1967): pp. 44–70, at p. 44.

[22]   Michael Harris, 'Sport in the Newspapers Before 1750: Representations of Cricket, Class and Commerce in the London Press', *Media History*, 4/1 (1998): pp. 19–28, at p. 24.

[23]   Robert C. Allen, *The British Industrial Revolution in Global Perspective* (Cambridge, 2009), p. 45; Francis Sheppard, *London: A History* (Oxford, 2006), p. 225.

[24]   McKendrick et al., *Consumer Society*, p. 24.

[25]   John Mullan and Christopher Reid, *Eighteenth-Century Popular Culture: A Selection* (Oxford, 2000), p. 19; Roy Porter, 'English Society in the Eighteenth Century Revisited', in Jeremy Black (ed.), *British Politics and Society From Walpole to Pitt 1742–1789* (Basingstoke, 1990), p. 39.

life [and] the domestic market hummed with activity'.[26] Changes in levels of consumption would be matched by changes in distribution, with proliferating shops becoming a regular feature of London life, competing and increasingly overtaking the importance of the market and fair.[27]

At the heart of this consumer society was the burgeoning press which demonstrated the increasing spending power of some groups. Newspapers were a celebrated attraction and feature of the coffee houses, themselves a signal of the increasing availability of 'luxury' items.[28] Moreover, the advertisements newspapers contained encouraged and maintained the material and commercial culture that was developing around them. By the end of the seventeenth century, the number of newspapers being produced had mushroomed, and it was during this time that the newspaper transformed in its presentation, style and tone.[29] Such growth had been encouraged by the lapsed Licensing (Printing) Act in 1695 and continued failures to establish a replacement in 1697, 1698, 1702, 1704 and 1712. Where the Printing Act required pre-publications to be approved by the King's licenser, its continuing failure to be reinstated or replaced with any meaningful laws meant that publishers had freedoms hitherto unknown. Investors were coming to realise that newspapers could offer profitable business.[30] The late seventeenth century saw a host of London papers, published weekly or thrice a week, which were available in the city and increasingly in the provinces. Shortly after in 1702 the *Daily Courant* was launched as the first daily newspaper.[31] This publication was followed by a surge of daily papers. With such a competitive and relatively unstable marketplace, publishers were realising that advertising could provide additional and welcome revenue to offset printing and distribution costs.[32] Advertisements for an ever-growing number of commercial products could be found in newspapers, and this in turn was changing how commercial products were presented to the public. The advertisement was crystallising around exaggeration, hyperbole and puffery.[33]

[26] T.H. Breen, '"Baubles of Britian": The American and Consumer Revolutions of the Eighteenth Century', *Past and Present*, 119 (1988): pp. 73–104.

[27] Dorothy Davies, *A History of Shopping* (London, 1966), p. 181; Mui and Mui, *Shops and Shopkeeping*; Wrigley, 'A Simple Model', p. 51; Breen, 'Baubles of Britain', p. 77.

[28] John Brewer, '"The Most Polite Age and the Most Vicious" Attitudes towards Culture as a Commodity', in Ann Bermingham and John Brewer (eds), *The Consumption of Culture: Image, Object, Text* (London, 1995), p. 348.

[29] Mullan and Reid, *Popular Culture*, p. 22.

[30] Jeremy Black, *The English Press: 1621–1861* (Stroud, 2001), p. 8.

[31] J.H. Plumb, *The Commercialisation of Leisure in Eighteenth-Century England* (Reading, 1974), p. 6.

[32] Mui and Mui, *Shops and Shopkeeping*, p. 222; J.M. Price, 'A Note on the Circulation of the London Press, 1704–1714', *Historical Research*, 31/84 (1958): pp. 215–24, at p. 218.

[33] McKendrick et al., *Consumer Society*, pp. 148–9.

The advertising of leisure, and in particular prize-fighting, would be influenced by the developments taking place around it. By the 1720s the bear gardens of the early modern period were facing closure and in their place emerged dedicated prize-fighting in fully commercialised venues. The shift from bear gardens to boxing amphitheatres offers an illuminating case study to track the growing commercialisation of leisure and their forms of promotion. This is not to say that the bear gardens were not commercial. Clearly their proprietors, publicans and bookies had been profiting from such events and from the venues for much of the early modern period, but the amphitheatre displays an increasingly sophisticated manipulation of the press, as well as displaying crucial changes in how its performers presented themselves to a wider public.

Amphitheatres

The bear gardens faced some of the earliest moral campaigns against blood sports. In 1724, newspapers were reporting that 'the Justices of the Peace for the City of Westminster and County of Middlesex, are about to suppress those publick and scandalous nusances the Bear-Gardens'.[34] Their closures did not signal the end of blood sports in the capital nor country.[35] They did, however, represent a changing attitude to animals in performance, with cruelty eventually being replaced by display and admiration, culminating with circus in the 1760s and 1770s.[36] Yet fighting between men and women remained a popular attraction. It also had enough support from the aristocracy to help it flourish in the commercial culture that was developing around them. Dedicated prize-fighting amphitheatres, perhaps with the help of loans from the wealthy, began to replace the older mode of performance. Figg's Amphitheatre appears to have been the first to be opened, and this was followed by Stokes' a few years later. Whether money was loaned to build these structures remains unclear, but there is evidence that Figg's amphitheatre was operated by the man whose name was given to the structure. In 1726 there was a hearing with the master of the rolls between Figg and his landlord, Mr Bouch, 'concerning the Amphitheatre built by the said Mr. Figg at his House ... without Leave or Lease from his said Landlord'.[37]

By this point, the human combatants were primarily the main attraction of the amphitheatres. From the 1730s, there was a shift away from sword-play and

[34] *Weekly Journal or British Gazetter*, 29 August 1724.
[35] See Douglas A. Reid, 'Beasts and Brutes: Popular Blood Sports c. 1780–1860', in Richard Holt (ed.), *Sport and the Working Class in Modern Britain* (Manchester, 1990), pp. 12–28.
[36] Marius Kwint, 'The Circus and Nature in Late Georgian England', in Rudy Koshar (ed.), *Histories of Leisure* (Oxford, 2002), pp. 45–60.
[37] *London Journal*, 26 November 1726.

weapons with an increased focus on fist-fighting, but its original pleasures – the thrill of watching individuals fight – remained unchanged. As grandiloquent as such venues may have sounded, the 'amphitheatres' were in fact semi-permanent wooden structures, 'a cross between a large fairground booth and a theatre'.[38] Byrom records in his journals that entrance cost 2s. 6d.,[39] the equivalent of about the average worker's day's wages.[40] For some critics this is proof that the prices were designed in order to keep the establishment exclusive[41] and there remains a wealth of evidence that Figg encouraged patronage from the upper classes, but its exclusivity is doubtable. Allen Guttman presents a number of diary extracts which suggest Figg's attracted audience members from across the classes.[42] Thomas S. Henricks maintains that most prize-fights in the capital offered differentiated admissions prices which separated the classes, with the cheapest in the pit 'to prevent the gentleman the inconvenience of having a performer fall off the stage into his lap'.[43] What is important to note is that all venues competed to provide a sense of comfort and safety to paying customers.[44]

The amphitheatres flourished in popularity and profit. Like other goods and services of the period, to sustain this popularity they relied on advertising to foster and sustain audiences. Newspaper promotion was not born at the amphitheatres, though. As the burgeoning press had grown, small notes promoting the forthcoming fights at the bear gardens became prominent in the classified advertisement pages, replacing the procession through the city as the primary form of promotion. One advertisement, with the text likely a word-for-word copy of the handbills handed out on the processions, declared:

> This present Tueseday, being the 26th of September, will be perform'd (at His majesty's Bear Garden in Hockley in the Hole) a trial of skill, between John Anderson the Famous highlander, and John Terrewest of Oundle in North-Hamptonshire, at all the usual weapons.[45]

Compared to what advertisements were to become the tone is subdued. The names are listed, as is one hometown, but otherwise there is little information to be taken. There is certainly no sense of personal resentment between the two men. The colour of the event itself – the blood, costume, characters and drama –

---

[38]   Brailsford, *Bareknuckles*, p. 4.
[39]   John Byrom, *Selections from the Journals and Papers of John Byrom: Poet – Diarist – Shorthand Writer, 1691–1763* (London, 1950), p. 66.
[40]   Guttmann, 'English Sports Spectators': p. 115.
[41]   Brailsford, *Bareknuckles*, p. 4.
[42]   Guttmann, 'English Sports Spectators': p. 115.
[43]   Henricks, 'The Democratization of Sport': p. 14.
[44]   Brailsford, *Bareknuckles*, p. 4.
[45]   *Post Boy*, 23 September 1699.

is absent. Over the next two decades promotion would gradually take on a more sensationalised tone and would litter the classified pages of daily and weekly newspapers. In the early 1720s, one newspaper advertisement for a prize-fight at the bear garden read:

> Whereas I Edward Sutton, pipe-maker, from Gravesend in the county of Kent, Master of the noble Science of Defence, thinking myself to be the most Celebrated master of the noble Science of Defence, thinking myself to be the most Celebrated Master of that kind in Europe, hearing the famous James Figg, who is call'd the Oxfordshire Champion, has the character to be the onliest Master in the World, do fairly invite him to meet me, and exercise at the usual Weapons fought on the stage, desiring no favour from the hero's hand, and not question in the least but to give such satisfaction, that has not been given for some years past by that Champion. I, James Figg, from Thame in Oxfordshire, Master of the Said Science, will not fail to meet this celebrated Master, at the place and time appointed; and to his request of no favour, I freely grant it, for I never did, nor will show any to no man living, and doubt not but I shall convince him of his own brave opinion.[46]

The challenge and acceptance that had been used on the stages of the bear gardens and transferred to the press in the early decades of the century now utilised a greater range of promotional hyperbole and ballyhoo. Sutton is convinced of his superiority where Figg implies his challenger is arrogant and egotistical. Dennis Brailsford has described that contests operated 'within the framework of challenges issued and accepted, with manliness, strength and courage held to be as much at issue as fighting skill'.[47] Within the columns of the newspapers, promoters were becoming more adept at capturing the drama audiences were used to seeing on the stage. Honour, in its melodramatic form, was used as a device to generate interest in the reading and listening public. Brailsford rightly suggests that if 'the build-up could give an impression of rancour between the fighters it was likely to whet more appetites and increase the takings'.[48] The added spice of rivalry that the promoters constructed in the press successfully maximised the profits of the promoters and pugilists, who benefited financially from larger attendances.

Such advertisements had become the accepted form of promotion for prize-fighting. Considering the fierce competition with other entertainment and commercial products, the pugilist's drive to promote the venture with ever-growing excitement becomes understandable. Other entertainments and material products were advertised with increasing frequency, and products needed

---

[46]   *Daily Post*, 10 April 1723.
[47]   Brailsford, *Bareknuckles*, p. 129.
[48]   Brailsford, *Bareknuckles*, p. 130.

an adequate definition of celebrity.[58] Fame and prestige clearly pre-date the period in question. His summary of the literature, however, does provide two important factors that are particularly pertinent for the study of prize-fighting in the early eighteenth century: the emergence of a (national) media and the development of a commodity culture.

Crucially, newspapers were able to report the events of an individual sporting star to a much larger audience than the small numbers in attendance at a particular event. Increasingly, an 'imagined community' of nation,[59] and some London papers clearly had a national readership in mind,[60] were able to keep up to date with the activities of individuals who they had likely never met. Francesco Alberoni has written that celebrity exists when 'each individual member of the public knows the star, but the star does not know any individuals'.[61] Some of the prize-fighters of the period appear to have partly met this definition. Newspaper reports and advertisements would have reached some households across England. Their fame, moreover, had surpassed simply those who had witnessed them fight first-hand. A poem by John Byrom claimed of Figg, 'To the towns, far and near, did his valour extend, And swam down the river from *Thame* to *Gravesend*'.[62] We might be critical of Byrom's reasons for extolling Figg, but his poem may have been attempting to capture a particular historical moment where fame was being distributed across the country with help from the press.

Similarly, just as newspapers were indicative of the commercial culture that was growing around them, many theories of celebrity posit that 'celebrity culture is irrevocably bound up with commodity culture'.[63] For Morgan a subject's marketability is the moment that marks modern celebrity: 'the point at which a public person becomes a celebrity is the point at which a sufficiently large audience is interested in their actions, image and personality to create a viable market for commodities carrying their likeness'.[64] In this reading, celebrities are products in themselves, used as a selling point in order to attract paying audiences to a particular entertainment. One of the reasons why the amphitheatres developed in that particular moment in time may have

---

[58]   Morgan, 'Celebrity': pp. 96–7.

[59]   Benedict Anderson, *Imagined Communities: Reflections on the Origin and Spread of Nationalism* (London, 1991); for a wider discussion of nation and celebrity see Jason Goldsmith, 'Celebrity and the Spectacle of Nation', in Tom Mole (ed.), *Romanticism and Celebrity Culture 1750–1850* (Cambridge, 2009), pp. 21–40.

[60]   T.R. Nevett, *Advertising in Britain: A History* (London, 1982), p. 17.

[61]   Francesco Alberoni, 'The Powerless "Elite": Theory and Sociological Research on the Phenomenon of the Stars', in Dennis McQuail (ed.), *Sociology of Mass Communications: Selected Readings* (Middlesex, 1972), pp. 75–98, here p. 79.

[62]   John Byrom, *Miscellaneous Poems Volume 1* (Manchester, 1773), p. 43.

[63]   Chris Rojek, *Celebrity* (London, 2001), p. 14.

[64]   Morgan, 'Celebrity': p. 97.

been because of the increasing attraction to named individuals in contrast to the earlier broader appeal of animal baiting. Celebrities are also devices to sell newspapers, periodicals and pamphlets. By the end of the century this had expanded to biographies and autobiographies. Finally, celebrities' images are used to create and sell merchandise for other products destined for the market. In the eighteenth century prints commemorating various sporting occasions and sporting celebrities were being produced by various entrepreneurs,[65] not least by the sportsmen themselves. On 19 January 1731 newspapers were advertising the publication of:

> *The Stage Gladiators: A Clear Stage and No Favour*, with the effigies of the Champions curiously engraven on copper. Printed for Messieurs Figg and Sutton, and sold by the Pamphlet-mongers of London and Westminster. Price 6d.[66]

The advert is interesting for three reasons. Firstly, Figg and Sutton were supposedly sworn rivals, yet here they were seemingly working in partnership to profit from their rivalry. We might posit that this is merely a business relationship, but there is the very real possibility that the sworn enemies presented in other advertisements were simply the products of promotion. In that case, the performers become closer to the fictional representation – or at the very least highly mediated performance of self – that would characterise celebrity in the coming centuries.[67] Secondly, it highlights an early example of the role of sporting celebrity in relation to commodity culture. Thirdly, it draws attention to the centrality of images in the distribution and dissemination of celebrity culture. Images, of course, allowed individuals to be recognised by those who had no personal interaction with the celebrity,[68] reinforcing the distance between performer and audience that was simultaneously being created by the press.

Images of boxers could be found elsewhere, not least in the trade cards distributed to promote their schools of arms. Trade cards were another important form of promotion of early eighteenth-century commerce, and though they advertised particular services, often spoke to a 'universe of commodities'.[69] James Figg's trade card has been a source of confusion, long thought to be the work of William Hogarth the work has more recently been credited to Anna

---

[65]	The selling of prints with cricket as the subject matter has also been noted by Harris, 'Sport in the Newspapers', p. 27.

[66]	*London Evening Post*, 19 January 1731.

[67]	Joshua Gamson, 'The Assembly Line of Greatness: Celebrity in Twentieth Century America', *Critical Studies in Mass Communication*, 9/1 (1992): pp. 1–24.

[68]	Elizabeth Barry, 'Celebrity, Cultural Production and Public Life', *International Journal of Cultural Studies*, 11/3 (2008): p. 253; Morgan, 'Celebrity': p. 103.

[69]	Berg, *Luxury and Pleasure*, p. 275.

Maria Ireland.[70] Mistakes about the designer's identity are easy to understand: Hogarth included Figg in his *Southwark Fair* print and designed the imagery for George Taylor's headstones. More importantly, perhaps, these trade cards were deliberately designed to reference 'images familiar across other types of print culture'.[71] Indeed, it might have been purposely designed to appear like a Hogarth. Such references not only highlight the vibrancy of that visual culture for the period but also the importance of a visual culture for celebrity.

Figg, and those who followed him in the years after his death, used trade cards, along with newspaper advertisements and their accompanying hyperbole, press conferences and performances, to create a brand,[72] a marketing concept that was itself becoming an important role in the commercial culture of eighteenth-century England.[73] The prize-fighter's brand was crucial to the promotion of the amphitheatre. Even when Figg was not fighting, like at the international match, his presence as a second was used in much of the promotion. The Figg brand was also used by performers to make profits in other ways: when the venues were not being used for exhibitions, it doubled as an equally extravagantly named 'school-of-arms'. At these schools, prize-fighters taught the use of weapons to upper-class patrons. Some spectators, then, were able to meet and train with these professionals in the amphitheatres as a training gym on days they were not being used as sporting arenas.

But this raises an important question to be asked about celebrity: to what extent did the desire to meet, mingle with or touch the famed pugilist – in other words the desire to overcome the distance created by the new forms of commercialised leisure – play in his school of arms' success? In every instance, products sold on the market promised, if only momentarily, to overcome the distance that a commercial leisure culture created. For those who could afford to pay for the school of arms this distance could be overcome by paying to train with the great master. Others could pay for a ticket to see the boxer in person. Most could potentially afford the prints featuring Figg and Sutton's likeness, and the price indicates the lower end of the market. By the end of the century these souvenirs had developed into pots and clay figures. What all three options provided was the opportunity for audiences and consumers to feel closer to the individual. The mechanisms of eighteenth-century capitalism placed sporting celebrities at a distance from audiences while at the same time providing the means of overcoming that distance through consumption.

---

[70] Stephen Hardy, Brian Norman and Sarah Sceery, 'Toward a History of Sport Branding', *Historical Research in Marketing*, 4/4 (2012): pp. 482–509, at p. 487.

[71] Berg, *Luxury and Pleasure*, p. 275.

[72] Hardy et al., 'History of Sport Branding': p. 487.

[73] Nevett, *Advertising in Britain*, p. 24.

Conclusions

To our modern eyes the sporting celebrities of the early eighteenth century seem modest. They do not exist in a world of 24-hour news cycles and endless gossip and speculation. But however modest they may appear, I have wanted to stress that this was a rich and vivid culture. The period did not merely sow the seeds of our own obsessions with fame and the famous but was itself blossoming. Boxers and their actions were regular fixtures of gossip and their exploits were as much part of the coffee-shop centred public sphere as conversations about politics. Figg and Broughton and the other names so often referenced in the sporting history books were active in the creation of their own fame. Pugilists used multiple mediums to spread their names and images across the country. Their entrepreneurial actions were a driving force in the creation of their own celebrity: they devised press conferences, used hyperbole and created public speculation in a manner akin to P.T. Barnum the following century. This was a celebrity culture, for better or worse, with its own peculiarities and specificities.

Yet it is also clear that to speak of a celebrity culture is also to speak of a commercial culture. The arrival of boxing amphitheatres and the celebrities they fostered were the consequences of the radical changes in society, in the economy and politics. The growth of newspaper networks and the development of industrial techniques all contributed to pugilists' successes and the manner in which they were able to publicise themselves. Celebrities and capitalism are tied together, and to understand the celebrities of the day is to understand culture and capitalism more broadly.

Chapter 6

An 'Art and a Science': Eighteenth-Century Sports Training

David Day

Introduction

Eighteenth-century industrialisation and urbanisation combined with substantial population growth to stimulate an entrepreneurial climate for leisure and sport within the rapidly expanding English cities. In London, innkeepers promoted cock-fighting, bull-baiting, horseracing, footracing, dancing contests and games of skill and strength. Sunday was the busiest day for inns on the outskirts of the city, many of which provided duck-hunting, dog-fighting and badger-baiting, while urban sporting houses and specialist facilities accommodated the gambling that was critical in moulding modern forms of sport.[1] Entrepreneurs like George Smith at the Artillery Ground promoted footracing and cricket, while the Peerless Pool was converted in 1743 by William Kemp into a pleasure bath where waiters attended to teach swimming. Thomas Higginson, who owned a fives court in St. Martin's Street, promoted fives, racquets or hand fives and offered tennis at his courts in the Hay Market and at High Holborn where there were also two billiard tables.[2]

Specialist arenas had previously been created for the rougher sports of the period and, by the end of the seventeenth century, Preston's Amphitheatre or Royal Bear Garden, situated near Hockley in the Hole in Clerkenwell, was presenting wrestling, boxing, cudgelling, fighting at back-sword, quarter-staff and bear-baiting.[3] The Amphitheatre was 150 by 200 feet, surrounded by tiered

---

[1]   John M. Golby and A. William Purdue, *The Civilisation of the Crowd: Popular Culture in England 1750–1900* (Gloucestershire, 1999); David Underdown, *Start of Play: Cricket and Culture in Eighteenth-Century England* (Harmondsworth, 2000); Dennis Brailsford, 'Religion and Sport in Eighteenth-Century England: "For the Encouragement of Piety and Virtue, and for the Preventing or Punishing of Vice, Profaneness and Immorality"', *British Journal of Sports History*, 1/2 (1984): pp. 166–83.

[2]   *Daily Advertiser*, 24 October 1743; 28 December 1743; 4 July 1744; *London Daily Post and General Advertiser*, 6 December 1743.

[3]   *A discourse upon the character and consequences of priestcraft, betwixt a Merry Andrew, a religious church-man, and Mr. Hickeringill* (London, 1705), p. 28; Vincent de Voiture, *The*

benches, and in the middle of the arena was a large stage for the human fighters, men like James Figg, Ned Sutton, James Stokes and John (Jack) Broughton,[4] all of whom subsequently promoted boxing through their own amphitheatres and then capitalised on their reputations by running teaching academies. Figg is credited with being the first to commercialise boxing when he set up a School of Arms in Tottenham Court Road in 1719 although he was best known as a teacher of gentlemen.[5] Ned Sutton and James Stokes developed an amphitheatre in Islington Road, which advertised boxing from the start of 1727, although Stokes had retired by 1731 to concentrate on commercial activities and on teaching, his pupils being 'equal in birth and fortune' to any in England.[6] After Figg retired, Thomas Sibblis took over his facility before George Taylor acquired the amphitheatre in 1734, subsequently enjoying considerable success as a manager, teacher and showman.[7] The best remembered of these boxing entrepreneurs was John (Jack) Broughton, a pupil of Figg's, who had appeared at Taylor's booth and fought at both Stokes's amphitheatre and at Sibblis's establishment in the 1730s. Broughton, considered as 'Champion' from the mid-1730s until 1750, brought a degree of offensive and defensive method into boxing, introduced some basic rules in 1743 and provided gloves, called mufflers, at his teaching academy to avoid physical damage to his gentleman amateurs.[8]

Footracing developed alongside boxing although there were important distinctions between the two since gentlemen might participate in pedestrian matches but they did not take part in prize-fights, although they supported and financed the fighters. Before gate money became important, the money for prizes, purses and training expenses normally came from these backers and patrons. Sometimes a subscription purse was organised to which many men contributed and sometimes athletes and their friends put up their own money

---

works of *Monsieur Voiture ... compleat: containing his Familiar letters to gentlemen and ladies.* Translated by Mr. Tho. Brown (London, 1705).

[4]   *Gazetteer and New Daily Advertiser*, 11 January 1788.

[5]   Nat Fleischer, *The Heavyweight Championship: An Informal History of Heavyweight Boxing from 1719 to the Present Day* (London, 1949), p. 4; *Daily Advertiser*, 15 June 1731.

[6]   *Weekly Journal or British Gazetteer*, 29 July 1727; 19 August 1727; 9 May 1730; *Daily Gazetteer* (London Edition), 11 July 1735; *Daily Advertiser*, 2 August 1731.

[7]   *Daily Journal*, 28 November 1732; John Godfrey, *A Treatise upon the Useful Science of Defence* (London, 1747), p. 40; An Amateur of Eminence, *The Complete Art of Boxing According to the Modern Method* (London, 1788), p. 48; *Daily Advertiser*, 12 March 1744; 23 April 1744.

[8]   *Daily Journal*, 23 November 1734; John Broughton, *Proposals for Erecting an Amphitheatre for the Manly Exercise of Boxing* (London, 1743), pp. 3–4; *London Daily Post and General Advertiser*, 25 January 1740. For further discussion of these boxing entrepreneurs see Dave Day, 'Entrepreneurial Pugilists of the Early Eighteenth Century', in Dave Day (ed.), *Sporting Lives* (Manchester, 2011), pp. 167–79.

but a wealthy patron was the most valued asset an athlete could have.[9] When Tyne and Mendoza engaged to fight for 100 guineas a-side in 1789 the former was backed by Lord Barrymore, the latter by Sir Thomas Apprice, and Mendoza declined a challenge in 1791 because of the absence of his 'friend' the Duke of Hamilton, whose permission he needed before he could fight.[10]

Although professional athletes like Mendoza had become increasingly visible during the course of the eighteenth century, they were not a new feature in the sporting landscape. In the Restoration period, many professionals had been paid retainers with grooms riding horses on behalf of their employers and liveried boatmen rowing matches to decide aristocratic wagers. Nobles engaged footmen for their speed and provided grounds and equipment for cricket as well as paying or employing professional players. Increasingly, however, the widespread promotion of sport as commercial entertainments meant that the best athletes were in demand from entrepreneurs, who wanted them because they would attract the crowds, while backers, cricket captains and racehorse owners needed them to defend their stake money. As a result, although wealthy patrons continued to employ the best performers, the freelance professional became commonplace by the end of the eighteenth century.[11] Many of these men extended their sporting careers by adopting training roles upon retirement when they drew on their own experiences, contemporary medical and scientific knowledge and an existing oral tradition surrounding training to devise their own, largely unrecorded regimes.

A significant influence on the creation of the trainer's role came from a reassessment of traditional ideas relating to the body during the Enlightenment leading to the belief that the application of science-based knowledge within systematic training programmes could enhance the performance of humans beyond their natural, God-given abilities. In addition to changes in attitudes towards the body, increasing industrialisation brought with it an emphasis on achievement through improved performance and sports started to resemble their modern forms as the English began systematically to quantify their sports and to move towards the invention of the sports record.[12] This emphasis on achievement highlighted the need to improve performance through application

---

[9] Peter Radford, *The Celebrated Captain Barclay: Sport, Money and Fame in Regency Britain* (London, 2001), pp. 60, 74–6.

[10] *Argus*, 19 November 1789; *Morning Chronicle*, 14 December 1791.

[11] Derek Birley, 'The Primrose Path: The Sports Pages Lecture 1995', *The Sports Historian*, 16 (1996): pp. 1–15; Dennis Brailsford, *British Sport: A Social History* (Cambridge, 1992), p. 49.

[12] Peter G. Mewett, 'From Horses to Humans: Species Crossovers in the Origin of Modern Sports Training', *Sport History Review*, 33 (2002): pp. 95–120; Alan Guttmann, 'English Sports Spectators: The Restoration to the Early Nineteenth Century', *Journal of Sport History*, 12/2 (1985): pp. 103–25.

and discipline, which brought training to the fore and made it an integral feature of sport with Figg, for example, taking responsibility for one fighter's 'Instruction and proper Diet' before a contest in 1725.[13] Thirty years later, *The Connoisseur* argued that the expanding competitive programme for boxers would lead gentlemen 'to keep champions in training, put them in sweats, diet them, and breed up the human species with the same care as they do cocks and horses'. Tellingly, the author believed that, as a result, this 'branch of gaming would doubtless be reduced to a science'[14] and gambling had much to do with stimulating training regimes. Backers who matched Perrins with Johnson in 1789 were prepared to wager up to £20,000 and they put Perrins into training to ensure a successful outcome.[15]

Analysing Performance and Identifying Talent

The constant search for improved performance by patrons and their hired trainers resulted in the development of training practices, a refinement of skills instruction and the systematic selection of talent. As training became more important, trainers began to incorporate contemporary scientific advances and technological innovations into their work. These initiatives were reflected in the instruction manuals produced by boxing enthusiasts, a common eighteenth-century practice that extended to manuals on angling and archery as well as hunting, horseracing, cocking, fencing and wrestling, which was covered comprehensively by Parkyns in 1713. The content considered technique, analysed with mathematical and theoretical principles that Parkyns credited partly to his association with Isaac Newton, fitness and diet, presaging some of the material presented in later boxing manuals. Parkyns selected middle-sized men, athletic, full-breasted, broad shouldered, brawny-legged and armed, yet clear-limbed, for wind and strength. If he liked a man's size and complexion he first asked whether or not his parents were still alive and, if not, at what age they died and then he explored their medical history and lifestyle, rejecting libertarians and men used to soft living. He also rejected 'sheep-biters' in favour of beef-eaters, who he believed had more robust, healthy and sound bodies, and he advised pupils never to exercise on a full stomach, to avoid excessive alcohol and to take only enough liquids to maintain the body's equilibrium and strength. Further suggestions were offered on suitable clothing and on the treatment of injuries with particular advice that sprains of the joints and tendons should be treated with cold water. For Parkyns, wrestling could be styled both as an 'Art

---

13   *London Journal*, 16 January 1725.
14   *Connoisseur* (Collected Issues), 22 August 1754.
15   *World*, 7 September 1789.

and a Science' and the more a wrestler exercised and practised the more those
experiences would develop his skills. His advice on boxing included soaping
one's hair if it were long and aiming the first blow with the head or fist at an
opponent's breast because this knocked the wind out of his body. Reflecting the
lack of regulation during this period, Parkyns also explained how to escape if an
opponent was thrusting his thumbs into the throat, grabbing the hair or pressing
his thumbs into the eyes.[16]

Defoe observed in 1720 that successful boxers were not necessarily stronger
but invariably had the 'longest breath'[17] and later authors not only distinguished
between technique, 'science' or 'art', and fitness, 'wind', as well as referring to
'bottom' but also assessed the relative value of each training component.[18] In a
seminal section on boxing in his 1747 book *A Treatise upon the Useful Science
of Defence*, Godfrey observed that the components of 'a Bottom' were wind,
improved by exercise and diet, and spirit, without which both art and strength
would be of little use. Strength was needed but a boxer would not succeed
without art,[19] a viewpoint confirmed by Lemoine in 1788 who suggested that
while boxing success was dependent upon a foundation of strength, combined
with manual dexterity, a lack of art would always be detrimental.[20] For Mendoza
and the author of *The Art of Manual Defence* good boxers needed strength,
courage, art, activity and wind, both of which could be acquired by practice
and could, therefore, be included under the heading of art. While recognising
that it was contentious, both authors considered strength more important than
art since a strong man could penetrate an adversary's guard and he would be
too powerful for his opponent to stop his blows effectually. His strikes would
have more impact than several hits from a weaker man and if fighters grappled
then the stronger man would have the advantage. Both texts suggested, however,
that no one should rely on strength without incorporating some knowledge of
technique, because this would always give a man the advantage over someone
with similar physical characteristics but who lacked science, and it gave a man

---

[16] Sir Thomas Parkyns, *Progymnasmata. The Inn-Play: or, Cornish-Hugg Wrestler*
(London, 1713), pp. 9–18, 37, 59.
[17] Daniel Defoe, *The Chimera: or, the French way of paying national debts, laid open*
(London, 1720), p. 3.
[18] Daniel Mendoza, *The Modern Art of Boxing as Practised by Mendoza, Humphreys,
Ryan, Ward, Watson, Johnson and Other Eminent Pugilists* (Little Britain, 1789 and 1790
editions), pp. 28–31; An Amateur, *The Art of Manual Defence; Or, System of Boxing:
Perspicuously Explained in a Series of Lessons* (London, 1799), pp. 68–91.
[19] Godfrey, *A Treatise upon the Useful Science of Defence*, p. 54.
[20] Henry Lemoine, *Modern Manhood, or, the Art and Practice of English Boxing*
(London, 1788), pp. 15–16, 26–7.

parity with those who were heavier and stronger. Strength, art and courage made a complete boxer but all these qualities were rarely found in one person.[21]

Table 6.1   The real scale of merit among the boxers

Boxers	W.	St.	A.	S.	B.
Perrings	10	10	n.k.	n.k.	n.k.
Johnson	8	9	6	5	6
Ward	6	7	10	9	10
Tring	8	8	4	3	8
Ryan	8	8	2	4	6
Dunn	7	6	4	4	8
Humphreys	5	5	8	6	8
Mendoza	4	4	10	10	6
Watson	4	5	9	4	9
Crabb	4	3	7	4	8
Martin	4	5	8	5	2
Big Ben	9	8	2	1	8
Doyle	5	6	0	0	8
Jackson	7	7	7	2	n.k.
Fewterel	9	8	0	0	5
Tyne	4	4	6	5	6
Bently	3	3	6	5	10

Note: The highest existing degree is 10. Where there has been no proof to judge by, they are marked n.k. not known. W. weight, St. strength, A. activity, S. skill, B. bottom.

Source: An Amateur, *The Art of Manual Defence* (London, 1799), p. 110.

Fewtrell argued in 1790 that it was still possible to be a good pugilist without having all the necessary attributes. The man who possessed more characteristics than his opponent would inevitably prove superior but in contests between equals a single component possessed by one man more than the other would give him an advantage. Strength, art, courage, activity, the ability to bear punishment, a quick eye and wind, were the constituents of a complete boxer. While it was impossible to display art properly without strength, Fewtrell's own experiences suggested that art was more critical than strength. Courage was essential, although

[21]   Mendoza, *The Modern Art of Boxing*, pp. 7–9, 28–31; An Amateur, *The Art of Manual Defence*, pp. 35–9, 68–91.

this varied even within the same man in different circumstances, and activity had become more important because shifting, the changing of ground and the moving away from an opponent, was now far more prevalent. The important attributes of quickness of eye and wind could be improved by constant practice. Fewtrell applied his analysis to his contemporary, Johnson, whose strength, science and bottom made him superior to everyone else although his greatest asset was that he always studied the strengths and weaknesses of opponents and used this knowledge to his own advantage. Other pugilists might be superior in strength, science or bottom but these abilities combined to form a complete boxer in Johnson.[22]

Science and Art: Technical Knowledge and Skill Development

Although there were differences in the level of importance allocated to the various components of performance there was unanimity that while some characteristics were naturally endowed others, especially 'scientific' skills, could be improved by frequent practice. The mechanisms explaining the complexity of animal and human motion had already generated interest among scientists and some of the earliest scientific experiments were concerned with muscle and its functions. Jan Swammerdam had shown in 1658 how he was able to contract a muscle by simple irritation, in 1666 Francesco Redi was the first to deduce that muscles generate electricity and in 1698, Dufay stated that the muscles of all living bodies produce electricity during motion.[23] Borelli, generally considered as the pioneer of modern biomechanics, studied running, jumping and skating, and it was the biomechanical paradigm he created in 1685, combined with the ideas emanating from Descartes' posthumous *Treatise on Man* (1662) and the industrialisation of the workplace, that stimulated the process of the instrumental rationalisation of the human body and its movement.[24] For London residents these scientific advances were being made readily accessible from the start of the eighteenth century by professional anatomy teachers who lectured to anyone who bought a ticket. Seen in the context of the Enlightenment enthusiasm for self-knowledge, anatomy was a legitimate component of a liberal education and

---

[22]   Thomas Fewtrell, *Boxing Reviewed; or, the Science of Manual Defence, Displayed on Rational Principles* (London, 1790), pp. 17–21, 61–5.
[23]   Jan Pieter Clarys and Katrien Alewaeters, 'Science and Sports: A Brief History of Muscle, Motion and ad hoc Organizations', *Journal of Sports Sciences*, 21 (2003): pp. 669–77.
[24]   Jacques Gleyse, Charles Pigeassou, Anne Marcellini, Eric De Léséleuc and Gilles Bui-Xuân, 'Physical Education as a Subject in France (School Curriculum, Policies and Discourse): The Body and the Metaphors of the Engine – Elements Used in the Analysis of a Power and Control System during the Second Industrial Revolution', *Sport, Education and Society*, 7/1 (2002): p. 7.

for those who wanted to understand something of anatomy without attending a dissection, there were anatomical waxwork exhibitions such as Rackstrow's public museum in the Strand.[25]

It has been argued that trainers were inevitably illiterate because they were generally drawn from the lower social classes but that underestimates the desire for literacy which emerged partly as a result of what Hobsbawm calls 'the meshes of the web of cash transactions' which spread in the eighteenth century.[26] As a result, the literacy rate in towns was high among urban tradesmen, retailers, skilled artisans, clerks and copywriters, all of whom required knowledge of reading, writing and calculating.[27] Sporting entrepreneurs certainly utilised these skills not least to produce their advertisements, many of which drew on the Enlightenment preoccupation with science. At the Gymnasium at Tottenham-Court at noon on Tuesday 29 January 1740 there was to be a

> Lecture in Manhood or Gymnastic Physiology, wherein the whole Theory and Practice of the Art of Boxing will be fully explained by various Operations on the Animal Oeconomy; and the Principles of Championism, illustrated by proper Experiments on the Solids and Fluids of the Body; together with the true Method of investigating the Nature of all Blows, Stops, cross Buttocks, &c, incident to Combatants. The whole leading to the most successful Methods of beating a Man, deaf, dumb, lame, and blind.[28]

The lecture syllabus was obtainable from 'Mr. Professor Broughton, at the Crown in Market-Lane; where proper Instructions in the Art and practice of Boxing are delivered without Loss of Eye or Limb to the Student' and Egan later asserted that Broughton had brought boxing to 'the rank of a science'.[29] However, Fewtrell argued in 1790 that boxing had advanced so significantly since Broughton's time that little more remained to be done to improve the science. Fewtrell's contemporaries, the 'moderns', were men possessed of every requisite to form a complete pugilist, thanks to a combination of talent and intense application. No 'labour, no expense had been spared to attain perfection and every manoeuvre, every finesse, which the mind could suggest, or the body

---

[25]   Alan W. Bates, '"Indecent and Demoralising Representations": Public Anatomy Museums in Mid-Victorian England', *Medical History*, 52 (2008): pp. 1–3.

[26]   Eric Hobsbawm, *Industry and Empire: From 1750 to the Present Day* (New York, 1999), p. 7.

[27]   John Lawson and Harold Silver, *A Social History of Education in England* (London, 1973), pp. 193–5, 237.

[28]   *London Daily Post and General Advertiser*, 25 January 1740.

[29]   Pierce Egan, *Boxiana; Or Sketches of Ancient and Modern Pugilism, From the Days of the Renowned Broughton and Slack, to the Heroes of the Present Milling Era* (London, 1812), pp. 7–16.

execute, had been attempted'.[30] It was this appeal to science that made the sport palatable to those who considered it 'cruel and unmanly' to enjoy watching a 'couple of fellows ignorant of boxing beat each other to pieces'. The pleasure that came from watching a skilful fighter originated from observing 'that done with ease which a man unacquainted with the science, would find it impossible to effect and the gratification amateurs received from beholding such contests, was an admiration of neatness and skill'.[31] Previewing the Humphries against Mendoza contest in 1788 one writer expected the fighters to show more science than on any previous occasion, which would satisfy amateur followers of this 'fashionable practice'.[32] By contrast, the Fewtrell and Jackson fight in June was devoid of science with Jackson, the eventual winner, repeatedly striking with his open hand and Fewtrell never standing up to his man.[33]

Fundamental to successful boxing was knowledge of human anatomy and fighters understood many basic anatomical principles, some of which influenced their fighting. In 1747, Godfery observed that a man's strength came from his muscles and that he could maximise this strength by the appropriate application of technique. Muscles were springs and levers that executed the different motions of the body but skill gave them additional force. To strike a hard blow, the fist should be shut as firm as possible since the flexors and extensors of the fingers would increase force to the arm in this position. By closing the left fist and clapping the right hand on that arm a man could plainly feel all the muscles swelling thereby demonstrating that muscles 'by nature designed for different offices, mutually depend on each other in great efforts'. The position of the body was important and the centre of gravity, which was dependant on the proper distance between the legs, was crucial because 'true equilibrium' of the body would allow it to stand much firmer against opposing force and enable it to deliver a more powerful blow. It was obvious, therefore, how a proper understanding of the art could make skilful men far superior to stronger men.[34] Godfrey's analysis was repeated almost verbatim over 40 years later by Lemoine, who also introduced phrases such as 'the tendons, and the nerves' and blows acquiring 'additional weight from the laws of gravity' into his text.[35]

Godfrey recorded that fighters were generally familiar with the most effective target areas on the body, particularly under the ear, between the eyebrows, and the stomach. The blow under the ear was believed to force blood both backwards into the heart, leading to a cardiaca or suffocation, and into the head, leading to the sinuses of the brain becoming so compressed that the man immediately

---

[30]   Fewtrell, *Boxing Reviewed*, pp. 42–6.
[31]   *Morning Chronicle and London Advertiser*, 28 March 1788.
[32]   *Morning Post and Daily Advertiser*, 7 January 1788.
[33]   *Morning Chronicle and London Advertiser*, 10 June 1788.
[34]   Godfrey, *A Treatise upon the Useful Science of Defence*, pp. 47–50.
[35]   Lemoine, *Modern Manhood, or, the Art and Practice of English Boxing*, pp. 16–17.

lost all sensation with blood often running from his ears, mouth and nose. Blows between the eyebrows caused a violent extravasation of blood, which fell immediately into the eyelids leading to their swelling almost instantaneously totally obstructing the sight and completely hoodwinking the opponent.[36] When Hunt beat the much heavier Slaughter-man in 1787, he 'directed every blow at the eyes, and won by completely sealing them up'.[37]

The 'mark', the pit of the stomach, was considered the most vulnerable target, since a severe blow here often caused instant sickness and an inability to continue.[38] Godfrey believed these blows hurtful because they affected both the diaphragm and the lungs, causing a painful convulsive state and lessening the cavity of the thorax, thus affecting the quantity of air retained in the lungs and causing great difficulty in respiration, which could only recover when the convulsive motion of the diaphragm ceases. The clever fighter reduced the impact of these blows by drawing in the belly, holding his breath and bending the thorax over his navel when he saw the blow coming. Lemoine (1788) later employed the term 'winding' to describe blows on the stomach.[39]

It is clear from comments in the early part of the century that a man hits more vigorously with his fist than with any other part of his arm because, being at the extremity, it carried more force,[40] that the basic mechanical principles relating to boxing were widely appreciated. In perhaps the most detailed exposition of boxing techniques produced in this period, the unknown author who called himself 'An Amateur of Eminence' described precisely the postures or attitudes in advancing, attacking, closely engaging and retreating. The advance, for example, was broken into three steps, the brace, the throw and the square. These fundamental steps, called the bar movements, were practised assiduously often to the beating of time.[41] Other authors were less prescriptive and confined themselves to advocating that in both advancing and retreating the boxer should step a pace forward with the leg that is foremost, and then with the hindmost foot, so as never to lose a stable position.[42]

The boxing literature addressed many techniques related to attack and defence. Blows from an adversary's left hand should be parried with the right

[36] Godfrey, *A Treatise upon the Useful Science of Defence*, pp. 50–52.

[37] *World and Fashionable Advertiser*, 27 September 1787.

[38] Mendoza, *The Modern Art of Boxing*, pp. 28–31; An Amateur, *The Art of Manual Defence*, pp. 68–91.

[39] Godfrey, *A Treatise upon the Useful Science of Defence*, pp. 53–4; Lemoine, *Modern Manhood, or, the Art and Practice of English Boxing*, pp. 21–6.

[40] William Machrie, *An Essay upon the Royal Recreation and Art of Cocking* (Edinburgh, 1705), p. 15.

[41] An Amateur of Eminence, *The Complete Art of Boxing*, pp. 1–16.

[42] Mendoza, *The Modern Art of Boxing*, pp. 28–31; An Amateur, *The Art of Manual Defence*, pp. 68–91.

arm or hand, and those of his right hand with the left, while fighters were advised against closing in with more powerful opponents, taking particular care to avoid the cross-buttock. Advice was often given about how to anticipate an opponent's attack and the advantages to be accrued from taking note of an opponent's modes of attack and defence and of their relative skills and strengths, in order to ascertain the movements necessary to 'stem the torrent of his ardour'. Particular attention should be paid to the direction of the opponent's eye and the inclination of his head, for as soon as the head inclined, the eyes were fixed upon the target and the arm raised to act. A quick and discerning eye allowed a fighter to anticipate attacks and it was important to look an opponent full in the face while taking his arms 'within compass of your view', peripheral vision as it would be called today, since the motion of eyes and hands would warn of where he was about to strike. When feinting, a fighter should direct his eyes away from his intended point of attack although this could expose a man to an attack.[43]

In 1788, the above mentioned author declared that by following the details included within his text a man's 'stage walk' would always enable him to advance or retreat at pleasure, and afford him superiority over those that may have double his strength but who had not had the benefit of learning his method of boxing. Discipline, reduced to general maxims and standing rules, rendered the art 'so easy and intelligent, that the adventitious combatant has but a poor stake against the initiated adept. Sleight in this science will accomplish what strength and resolution cannot'.[44] However, the rigid nature of his advice was contested by others. In 1790, Fewtrell declared that to point out any attitude as the best in every case would be ridiculous. Everyone should adopt his mode of defence according to his own powers, of which, after some practice, he would be the best judge. His only recommendation was that when a person, after mature deliberation and some experience, had adopted a particular guard, he should not easily relinquish it but should focus on its improvement instead.[45]

All commentators agreed that practice was essential to ensure a perfect knowledge of the science of boxing and that it should never be neglected since appropriate practice could increase both strength and activity. A mirror enabled a man to strike the right poses and to practice lessons and the same use could be made of a candle, by standing between its light and the wainscot, on which a man's shadow could be observed. If neither candle nor mirror were available boxers could practice by striking forward with each arm successively which would improve the capacity to strike more often and more quickly. The same could be done with a pair of dumbbells in the hands, of a weight just adapted

---

[43]   An Amateur, *The Art of Manual Defence*, pp. 39–42; An Amateur of Eminence, *The Complete Art of Boxing*, pp. 1–16.

[44]   An Amateur of Eminence, *The Complete Art of Boxing*, pp. 1–16.

[45]   Fewtrell, *Boxing Reviewed*, p. 30.

to age and strength. The best practice of all was to have a companion to spar with because this allowed a man to unite practice with theory. Sparring, boxing practised merely as an art or exercise by two persons without any intention of hurting each other, was vital in forming a complete pugilist. It was the only proper introduction to boxing, a method of assessing whether the pupil had absorbed the relevant lessons, and a means of trying out new strategies. It also enabled a man to assess the effectiveness of his professor's lessons and allowed him to exercise his mental faculties, which was not always possible in an actual contest.[46]

Training and 'Wind'

While technique was developed by the boxing professors in their schools and academies, the attributes of wind, activity and bottom were improved through training regimes under the supervision of expert trainers. Mewett argues that, at the start of the nineteenth century, these men drew from the training procedures already in place for other species, notably of horses, and that Classical training regimes had little influence on emerging training practices but the evidence suggests otherwise. The importance of exercise, described variously as 'all that motion or agitation of the body, of what kind soever, whether voluntary or involuntary' or as 'an agitation of the body, a system of tubes and glands admirably adapted throughout as a proper engine for the soul to work with, which produced salutary effects', had long been recognised.[47] Many authors drew on Classical examples, in some cases to point out the dangers of uneven development resulting from specialised training since, in 'every exertion beyond that what is gained in one part is inevitably lost in another'. In addition, the profuse sweating induced by such practices could 'debilitate the human body by depriving it of a great part of the juices necessary to its preservation'.[48] In 1634, Peacham recommended running and leaping as being healthful for the body[49] and systematic training programmes for humans were clearly operating in the seventeenth century since Stubbe observed in 1671 that bodies which were dieted and 'brought up to an Athletick habit, do soonest of all decline into

[46]   Fewtrell, *Boxing Reviewed*, p. 14; Mendoza, *The Modern Art of Boxing*, pp. 28–31; An Amateur, *The Art of Manual Defence*, pp. 68–91.

[47]   Francis Fuller, *Medicina Gymnastica: Or, a Treatise concerning the Power of Exercise with Respect to the Animal Oeconomy and the Great Necessity of it in the Cure of Several Distempers* (London, 1705), pp. 231–54; A Friendly Traveller, *The Ensign of Peace Shewing how the Health, Both of Body and Mind, May be Preserved* (London, 1775), pp. 13–14.

[48]   *The Scots Magazine*, March 1790, pp. 107–9.

[49]   Henry Peacham, *Compleat Gentleman 1634: With an Introduction by G. S. Gordon* (Oxford, 1906), vol. 4, pp. 215–18.

sickness and premature old age'.[50] Likewise, Tillotson, in 1710, declared that an athletic constitution and perfect state of health was considered by physicians to 'verge upon some dangerous disease, and to be a fore-runner of it'.[51]

Five years earlier, medical man Francis Fuller had been much more positive when proposing gymnastics as practiced by the ancient Greeks as the most effective form of physical training in his *Medicina Gymnastica*. His sources included Galen and Mercurialis, who had argued that exercise should be individualised according to a person's constitution and level of fitness, as well as contemporary medical and scientific knowledge.[52] In 1725, George Cheyne reflected on the current state of knowledge in his *Essay of Health and Long Life* and outlined many of the basic principles of health and exercise that underpinned the training regimes developed during the eighteenth century. He reflected on the importance of those 'non-naturals' which were necessary 'to the subsistence of man', namely, air, meat and drink, sleep and watching, exercise and rest, evacuations and their obstructions, and the passions of the mind, which had a greater influence on health than most people were aware of. His advice included giving more food to strong men, those of a large stature and those involved in hard labour, avoiding going to bed on a full stomach, always ensuring full evacuation of the bowels with one regular stool a day, and walking as a most useful and natural exercise. He also observed that the organs of labouring men were strengthened by their employment. The legs, thighs and feet of chairmen, the arms and hands of waterman, the backs and shoulders of porters all grew thick, strong and powerful over time. He concluded that using any organ frequently and forcibly brought blood and spirits into it and made it grow plump and brawny. He then argued that there were four conditions necessary for beneficial exercise. It should be carried out on an empty stomach, it should not be carried out to a depression of spirits or a melting sweat, post-exercise recovery should be in a warm room to avoid a rheumatism fever or cold and, lastly, being judicious in exercise to avoid overexertion. He also recommended cold bathing and the flesh brush as an exercise for promoting a full and free perspiration and circulation.[53] In the training advice they offered, eighteenth-century texts drew on these basic principles along with the medical knowledge of the period which remained centred on humoral theory. The work of the trainer was to identify any humoral imbalances in their athletes and

---

[50]   Henry Stubbe, *An Epistolary Discourse Concerning Phlebotomy in Opposition to G. Thomson Pseudo-chymist, a Pretended Disciple of the Lord Verulam* (London, 1671), p. 96.

[51]   John Tillotson, *The works of the Most Reverend Dr. John Tillotson ... containing fifty four sermons and discourses, on several occasions* (1710), p. 481.

[52]   Fuller, *Medicina Gymnastica*, pp. 231–54.

[53]   George Cheyne, *An Essay of Health and Long Life* (Dublin, 1725), pp. 38, 45, 49–53, 72, 88.

redress them through a programme of diet, exercise and medication.[54] Even though medical knowledge progressed significantly during this period and new explanations of how the body functioned emerged, humoral theory continued to exert a powerful influence.

While there had been differences in the level of importance allocated to the various aspects of performance there was unanimity among authors that wind could be improved by regular and specific training. Violent exertions could cause a man to become out of breath and a man was considered to have good wind when he displayed powers of respiration and an ability to maintain activity. Bad wind resulted in a man being quickly disabled by the fatigue of personal exertion.[55] Good wind was enhanced by proper exercise or 'training', and, if impaired, it could be recovered by training and regularity of living.[56] In 1726, Thomas Tryon emphasised that individuals should not pass immediately from a 'disordered kind of life' to a strict exercise programme but should do it little by little since doctors believed that it was dangerous to abandon one's traditional lifestyle. He also drew attention to the appropriate methods of preparing the body, declaring that the body should be well purged and cleared of all ill humours by gently taking medicines over two or three days. The first day purged the bowels, the second the liver, and the third the 'reins' in which lay the 'drain' of the ill humours. As to diet, beef gave strength to those who were physically active enough to digest it properly, while the best ale was neither too new or too old, nor too stale, but was clear and well brewed.[57] The association between boxing, beef and the English was an enduring one. In the 1750s, one writer observed that the sturdy English were as much renowned for their boxing as their beef, both of which were unsuited 'to the watry stomachs and weak sinews of their enemies the French'. Beef and boxing underpinned the 'long-established maxim, that one Englishman can beat three Frenchmen'.[58]

Later writers were clear that aliment, whatever was capable of nourishing the animal body, was principally of bread with farinaceous substances such as beans, peas and lentils, although their constant use could cause obstructions. Fish was the least nourishing of animal foods while older animals were better than younger ones even though the flesh was tougher and harder to digest. Roasted meat contained an excellent nourishing juice and water was essential for life, although too much of it relaxed and weakened the solids and it should not be

---

54   Mewett, 'From Horses to Humans': pp. 95–120.

55   An Amateur, *The Art of Manual Defence*, pp. 68–96; Mendoza, *The Modern Art of Boxing*, pp. 28–31.

56   Fewtrell, *Boxing Reviewed*, pp. 17–21; A Friendly Traveller, *The Ensign of Peace*, pp. 2–6.

57   Thomas Tryon, *The Way to Health and Long Life or a Discourse of Temperance* (London, 1726), pp. 26, 38, 46, 50.

58   *The Connoisseur*, 1/30 (1755–1756): pp. 177–80.

drunk cold when the body was hot. Perfect digestion was always the best rule especially if one was planning to be particularly active after a meal.[59] In 1789, Dr Fothergill noted that bread taken in considerable quantities was suitable for labourers, whose strong organs ensured they could digest it properly, and that the main constituents of the diet should be animal food. Rich, sweet puddings, especially baked, and fruit after meat were 'unnatural and improper' while mild, well-brewed beer was acceptable as a beverage.[60]

Training to improve wind took athletes away from their usual routines and put them under the control of experts for periods of time that differed according to the authority consulted. Following Slack's challenge in 1750, Broughton noted that since Slack had been 'in keeping' for some months and he himself was not immediately prepared for competition, he declined the fight until he had had a month's training.[61] While the so-called 'Amateur of Eminence' (1788) believed in 10 days or a fortnight of preparation,[62] Mendoza noted that this could extend to three weeks although others like Humphreys normally took at least six weeks to prepare.[63] Tryon observed in 1726 that the best air was pure and free from all pollution, 'breathing sweetly with pleasant Gales, and sometimes moisture as with wholesome showers'.[64] Since it was generally accepted that the best quality air, 'void of all bad exhalations' and not too hot, cold, dry or moist,[65] was to be found in rural areas, trainers normally took their men out of towns when preparing for fights. When Belcher and Burke were matched for 200 guineas a-side by Captain Fletcher and Fletcher Reid, in 1802, Belcher, accompanied by Joe Ward, set off six weeks before the fight to Yorkshire to put himself into training while Burke trained in Newmarket. Reflecting on the failure of this fight to materialise, Burke said that he 'had been in training seven weeks at Middleham, and was never in better condition. I ran and leaped with many people, and always beat them'.[66]

When 'in training' contestants lived with their trainers, who supervised all aspects of their daily lives and whose success was ultimately assessed not only in terms of the competitive outcome but also in relation to their athlete's physical appearance. The gaze of the spectators was an important measure of whether it was thought that the training had been properly conducted and the 'ceremony

---

[59]   A Friendly Traveller, *The Ensign of Peace*, pp. 2–6.

[60]   Dr Fothergill, *Interesting Observations on Diet* (New London Magazine, July 1789), pp. 325–90.

[61]   *London Evening Post*, 13 March 1750.

[62]   An Amateur of Eminence, *The Complete Art of Boxing*, pp. 17–21.

[63]   Mendoza, *The Modern Art of Boxing*, p. 24; An Amateur, *The Art of Manual Defence*, pp. 88–94.

[64]   Tryon, *The Way to Health and Long Life*, p. 19.

[65]   A Friendly Traveller, *The Ensign of Peace*, pp. 2–6.

[66]   *The Aberdeen Journal*, 19 May 1802; *Jackson's Oxford Journal*, 17 July 1802.

of peeling', the stripping-off of garments before an event, was normally the first indication as to the condition of the fighters.[67] On peeling before his fight with Humphreys in 1790, Mendoza appeared

> the largest and heaviest man; a circumstance arising partly from his increase in bulk, and partly from the mode of training adopted by Humphries, apparently more for the purpose of rendering him light and active than of adding to his weight. The odds on stripping were five to four on Mendoza.[68]

In 1788, the author of the *Complete Art of Boxing* remarked that a sinking of the spirits often betrayed a champion into actions unworthy of himself, creating fear, shame and disgrace, and that in order to keep up his animal spirits an athlete should prepare as much as he judged necessary. During training, he should follow a disciplined programme, beginning with an evening's warm bath for the feet, legs and the small of the thighs. After he was cool again, he washed his loins, face, hands and arms with cold spring or pump water making sure that no soap was used in any ablutions. Following a supper of runnet milk, or milk-pottage and a little bread, butter or salt, the man should retire early. Each morning meal should be runnet whey and hard white biscuit, without seeds, while dinner alternated between stewed veal with rice and well-fed fowls, with a melt or two, boiled to a jelly. No tea should be taken in the afternoon but a rusk and chocolate taken early in the evening followed by supper as before. As for drinking, only a glass or two of red wine diluted with water was allowed after dinner with no porter, table-beer, ales or spirits. Before dinner, half a pint to a pint of mulled wine would do no harm, provided a glass or two of strong jelly was eaten beforehand and a rusk or a well toasted crust taken with it. Salts or acid juices were to be avoided although lump sugar was allowed and, 'if the habit requires it', half a pint of mulled claret at night, with plenty of lump sugar, was recommended. As for the non-dietary regimen, disciplined hours of rest and recreation were to be observed throughout the training period with a man retiring to bed exactly at nine and rising at five. Breakfast was taken at seven, rusk and wine at eleven, dinner at one, chocolate at four, supper at seven, and from then until bedtime the athlete should be entertained, if possible, with martial music. This would help a man form an 'heroic state of spirits', make his dreams agreeable and add to his 'vivacity and serenity of thought'. The mind must not be 'ruffled or agitated' but everything should be conducted with 'harmony and liveliness'. The mornings should be spent in an early walk, not exceeding a mile, after eating a single gingerbread nut (steeped in Hollands Geneva [gin]),

---

[67]   Mewett, 'From Horses to Humans': pp. 95–120.
[68]   *Diary or Woodfall's Register*, 2 October 1790.

and returning very slowly to avoid heating the body. It was important to avoid overheating so men were advised to 'lay cool at night'.[69]

In *The Modern Art of Boxing* (1789 and 1790 edition), Mendoza repeated much of this advice, regarding these training methods as having been 'laid down and approved by many scientific men'. It was emphasised that while in training no bloodletting or physic should be employed because the cooling of the body, and at the same time the strengthening of the fluids, could not be effected if either method were used. The evening exercise could be any cheerful indoor amusement, or a walk, before retiring. However, Mendoza also offered an alternative, less prescriptive, regime. Boxers should live temperately, but not abstemiously, taking exercise but not to the point of fatigue. The fighter and his trainer were particularly advised to take care to avoid excess in food, wine or women. Good air was recommended and men should train in the country, going to bed about ten, rising about six or seven, having a cold bath if possible, followed by a dry rub, some muscular exercise and a walk of a mile or two. On returning, they should eat a good breakfast, take the air again, then practice sparring and any other moderate exercise until dinner, when they must avoid eating much. Beverage at dinner should be wine and water, and a glass or two of old hock afterwards. The afternoon should be spent riding or walking and about eight o'clock a supper taken of any light nourishing food. If possible, the man should exercise again, maybe utilising the dumbbells, until retiring to bed.[70]

As for the day of competition, Godfrey advised fighters to avoid too much food (aliment) because this would help avoid compression on the *Aorta Descendens* and preserve their stomachs from the blows, which they would be more exposed to if distended with food. The result would be a vomiting of blood, caused by the eruptions of some blood vessels, from the overcharging of the stomach. He advised fighters to take a little cordial water upon an empty stomach, which would be helpful in 'astringing the Fibres, and attracting it into a smaller Compass'.[71] Other texts advised eating no more than a single slice of bread, well toasted without butter, or a hard white biscuit toasted, and about a pint (Mendoza suggested a half pint) of best red wine mulled, with a tablespoonful of brandy, to be taken an hour before dressing. On the stage, drinks should consist of Hollands, bitters and Fine China orange juice, with dissolved lump sugar, mixed at a strength suitable for the individual fighter.[72]

[69]   An Amateur of Eminence, *The Complete Art of Boxing*, pp. 17–21.

[70]   Mendoza, *The Modern Art of Boxing*, pp. 24–7.

[71]   Godfrey, *A Treatise Upon the Useful Science of Defence*, p. 53.

[72]   An Amateur, *The Art of Manual Defence*, pp. 88–94; An Amateur of Eminence, *The Complete Art of Boxing*, pp. 17–21; Mendoza, *The Modern Art of Boxing*, p. 27.

Some Reflections

A description of a Mr Montague in 1777 recorded that he danced, fenced, walked, rode, played cricket and shot better than anyone in the surrounding district. He had also been tutored 'in the less gentleman-like exercises of quarter-staff, boxing and wrestling, exercises which were calculated to increase courage'.[73] Clearly, the science of manly defence had become an integral part of a gentleman's education and boxing schools were established by prize-fighters like Mendoza, who had premises in Houndsditch and who added P.P. ('Professor of Pugilism') to his name in 1789.[74] Among his contemporaries, Humphreys was 'the instructor of most of the young men of fashion for a guinea for six lessons' at his school in London, which was opened in 1788 and much frequented by the Westminster boys and patronised by some of the first people in this country who 'will probably soon procure him a comfortable independence'.[75] Ward was teaching in Bristol where he was allowed 16 shillings a week by his patrons, on condition that he fought no one without their agreement.[76]

Many practitioners embarked on careers as trainers, often using their experiential knowledge to prepare rowers and pedestrians in addition to fellow pugilists. Previews of the Wood versus Barclay pedestrian match in 1807 recorded that Barclay was training at Newmarket under the guidance of the 'noted pugilists, William Ward and son, Crib and Gulley'.[77] Their training advice displayed considerable longevity, underpinning practices across all professional sports for much of the nineteenth century. Part of the reason for this permanency was that these regimes had proved to be extremely effective in developing athletes well beyond the normal capacities of their contemporaries. In 1789, Ward was found guilty of manslaughter after being challenged by a local blacksmith, a remarkably strong man, fond of fighting and the best bruiser in his neighbourhood. Ward initially refused to get involved but eventually they had four rounds during the last of which the blacksmith received a blow on the right temple that killed him.[78] Two years later while Mendoza was sparring at Norwich, a tall dragoon discarded his mufflers and demanded that he box in earnest. Mendoza removed one glove and, although he only used one hand, within three minutes his opponent could not find his way out of the room, both

---

[73]   Frances Brooke, *The Excursion. In two volumes* (Dublin, 1777), vol. 1, p. 101.

[74]   *Morning Chronicle and London Advertiser*, 6 January 1789; World, 17 June 1789.

[75]   *Public Advertiser*, 24 January 1788.

[76]   *World and Fashionable Advertiser*, 21 September 1787.

[77]   See following for details of this contest. *Hampshire Telegraph and Sussex Chronicle* etc., 31 August 1807; *The Morning Chronicle*, 2 October 1807; 8 October 1807; *The Ipswich Journal*, 10 October 1807; *The Hull Packet and Original Weekly Commercial, Literary and General Advertiser*, 13 October 1807; 3 November 1807.

[78]   *World*, 7 May 1789; 8 May 1789.

his eyes being closed.[79] Paradoxically, this level of expertise contributed to the declining popularity of bare-knuckle boxing as expert training and improved techniques made the sport a brutal affair. James, fighting Gamble in 1800, had his nose cut dreadfully in the fourth round, his collarbone broken in the twentieth, his jaw broken in the twenty-first and yet he still fought four more rounds before yielding.[80]

The proliferation of boxing manuals in the last quarter of the eighteenth century reflected a desire of participants and observers to record the essential elements of this martial 'science'. While this term had been used in conjunction with similar activities throughout the century and while training had been undertaken by professional athletes for at least as long, it was only now that contemporaries believed a full understanding had been achieved of the importance of 'wind', 'bottom' and 'science'. There was general unanimity about the content of training regimes, which is not surprising given the limited and exclusive circle that surrounded professional athletes. As this cadre of sportsmen subsequently extended their sporting interests, many pugilistic training methods, with some sports specific amendments, became the standard modes of preparation for other gambling focussed activities such as rowing and pedestrianism. At the beginning of the new century, some of the oral traditions and practices of these trainers were recorded and published although it was not easy to obtain information from individuals who relied on their training knowledge for their regular employment and who often kept the details of their methods within their own family. Sir John Sinclair's *A Collection of Papers, on the Subject of Athletic Exercises* (1806), outlined the thoughts of some of these men, and he observed 'the almost incredible perfection, to which those whose profession it is to train men to athletic exercises, have brought to their respective art'.[81]

Sinclair's subsequent four-volume *Code of Health and Longevity; or Concise View of the Principles Calculated for the Preservation of Health and the Attainment of Long Life* in 1807 drew further upon ancient sources, contemporary physicians, sports trainers and published boxing manuals to explore the current state of athletic training.[82] The training regimes described here by Sinclair represented a refinement, not a replacement, of the training programmes offered in the last half of the eighteenth century and emphasise that any form of training occurs within a specific social and historical context and builds on previous knowledge,

---

[79]   *Gazetteer and New Daily Advertiser*, 6 December 1791.
[80]   Pierce Egan, *Pancratia, or a History of Pugilism* (London, 1812), p. 132.
[81]   John Sinclair, *A Collection of Papers, on the Subject of Athletic Exercises* (London, 1806), p. 8.
[82]   John Sinclair, *The Code of Health and Longevity; or, a Concise View of the Principles Calculated for the Preservation of Health and the Attainment of Long Life* (Edinburgh, 1807), especially pp. 39–150 and the Appendix which considers training methods.

as do all human activities. As a result it behoves the modern commentator to avoid being judgmental. Nietzsche was scathing of those 'who write history in the naive faith that justice resides in the popular view of their time'[83] and it would be arrogant of twenty-first-century contemporaries to be critical of the efforts of eighteenth-century trainers. Even when training programmes changed in the later stages of the Victorian period, they continued to address the key essentials of diet, exercise, psychology and technique, as identified by these men, training elements that remain the cornerstones of athletic preparation for the modern Olympian.

---

[83]　Friedrich Nietzsche, *The Use and Abuse of History*, trans. A. Collins (New York, 1957), p. 38.

PART III
Promoting Health or Danger?
Physical Exercise under Scrutiny

Chapter 7
Exercise for Women

Alessandro Arcangeli

Sports and Physical Exercise: Gendered Definitions

Women played a very specific role in the physical culture of early modern Europe, as documented in both theory and practice. I believe that the incorporation of 'physical exercise' and 'motion' in the title of the present volume to complement the basic key word 'sport' is positively helpful with particular reference to the topic of my contribution considering that the term has rarely been applied to activities in which women actively participated in the past. Both the progress of sport for women and the increasing part women play in sports studies are predominantly twentieth-century phenomena.[1]

Physical Exercise for Women: Preparation for Birth and Preserving Beauty

It is difficult to discuss women and the Renaissance period without at least some reference to Baldassarre Castiglione's *Book of the Courtier*. It is noticeable that, although with understandably less space and detail than for his courtier, Castiglione reserves some room for the topic of physical exercise for women, too. At the beginning of Book Three, he constructs the ideal of the *donna di palazzo* by distinguishing between qualities required of men and women alike, and those which are gender-specific; a pattern he readopts in his discussion 'of the exercises of the bodye' in particular (III.4).[2]

In his opening essay within the volume on *Women in Italian Renaissance Culture and Society* edited by Letizia Panizza, Dilwyn Knox also, understandably, considers the *Cortegiano*. After quickly summarizing Giuliano de' Medici's

---

[1]   Although the literature on women and sport has grown significantly over the past few decades, not many books offer much information and insights for periods prior to the last two centuries. For a historical survey: Allen Guttmann, *Women's Sports: A History* (New York, 1991). On the issue of sport and the construction of gender: Sandra Günter, *Geschlechterkonstruktion im Sport: eine historische Untersuchung der nationalen und regionalen Turn- und Sportbewegung des 19. und 20. Jahrhunderts* (Hoya, [2004]).

[2]   Baldassare Castiglione, *The Book of the Courtier*, trans. T. Hoby [1561], ed. V. Cox (London, 1994), p. 213.

presentation of diverging male and female models, however, Knox adds the interesting remark that Castiglione's solution is not as stereotypical as one may expect, and in the previous literature – typically in Leon Battista Alberti's *Libri della famiglia* – modesty had played central role; a virtue, he adds, that at least for part of its cultural history was not highly gendered, being a moral requirement for both women and men.[3] Castiglione therefore presents gendered as well as non-gendered ideals of motion.

Now that we are aware of this specificity of Castiglione's model construction, let us check its actual contents, bearing in mind that the *Book of the Courtier* is written in the form of a dialogue, exploring a wide variety of ideological orientations. Among Castiglione's characters, Giuliano de' Medici is the author's spokesperson in Book Three; his first references to exercise are generic, limited to a recommendation on how to perform them: 'the exercises of the body comlie for a woman shall she do with an exceading good grace' (III.4).[4] His interlocutors are not satisfied with this level of information, and press for a list of commendable physical activities. One of the most misogynous personae, Unico Aretino, addresses the topic with a provocative reference to past customs: 'Emonge them of olde time the maner was that women wrastled naked with men, but we have lost this good custome together with many mo[re].'[5] Cesare Gonzaga reinforces his point by adding: 'And in my time I have seene women play at tenise, practise feates of armes, ride, hunt, and doe (in a maner) all the exercises beeside, that a gentilman can do.'[6] Giuliano will not allow such blurring of gender roles, and replies:

> Sins I may facion this woman after my minde, I will not onelye have her not to practise these manlie exercises so sturdie and boisterous, but also even those that are meete for a woman, I will have her to do them with heedefulnesse and with the soft mildenesse that we have said is comelie for her. And therefore in daunsynge I would not see her use to swift and violent trickes, nor yet in singinge or playinge upon instrumentes those harde and often divisions that declare more counninge then sweetenesse.[7] (III.8)

3   Dilwyn Knox, 'Civility, Courtesy and Women in the Italian Renaissance', in Letizia Panizza (ed.), *Women in Italian Renaissance Culture and Society* (Oxford, 2000), pp. 2–17.

4   Castiglione, *The Book of the Courtier*, p. 217 (NB: in all quotations, in the wording of Thomas Hoby's sixteenth-century translation).

5   Castiglione, *The Book of the Courtier*, p. 218. For a comparative perspective, consider the near-naked women wrestling at the court of the Japanese emperor in the fifth century CE, or women imagined to play team ball games dressed as kickball players in a text of the early fourteenth century – though apparently a rare sight in the Orient too: Allen Guttmann and Lee Thompson, *Japanese Sport: A History* (Honolulu, 2001), pp. 14–15, 29–30.

6   Castiglione, *The Book of the Courtier*, p. 218.

7   Castiglione, *The Book of the Courtier*, p. 218.

The subsequent passage contains a well-known distinction between the musical accomplishments suitable or not for a lady; for music and dance alike, Castiglione's spokesman insists on manners of performing them, such as attire and letting oneself be invited with insistence before accepting to display skills. Furthermore, there would be activities which women were not supposed to practice, nevertheless it was expected that they were sufficiently familiar with them to be able to judge if men performed them skilfully: 'and in those exercises that we have saide are not comelye for her, I will at the least she have that judgement, that men can have of the thinges which they practise not' (III.9).[8]

Thus notions of manliness and femaleness clearly influenced shared understandings of the decency of certain sports for each sex; reciprocally, customs and bodily practice could actively reinforce those gendered notions. The 'fair sex' was supposed to move softly and rarely. This distinction based on gender has operated along a variety of strategies, in discourse as well as in actual rules and prohibitions: two very general ones are for example the consideration of some activities as not befitting women altogether (e.g. for the postures and gestures they involve) and a policy of segregating the sexes as certain physical activities and games were seen as improper for mixed-sex groups. Thus skittles and badminton featured among suitable entertainments for well brought-up seventeenth-century French ladies.[9]

With reference to the English regimen for health between the sixteenth and the seventeenth century, Andrew Wear has suggested that this textual output devoted a limited attention to women, a fact for which we may find a variety of explanations: following the ancient tradition of health advice books, such works were written by men for an implicitly male readership, took man as the archetype of humanity, and possibly regarded the life of men more valuable than that of women.[10] The main roles in which the health of women mattered for the development of the archetypical man were as mothers and wet-nurses. Therefore, it is not surprising that we come across dietary rules for women within

---

[8]   Castiglione, *The Book of the Courtier*, p. 219. See also Ruth Kelso, *Doctrine for the Lady of the Renaissance* (Urbana, 1956), pp. 217–22; José Guidi, 'De l'amour courtois à l'amour sacré: la condition de la femme dans l'oeuvre de B. Castiglione', in José Guidi, Marie-Françoise Piéjus and Adelin-Charles Fiorato (eds), *Images de la femme dans la littérature italienne de la Renaissance: préjugés misogynes et aspirations nouvelles. Castiglione, Piccolomini, Bandello* (Paris, 1980), pp. 9–80, at pp. 71–4; Guttmann, *Women's Sports*, p. 57.

[9]   Georges Vigarello, 'S'exercer, jouer', in Alain Corbin, Jean-Jacques Courtine and Georges Vigarello (eds), *Histoire du corps* (3 vols, Paris, 2005–2006), vol. 1, *De la Renaissance aux Lumières*, pp. 235–302 (paperback edn, 2011: pp. 247–317). Among Vigarello's main sources are Jean-Baptiste Thiers, *Traité des jeux* (Paris, 1687) and Jean Barbeyrac, *Traité du jeu* (Amsterdam, 1737).

[10]   Andrew Wear, *Knowledge and Practice in English Medicine, 1550–1680* (Cambridge, 2000), pp. 164–5.

the literature on the preservation of health mainly in such roles. A chapter on the regimen of the wet-nurse can already be found in Galen's *De sanitate tuenda* (I.9), which served as a role model for later publications.[11]

During the sixteenth century, the Italian physician Girolamo Mercuriale collected the ancient medical knowledge on the subject of exercise with a focus on gymnastics. Book IV, Chapter 9 of his *De arte gymnastica* deals with exercise for the healthy, and discusses the issue with reference to humoral balance. Those who have a predominantly wet temperament receive great benefit from 'exercise and work' (here not distinguished at all in their implications for health): 'Hence among women, who are generally endowed with a moist temperament, it is those who work and exercise longer and more vigorously who live a healthier and less troubled life'; the argument continues, with reference to Aristotle's *De generatione animalium* (Book IV), on specific issues stating the benefit of hard work for a woman when she gives birth.[12] It was received wisdom of ancient gynaecology that exercise makes for easy labour and well-being of the fetus, while idleness is a cause of difficult labour.

Commenting on this piece of traditional advice, the Veronese physician Bartolomeo Paschetti, in his book on the preservation of the health of the Genoese, published in 1602, discussed the issue of the amount and sort of exercise recommended for women, too. The book belonged to a specific subgenre, that of the consideration of the health for the dwellers of given cities, an early modern development of the late medieval texts concerned with public health in time of plague. Written in dialogue form, the book when discussing the amount of exercise appropriate for each complexion repeats Aristotle's argument that those women who have exercised and eliminated superfluities by avoiding staying at home and lying in bed all the time will live longer and healthier lives, and particularly bear children more lightly and suffer less when giving birth. At this point one of the patricians who takes part in the fictional conversation, Giulio Pallavicino, wittily comments on local social customs, suggesting that Genoese women 'who so willingly, and so often, go out, will therefore enjoy healthy and long lives'.[13] However, the physician plays his role as an expert and an outsider

───────────────

[11]   *A Translation of Galen's Hygiene* (De Sanitate Tuenda), trans. and ed. R.M. Green (Springfield, 1951), pp. 29–30.

[12]   Girolamo Mercuriale, *De arte gymnastica*, ed. C. Pennuto, trans. V. Nutton (Florence, 2008), pp. 490–91: '[Qui ab his humidam corporis temperiem possident, nullum nocumentum, quinimmo egregiam utilitatem] ab exercitationibus et laboribus [perpiciunt]. Atque hac ratione ex mulieribus humida temperie in universum praeditis illae saniorem et minus molestam vitam degunt, quae diutius et valentius elaborant et exercentur.' [Parts in brackets are not quoted in the text.]

[13]   Bartolomeo Paschetti, *Del conservare la sanità, et del vivere de' genovesi* (Genoa, 1602), pp. 171–2: 'Dunque –soggionse il Pallavicino – le nostre donne, che così volentieri e così spesso escono di casa goderanno sana e lunga vita?' Paschetti was a pupil of Mercuriale.

by commenting that this would be the case, should women not use sedan chairs all the time. He goes on with a historical digression recalling how this practice was first introduced into Genoa, by taking the place of horse riding and other previous forms of transport between the city and its immediate surroundings; alas, nowadays it has become a status symbol ('per certa vana grandezza'), and every young woman, even if fit, would use it for going around town, to church, or to visit friends and relations, thus ending up not exercising at all.[14]

Perhaps the comment that this was not really exercise was slightly harsh: being carried on a sedan chair, coach or boat, rather than moving by oneself, exemplified an existing medical notion, that of *agitatio* or passive exercise – a moderate form of motion which was regarded as befitting women, children and the elderly. The salutary effects of rocking movements are praised within Plato's *Laws* (VII, 389 Bff.) and appear to be favoured by at least part of the ancient medical tradition (among others, Asclepiades and his followers). In the context of a work such as Soranus of Ephesus' *Gynaecology*, for instance, their recommendation is linked to a mechanistic understanding of the body and of its functioning. Soranus recommended passive exercise at particular stages, like the eighth month of pregnancy, or, combined with other forms of motion, in given conditions, such as *pica*, a pathological craving by the expectant mother for substances unfit for food. For the wet-nurse, he endorsed it together with more active forms of exercise (including ball games); the issue, here, is that nourishment needs to be carried to the upper parts of the body, and eventually to the breasts. Needless to say, eventually rocking would be befitting the new-born, too.[15]

Agitatio is again on the agenda in Mercuriale's book. From the second, enlarged edition, it was published with a set of illustrations based on drawings by Pirro Ligorio, an artist and antiquarian who belonged to the Roman circle of Cardinal Farnese. The images are well known and significantly contributed to the success of the book. The one that portrays exercise for women has a young woman hanging on a swing while being gently rocked by two female helpers by the pulling of ropes (see Figure 7.1).[16] The idea is that the scene, together with all the others, represents a practice common in classical antiquity. However, one should bear in mind that Ligorio was an unrepentant forger of Latin inscriptions, and can hardly be trusted as a testimony to the iconography of his past. What he certainly testifies to is the Renaissance imagination of antiquity. In this sense, he was also influential in the diffusion of pictorial models, for instance as an adviser

---

[14]   Paschetti, *Del conservare la sanità*, pp. 171–2.

[15]   *Soranus' Gynecology*, ed. and trans. O. Temkin (Baltimore and London, 1956, repr. 1991), p. xxxiv and *passim*.

[16]   Mercuriale, *De arte gymnastica* (also for the original drawing).

164   L I B E R

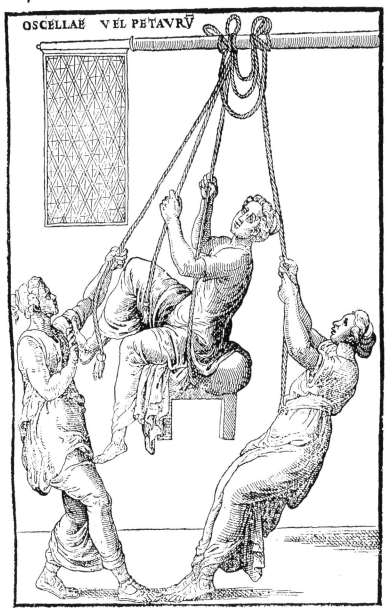

Figure 7.1 Swing or *petaurum*

Source: Hieronymus Mercurialis, *De arte gymnastica libri sex* (Venice, 1587), p. 164. By permission of the Ministry of Cultural Heritage and Activities and Tourism – Marciana National Library.

to the designing of the fresco decoration on the subject of games in the guest apartment of the Este Castle in Ferrara.[17]

Within the context of a conceptualization of the body as dominated by fluids, intensive exercise was considered as a cause of their absorption with detrimental effects on menstruation, and consequently on fertility and general health: a regularly mentioned example for this problem was the ballerina as evoked by the Portuguese physician Rodrigo de Fonseca, professor of medicine at Pisa at the beginning of the seventeenth century.[18] The awareness that violent exercise could also be responsible for problems regarding pregnancy is already explicit in the ancient text of Soranus, who listed energetic leaping and carrying heavy weights as short cuts for miscarriage.[19]

While Paschetti, in his reprimand against sedan chairs, seemed nostalgic of times in which women travelled by riding properly, there are contemporary medical authors who testify that the practice had not been abandoned, or quite the contrary that it was just being established. For example, Giulio Alessandrini, physician to three Holy Roman Emperors, discusses in the chapter *de exercitatione ab extrinseco* (that is, precisely, being carried rather than moving on one's own right and energy) of his books *de sanitate tuenda* the various types of horse riding, concluding that 'nowadays, women happily make use of horses (something I do not recall we read of the ancient, unless perhaps we want to consider the Amazons) for accomplishing often long journeys, many in a manly way also in running, jumping and hunting'.[20] The context seems to suggest that it is the horses – rather than the women themselves – that run and jump; even so, the implication is that of a vigorous exercise, and the historical comparison records a development towards a widening of the practice across the gender barrier.

As well as for the swing, Mercuriale also mentioned women – together with children – as a category for which frequent dancing is documented in antiquity; he advises, however, that it may be harmful in pregnancy. Dance played a dominant part in the early modern discourse on exercise, and particularly whenever a

---

[17]   Arcangeli, *Recreation in the Renaissance*, pp. 25–9.

[18]   Rodericus a Fonseca, *De tuenda valetudine et producenda vita* (Florence, 1602), p. 87; cf. the Italian version Roderigo Fonseca, *Del conservare la sanità* (Florence, 1603), p. 103. I retraced this reference with the kind help of Massimo Rinaldi.

[19]   *Soranus' Gynecology*, pp. 45–6. Fonseca (*De tuenda valetudine*, p. 12; cf. Fonseca, *Del conservare la sanità*, pp. 13–14) also derived from Hippocrates a variety of lifestyle caveats for the various stages of pregnancy. Generally speaking, women in such condition were encouraged to travel by sedan chairs and boats, not horse carriages.

[20]   Iulius Alexandrinus, *Salubrium sive De sanitate tuenda* (Cologne, 1575), VI, 11, p. 156: 'Itaq; temporis nostri foeminae (quod legisse apud veteres, nisi fortè Amazonas velimus, non memini) equo utuntur feliciter, ad conficienda itinera saepe magna, multaeque viriliter in cursu etiam, in saltu, in venatione.'

specific consideration was given to women. The latter point is far from obvious if one takes into account that, as a social practice, it was usually promiscuous, not gender-specific. However, it tended to be regarded as the pastime characteristic of women, in the same way in which hunting was for men.[21] Its discussion is ubiquitous. In 1669 Michel Bicaise, a Provençal physician who examined dance at length, linked its benefit to humoral explanation: the expulsion of superfluous fluids is particularly useful for the health of women and dance, by shaking the whole body, stimulates transpiration.[22]

It should be mentioned here that Renaissance dancing developed a textual tradition of its own. The fifteenth-century treatise by Guglielmo Ebreo da Pesaro *On the Practice or Art of Dancing* – one which is preserved in several variants and manuscripts – contains a specific chapter of 'rules for women'. However detailed in terms of posture, gesture and aesthetics, they tend to reinforce the moral discourse on conduct rather than allowing us a glance over the dancing body: 'It behoves the young and virtuous woman who delights in understanding this discipline and art, to behave and conduct herself with far more discretion and modesty than the man ... Her bearing should have the proper measure and an airy modesty, and her manner should be sweet, discreet, and pleasant.' Among the precise instructions one reads that 'she should carry [her head] upright' in a position of which is suggested that it is taught to us by nature itself (in a game of constructing what is culturally supposed to be perceivable as a natural posture and gait). At the end of the dance, she should bow to the man (the text here is providing us with nothing short of an invention of the dancing couple), by turning her 'sweet gaze' ('dolce riguardo') on him.[23] Over a hundred years later, a derivative of this can be found in the rules opening Fabritio Caroso's *Nobiltà di dame*: by the time of this text, though, what we are facing are rules partly preceding dance proper and governing behaviour and attire (including the use of appropriate dancing slippers); on the whole, much etiquette and very little sport in any ordinary or indeed acceptable sense.[24]

Nicolas Abraham de La Framboisière, a physician and counsellor to the King of France Henry IV, authored a different example of a health advice book. His treatise, *Le gouvernement necessaire à chacun pour vivre longuement en santé* was published in Paris in 1600 and devoted a specific book to 'le gouvernement

[21]   For perspectives on women in dance history: Lynn Matluck Brooks (ed.), *Women's Work: Making Dance in Europe before 1800* (Madison, 2007).

[22]   Michel Bicais, *La manière de regler la santé* (Aix, 1669), pp. 280–88.

[23]   Guglielmo Ebreo of Pesaro, *De practica seu arte tripudii. On the Practice or Art of Dancing*, ed. and trans. B. Sparti (Oxford, 1993), pp. 108–11 ('Capitulum regulare mulierum/Rules for women').

[24]   Fabritio Caroso, *Courtly Dance of the Renaissance: A New Translation and Edition of the* Nobiltà di dame *(1600)*, ed. J. Sutton, 2nd edn (New York, 1995).

des dames'.[25] This text, which deals with female health in a more general way, allows us to reassess the aforementioned view on women's exercise. It provides a more comprehensive perspective than the ones dominated by male concerns for reproduction.

The choice of the vernacular as the first language of writing and publication for a medical text, rather than one of secondary translation and divulgation, is made by La Framboisière for the first time for this treatise, and he claims to have made it at the express request of the king. His book is therefore an important testimony that authors of health advice books turned more and more to a lay audience. The specific book on women is dedicated to Catherine de Lorraine, Duchess of Nevers, granddaughter of Henry II and of Catherine de' Medici. The first subject brings to the fore of the author's and expected readership's concerns the issue of the preservation of female beauty. *Beauté* is asserted as depending on both the right proportion of limbs and good bodily temperament. The author does not abstain from recommending lengthy remedies for beautifying women's faces and hair by providing specific instruction on how to preserve the beauty of teeth and whitening them, or giving advice in matter of suitable jewellery, and even colours to wear ('Green, blue and purple delight the sight').[26] However, the core discussion is Hippocratic in terms of recommendations on suitable air, foodstuff, and the remaining traditional components of a regimen. When he arrives at exercise, he suggests a moderate use, and explains its benefits. In his advice on the actual type of exercise, he follows tradition: 'dance is particularly appropriate for them'. Hot baths and a special attention to the hygiene of the head ('because their brains are very humid') complete the passage.[27] The discussion of the passions as traditionally the last category of non-naturals offers La Framboisière the opportunity for a further recommendation that is relevant for a history of leisure and pastimes: while troubling emotions such as anger, fear and sadness should be altogether avoided, he suggests 'that they apply their minds to sing music, play instruments and other pleasant things in order to rejoice and keep themselves always in cheerful humour'.[28] Further, specific consideration of the regimen for pregnant women includes the usual advice to avoid violent agitation of both body and spirit. Once more, a section deals

---

[25]   Nicolas Abraham de La Framboisière, *Le gouvernement necessaire à chacun pour vivre longuement en santé* (Paris, 1600), pp. 201–46. The author was also head physician for the army and professor and dean of the faculty of medicine at the University of Reims.

[26]   La Framboisière, *Le gouvernement*, p. 206: 'Le vert, le bleu et le violet resjouissent la veue.'

[27]   La Framboisière, *Le gouvernement*, p. 208: 'la danse leur est singulièrement propre'; 'd'autant qu'elles ont le cerveau fort humide'.

[28]   La Framboisière, *Le gouvernement*, p. 209: 'qu'elles appliquent leurs esprits à chanter la musique, sonner des instruments, et autres choses plaisantes, à fin de les resjouir, et les tenir tousjours en gaye humeur.'

with the wet-nurse (she needs to take some exercise at mealtimes, for instance, but not afterwards, if her milk is too thick; while she should avoid working and exercising too much, if it tastes sour).

Exercise, Pleasure and Work

With its emphasis on beauty, La Framboisière's book signals intertextual relations with contemporary literature on and/or for women, which range from the editorial output on cosmetics[29] to works on such issues as the *Plaisirs de dames*. A book by that title was published in 1643 by the French writer François de Grenaille; it contained a chapter on *Le bal*, as well as others on *Le bouquet, Le cours, Le miroir, La promenade, La collation* and *Le concert* (dance, the bouquet, the mirror, strolling and the promenade, banqueting and concerts, with the addition, in a subsequent German adaptation, of the topics of *Die Bekleidung, Die Schönheit* and *Der Ehestand* – dress, beauty and marriage).[30] 'Pleasures' is obviously not the same category as sports, and includes much less physical occupations. However, it is precisely this multiplicity of forms by which human activities were conceptualized that it is interesting to investigate, since it sheds light on the contemporary interpretation of the varieties of social practice. Within the spectrum of human activities, pastimes would be deliberately undertaken as pleasurable and their varying physical involvement was perhaps a factor understood and appreciated precisely because it was variable, that is it allowed to alternate more tasking with more relaxing occupations. Hence physicians too, according to their preference for lighter or more dynamic genres of exercise, as well as to the varying complexions of the individuals they considered, had the opportunity to recommend some and warn against others.

That Grenaille dedicated two chapters to promenading is revealing as to the place walking in public had acquired within the spectrum of contemporary forms of sociability. As the aim of the French author was moral instruction, each of his chapters includes an open critique of the social practices it describes and discusses. As a rhetorical device, each chapter is constructed by juxtaposing a series of arguments in its favour and reasons for concern and caution, if not its straightforward rejection. Thus we first learn that promenading could be physically beneficial; and that it would be commendable as both an escape from

---

[29]   In Jean Liébaut's *Trois livres de l'embellissement et ornement du corps humain* (Paris, 1582), pp. 28–9, however, one can only find generic instructions on who should exercise and when, drawn from Hippocrates. Both La Framboisière's and Liébaut's texts are available online in the Bibliothèque numérique Medic@ at http://www.biusante.parisdescartes.fr/histmed/medica.htm.

[30]   François de Grenaille, *Les plaisirs des Dames* (Paris, 1641); François de Grenaille, *Frauenzimmer Belustigung* (Nuremberg, 1657).

the urban environment, and a form of social interaction with some companions. However, Grenaille warns especially women against vanity and challenges to their modesty when promenading; and their very need for any form of relaxation is questioned by him when considering that they are not the gender whose ordinary occupation is tasking and fatiguing.[31]

The fact that the most popular forms of early modern sociability comprised a multiplicity of activities of varying physical impact, and those associated with women in particular tended to be more gentle and require limited effort, ensured that favoured *plaisirs* could be far less dynamic than promenading. When the French historian Emmanuel Rodocanachi published, in 1907, his *La femme italienne à l'époque de la Renaissance*, conversation, parlour games, playing cards and – unfailingly – dance filled the private life section devoted to *divertissements*. Among more dynamic deeds he records, for eighteenth-century Siena, is the detailed description the French traveller Guyot de Merville provided of ladies engaged in snowball fights.[32]

Let us return to the distinction between exercise and physical work, and the comparative assessment of their benefit for health. A classic reference for our period is provided by Robert Burton's recommendations for melancholic women. For a start, it may be worth recalling that the Oxford academic lists leisure and the care for pastimes among the *causes* of the physical and psychological conditions of both aristocratic men and women. Later on in the book, as contradictory as it may seem, Burton recommends within his discussion of remedies for melancholy a moderate use of recreations, well aware that some of them are physical, others spiritual. While study, in his opinion, only befits men, women have their own occupations which range from needlework, spinning, cushion making and the preparation of jams, to gentle gardening, flower arrangement, gossip and prayer. These stereotypical references are of particular interest here for the ambiguity of their status and function. For a start, Burton just records what women do anyway, rather than prescribing any corrections to their behaviour. For him, the somewhat alien female world spans across a range of activities involving a

---

[31] Grenaille, *Les plaisirs des Dames*, pp. 40–57, 161–233; Laurent Turcot, '*Les plaisirs des Dames* (1641) de François de Grenaille: du Cours à la promenade', Études françaises, 47/2 (2011): pp. 165–81 (a study in which Grenaille's double-faced argumentation is not fully accounted for). For context and developments Laurent Turcot, *Le promeneur à Paris au XVIIIᵉ siècle* (Paris, 2007). From a comparative perspective see also: Laurent Turcot, 'Entre promenades et jardins publics: les loisirs parisiens et londoniens au XVIIIᵉ siècle', *Revue belge de philologie et d'histoire/Belgisch Tijdschrift voor filologie en geschiedenis*, 87 (2009): pp. 645–62; Christophe Loir and Laurent Turcot (eds), *La promenade au tournant des XVIIIᵉ et XIXᵉ siècles (Belgique -France -Angleterre)* (Brussels, 2011).

[32] Emmanuel Rodocanachi, *La femme italienne à l'époque de la Renaissance* (Paris, 1907), pp. 187–211; other entries in the volume's index are of some interest, as for instance *equitation*.

variety of physical effort. The predominant rationale seems to be that women – as well as men, though in their own ways – need to keep themselves occupied, which has more a psychological dimension of keeping their mind engaged and distracted by an activity, rather than necessarily being very dynamic. After the initial tirade against the idleness of the nobility, the distinction between work and leisure in Burton's therapeutics seems to blur: it is irrelevant in respect of the effects human activities have on their performers.[33]

A variation on the consideration of the place given to women within social groups and occupation-related issues of health is offered by the above-mentioned Fonseca, who explicitly regarded the lives of better-off women as comparable to those of servants. Since they are stuck at home most of the time, women do not get the chance to exercise properly. However, they manage some beneficial physical effort by sweeping, adorning their houses, bread making, washing, strolling and walking up the stairs. They should not, in his opinion, engage excessively in sewing and spinning, as such activities are not helpful for their sight and general health. Weaving has the advantage of requiring movement from all body limbs; however, it does not make women change location, and from that respect hardly deserves the label of exercise.[34]

In his 1553 *Libro del ejercicio corporal y de sus provechos*, the Andalusian physician Cristóbal Méndez addressed the issue of women, exercise and work in greater detail and in relation to rank and ethnicity. In the chapter 'del exercicio particular de las mugeres', he acknowledged that for many women physical activity was far from lacking from daily life. Those who helped their husbands in their labours, both in the towns and in the countryside, would not need to worry. He even quotes Ptolemy's *Cosmography* when stating that in most of Spain women not only worked as well, but rather that they often did so instead of the men, the latter lazing about (*holgando*) all the time – although Méndez felt the need to correct his source and to repeat that it is matter of collaboration between sexes. Therefore, it was specifically wealthy *señoras* – as the author also experienced during the time he spent in Mexico – who were in need of occupying themselves with *pasatiempos*, here again centred on sewing and on a variety of other tasks in the production of textile artefacts. Since these occupations tend to be sedentary, he recommended long walks to them for the exercise of the legs, suggesting that they could start by strolling the length of their own house. A short, final paragraph also praised the benefits of singing for nuns. That may sound peculiar to the modern ear. Nevertheless, a tradition that went back to the Hippocratic *De diaeta* took sight, hearing, voice and thought into serious

---

    [33]   Robert Burton, *The Anatomy of Melancholy*, eds N.K. Kiessling, T.C. Faulkner and R.L. Blair (6 vols, Oxford, 1989–2000), vol. 2, p. 95.
    [34]   Fonseca, *De tuenda valetudine*, pp. 18–19; see Fonseca, *Del conservare la sanità*, pp. 21–2.

consideration as fields of beneficial exercise. Still, Méndez found nuns could also do with a walk.[35]

Surprising as it may appear, nuns as an occupational category featured significantly in the medical literature of the time. Bernardino Ramazzini, who published the first systematic survey on occupational illnesses (*De morbis artificum*, 1700), was aware of them as a type of patient with their own specifications. For instance, he found their cells wanting fresh air. In the edition of 1713, Ramazzini added a special dissertation on how to preserve the health of nuns, which was advertised on the title-page as one of the new features of the revised publication. This text also had an independent editorial life. Among its characteristics is the choice to discuss preventive rather than curative medical treatments, contrary to all the chapters and occupational categories of Ramazzini's book. This might be why a more prominent role was given to exercise, a topic medical literature tended to include much more frequently within the discourse of health preservation rather than in the actual cure of illnesses. Inactivity is here once more the key source of preoccupation: he regrets that apart from reading and singing, the only more vigorous exercise in which nuns seem to be constantly engaged is bell-ringing, which annoys the neighbourhood. The dissertation on nuns is not the only section of the *De morbis artificum* that deals with women: Ramazzini also discusses midwives, wet-nurses and laundresses, as well as mixed-sex categories such as weavers.[36]

Beyond Theory: Women and Physical Exercise in Practice

Obviously practice did not always follow theory, and even the normative literature testifies of transgressions, thus providing information on women's engagement in lively sports. This is for example the case for a race of women that was traditional in Ferrara, on the occasion of the feast of the local patron saint, St George. Ugo Trotti, a jurist who writes in 1456 one of the earliest juristic treatises *de ludo* (one that remained manuscript), mentions it at the crossroads between law and Christian ethics as a custom whose participants inevitably committed sin.[37]

---

[35] Cristóbal Méndez, *Libro del ejercicio corporal y de sus provechos*, ed. E. Álvarez del Palacio (León, 1996), pp. 315–18 (see also pp. 184–5).

[36] Bernardino Ramazzini, 'The Diseases of Workers', in Bernardino Ramazzini, *Medical and Physiological Works*, eds F. Carnevale, M. Mendini and G. Moriani (2 vols, Verona, 2012), vol. 1, pp. 43–307, esp. pp. 281–7 ('Dissertation: The Care of the Health of Nuns').

[37] Alessandro Arcangeli, 'Danza e spettacolo nel diritto comune', in F. Mosetti Casaretto (ed.), *La scena assente. Realtà e leggenda sul teatro nel Medioevo* (Alessandria, 2006), pp. 175–92, here p. 184; Deanna Shemek, *Ladies Errant: Wayward Women and Social Order in Early Modern Italy* (Durham, NC and London, 1998), pp. 17–44.

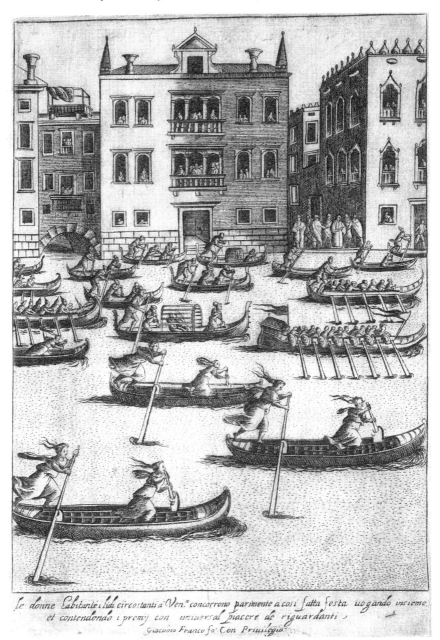

le donne l'abitante i lidi circostanti a Ven.ª concorrono parimente a così fatta festa uogando insieme et contendendo : premij con uniuersal piacere de riguardanti .

Giacomo Franco fo Con Priuilegio

Figure 7.2 Women from the Venetian area compete in a festive rowing contest

Source: Girolamo Franco, *Habiti d'huomeni et donne venetiane* (Venice, 1610), fol. 25r.

Races and festivals point in a direction in which we do find information about women occasionally (locally and/or periodically) engaged in more vigorous physical activity than was usually considered fit for them. Whether we regard such customs and episodes as a challenge to social norms is to some extent a matter of choice. However, one should never forget that a carnivalesque reversal of convention can barely be regarded as a threat to the status quo unless contextual information suggests that it was performed with subversive intentions (or unless the modern interpreter applies freely the category of subversion regardless the historical agents' perception). Once again, the festival setting places these activities within a context that is clearly distinguishable from the subsequent developments of sport in terms of social meaning if not in terms of actual patterns of movement and personal interaction; gender relationships, together with the rest of social distinctions, worked in a particular way in the world of the festival.

For instance, numerous regattas in which women competed are recorded in Venice between the late fifteenth and the late eighteenth century. They were organized on a variety of occasions including the welcoming of important visitors, and saw in particular the participation of working women from the neighbouring beaches, used to rowing when transporting goods. (see Fig. 7.2) The comments left in historical records seem to suggest that the entertaining power of the spectacle contained an element of mockery or the exotic – not to mention the voyeurism we have already encountered in Castiglione's misogynistic characters.[38] Rules concerning the participation of women in public contests could vary within comparatively short distance. While, for instance, a male-only audience was considered for the *gioco del pallone* in Verona, women could take actively part in the game in eighteenth-century Venice.[39] Within the preface (*proemio*) to his *Trattato del giuoco della palla* (1555), the Italian writer Antonio Scaino mentioned women practising a variety of ball games from a mythical past (Homer) to a more concrete present (the Italian cities of Udine and Ferrara). One feels nevertheless that, within an introductory text that is addressing his dedicatee and plays the rhetorical game of testifying the antiquity and broad interest of the practice, the author's logic is to show how even the less predictable subjects have enjoyed it.[40]

---

[38] Luigi Roffaré, *La Repubblica di Venezia e lo sport* (Venice, 1931), pp. 214–31; 2nd edn as *Lo sport a Venezia* [Venice, 1999], pp. 110–18. Cf. Bianca Tamassia Mazzarotto, *Le feste veneziane* (Florence, 1961), pp. 57–60; Wolfgang Behringer, *Kulturgeschichte des Sports* (Munich, 2012), pp. 170–71.

[39] Tamassia Mazzarotto, *Le feste veneziane*, p. 151.

[40] Antonio Scaino, *Trattato del giuoco della palla*, ed. G. Nonni (Urbino, 2000), pp. 13–14.

The working class, in general, is considered to have been characterized by a distinctive physical experience in which women were not totally excluded. Summarizing the work of other sport historians, Neil Tranter wrote:

> All historians are agreed that the Victorian and Edwardian 'revolution' in sport was predominantly a male phenomenon in which females, and working-class females especially, had relatively little part. Fragmentary though it is, there is sufficient evidence to suggest that in earlier ages working-class women were more frequent participants in sport. At various times between the seventeenth and early nineteenth centuries they were regularly recorded among the crowds at horseraces, cricket matches, rowing and pedestrian events and at animal blood sports like bull-baiting and combat sports like prize-fighting, wrestling, sword-fighting and cudgelling. In the sports of football, rowing, cricket and, occasionally, prize-fighting some even participated actively. Because of the scattered and imprecise nature of the evidence, the extent of this participation cannot be quantified exactly. But the general assumption is that it was more extensive than it was to be in Victorian and Edwardian times.[41]

Equally interesting is what we can see at the opposite end of the social spectrum. It has convincingly been observed by Allen Guttmann among others that class could often operate as a more powerful distinction than gender in defining who should and who should not practise specific leisure activities. Thus, we can find documentation of elite women participating in pastimes which were denied to folks of lower rank.[42] For example, we do find women belonging to the ruling classes engaged in hunting.[43]

However, for late eighteenth-century Anglo-American middle- and upper-rank women a shift can be recognized from an earlier higher degree of women's participation into male sporting life to a privatization of women's physical activity, confined within ideals of domesticity and concerns for health, while the public sphere was left as an arena for men only; an observation that has perhaps a validity beyond those regional and cultural borders (and not inconsistent with what we have just registered for the British working classes).[44]

---

[41] Neil Tranter, *Sport, Economy and Society in Britain 1750–1914* (Cambridge, 1998), p. 78.

[42] Guttmann, *Women's Sports*, p. 81 (with reference to field sports).

[43] Vigarello, 'S'exercer, jouer', p. 276 (paperback edn: pp. 290–91).

[44] Nancy L. Struna, '"Good Wives" and "Gardeners", "Spinners and Fearless Riders": Middle- and Upper-Rank Women in the Early American Sporting Culture', in James A. Mangan and Roberta J. Park (eds), *From 'Fair Sex' to Feminism: Sport and the Socialization of Women in the Industrial and Post-Industrial Eras* (London, 1987), pp. 235–55. Needless to say, even during colonial times women tended to take part in public sport events as observers rather than contestants. Anyway, 'the physicality of women was not an item for

One strand of the medical discourse was also concerned with the physical development of children. Considering that exercise was not often the subject of extensive treatment; even less interest was taken in the specific physical needs of girls. An exception to this rule is represented by a chapter in the book of the Parisian physician Desessartz from the middle of the eighteenth century. His point of departure is the consideration – fairly unusual within his profession – that the peculiarity of female bodies as opposed to male ones derives not wholly from nature; rather it is partly the result of nurture, as demonstrated by the gap distancing 'modern' upper-class women from both their ancient and their socially inferior counterparts in diet and physical activity alike. The delicateness of the women of rank is exhibited as a status symbol: idleness is responsible for their weakness. Women should try to correct such tendencies by periodically resorting to promenading, moderate dancing, singing and horse riding; within a reference to summer rustication, Desessartz also expressly mentions fishing and hunting.[45] While this awareness had not produced a systematic physical education for girls during the early modern period, this consideration would enter the agenda by the following century. Despite the pleas for a balanced development of body and mind repeatedly subscribed by humanist educationists, the programme of physical education for boys as conceived by Richard Mulcaster in Elizabethan London had to wait some time to find its female counterpart.[46]

---

public consumption; indeed, no evidence indicates that women displayed the physical aggressiveness inherent in public sporting contests' (Struna, 'Good Wives', p. 237).

[45] Jean-Charles Desessartz, *Traité de l'éducation corporelle des enfants en bas age* (Paris, 1760), pp. 406–19; available online in the Bibliothèque numerique Medic@. Rousseau was familiar with this treatise and the *Émile* was published only two years later.

[46] The above-mentioned Bibliothèque numerique Medic@ includes the title Napoléon Laisné, *Gymnastique des demoiselles à l'usage des Écoles normales, des lycées et collèges de jeunes filles, des pensions et des écoles*, wrongly dated 'Paris, circa 1660' though clearly a nineteenth-century publication. On humanism: Eleanor B. English, 'Women and Sport during the Renaissance', in Jan Borms, Marcel Hebbelink and Antonio Venerando (eds), *Women and Sport* (Basel, 1981), pp. 24–30.

Chapter 8

Healthy, 'Decorous' and Pleasant Exercise: Competing Models and the Practices of the Italian Nobility (Sixteenth to Seventeenth Centuries)[1]

Sandra Cavallo and Tessa Storey

Italy played a key role in the development of the new physical arts that became fashionable in the early modern period such as fencing, dancing, dressage and various types of ball games. Their importance can be measured both through the number of treatises published on these subjects and the proliferation of teachers and schools offering a training in these sports.[2]

From the late fifteenth century Italy also witnessed an extraordinary proliferation of medical literature in the vernacular, directed to a wide audience, which disseminated advice on how to keep healthy. The impact of physical activities on health was a central theme in these texts, and it also appeared in instruction manuals devoted to explaining the new sports.[3] Scaino, for example, in his treatise on ball games, includes a full section on the humoural rationale behind physical activity.[4] His discussion of the complexions and ages most suited to certain types of exercise and the seasons in which these should be practised is also justified entirely in medical terms.[5] However, health was not the only consideration when it came to determining what exercises were appropriate to whom. Even in Scaino, certain activities were associated with social status, occupation and specific age groups for complex reasons that this chapter is going

---

[1]   In this study we present new textual and archival material to develop some of the ideas discussed in our *Healthy Living in Late Renaissance Italy* (Oxford, 2013), and extend the analysis to the practice of hunting which was not considered in the book.

[2]   Claudio Bascetta (ed.), *Sport e giochi, trattati e scritti dal XV al XVIII secolo* (Milan, 1978), esp. pp. 113–20, 196–8, 201.

[3]   We trace the development of this literature (regimens) and its characteristics in our *Healthy Living*, chapter 1.

[4]   Antonio Scaino, *Trattato del gioco della palla diviso in tre parti* (Venice, 1555), pp. 296–7.

[5]   Scaino, *Trattato del gioco*, pp. 305–7.

to untangle.[6] During the sixteenth century a certain degree of tension is visible therefore between traditional medical principles and the new views of the body that developed in courtly and urban environments, and later in clerical thought. Moreover, these competing discourses also collided with the revival of traditional ideas of noble virtue which, for example, manifested itself in hunting practices. Drawing on preventive medical literature and on various types of didactic text, as well as on the lay accounts available in contemporary correspondence, the following pages will examine these different understandings of exercise and how these divisions were addressed and eventually reconciled.

Medical Advice and Decorous Exercise

The importance of exercise in sixteenth- and seventeenth-century medical accounts was explained by its relation to the sequence of changes in the body which were prompted by some degree of movement. Movement was understood to increase the body's natural or inner heat on which all health and indeed life depended. Galenic medicine envisaged this in terms of an inner flame or fire which, burning constantly, needed to be provided with fuel (food and drink) and to be kept burning at an optimal temperature for that particular individual. Equally important was the maintenance of the body's so-called 'radical' or innate humidity, which was also facilitated by movement and ideally one should do sufficient exercise to gently distribute heat and nourishing, humidifying blood around the body. The ultimate aim of much of the health advice in regimens was to explain to the reader how to prolong youth and defer the ageing process by maintaining the body's natural heat and preserving its natural inner humidity for as long as possible, since ageing, and ultimately death, were associated with the gradual loss of both these qualities, as the body got colder and drier.[7]

Exercise conferred many more benefits than this, however. By increasing one's inner heat the digestive system, envisaged in terms of a stove, was able to speed up the process known as 'concoction' and process the resulting waste products more efficiently. Several of the so-called 'excrements' which it produced were visible, such as semen, excrement expelled via the intestines, sweat expelled through the pores, and the hair and nails which were themselves considered to be waste products pushed out of the body. Other residues were invisible: one was a smoke excreted from the heart and exhaled in the breath, another was a subtle vapour

---

  6   Scaino, *Trattato del gioco*, p. 314.

  7   On this association see for example Lampridio Anguillara, *Vaticinio et avertimenti per conservare la sanità et prolongar la vita humana* (Ferrara, 1589), p. 9, or Alessandro Trajano Petronio, *Del viver delli Romani, et di conservar la sanità ...* (Rome, 1592), pp. 272, 275.

transpired through the pores.[8] The heat generated by movement facilitated the expulsion of all these excrements in different ways. It 'softens hard things' which might otherwise block the body's exits; but it also, crucially, opened up the pores, allowing sweat and the invisible vapours to escape more easily, even pushing them out. Without this 'encouragement' the pores alone were insufficient for the purpose and these waste products would be retained within the body. The consequences were understood to be varied and often dramatic. For example, they could suffocate the inner flame itself, even extinguishing it.[9]

The re-invigoration of internal heat meant that it was drawn to the surface of the body thereby enabling digested food to travel round the body more swiftly to each limb. However, this heat only moved in those limbs or body parts which had themselves been exercised, so the benefits of movement were extremely localised. This partly explains why one was expected to exercise not just the limbs, but also discrete muscles such as the voice, tongue and even the sense organs. Indeed, this requirement also affected the imagination, the mind and the soul, both in order to rid the brain and heart of 'insensible excrements' and to 'strengthen the virtues'.[10] Some doctors also outlined the kinds of exercises one could do for these parts of the body, such as 'speculating', singing psalms and listening to theology.[11]

Not all exercise was good, however, and fears that overexertion could damage one's health were traced back to antiquity and seem to have increased over the sixteenth century. These concerns were analysed in great detail by Doctor Paschetti in his 1603 regimen. One of the criticisms levelled at exercise was that it made one tired; and fatigue was to be avoided, since it dissipated or destroyed one's 'spirits'.[12] More specifically, and more worryingly, violent exercise was believed to produce too much heat in the body, going beyond merely 'consuming' superfluous humours, but actually drying up its inner humidity, which, as we have already seen, was considered to be the main cause of ageing. A number of other issues could also be raised – such as the dangers of first overheating and then suddenly cooling down – so that overheating provided a sufficient basis for widespread anxiety about the potential drawbacks of overexertion. As part of this anxiety particular mention was made of the dangers of exposing the head to excessive heat, since a balanced temperature of the brain was indispensable

---

[8]   See for example Viviano Viviani, *Trattato del custodire la sanità* (Venice, 1626), pp. 112–16.

[9]   Bartolomeo Paschetti, *Del conservar la sanità* (Genoa, 1602), pp. 148–9.

[10]   Viviani, *Trattato*, 186, and Elici Frediano, *Arca novella di sanità* ... (Lucca, 1656), p. 167.

[11]   For example Castor Durante, *Il tesoro della sanità* (Venice, 1586), p. 20.

[12]   Paschetti, *Del conservar*, pp. 145–8.

to health.[13] As a primarily cold damp organ, the fear was that excessive motion (especially if coupled with exposure to the hot sun) could easily overheat the brain, leading to various disorders: over-rapid movement of the spirits of the intellect led to frenzies. On the other hand if allowed to become too cold, these spirits froze and the intellect was made sluggish.[14]

In view of these concerns, it is interesting to find that in the health advice that a seventeenth-century noblewoman dispensed to family members, there were recurrent recommendations to avoid overheating, especially of the head. This emerges from the letters that Maria Spada, reputed for her medical wisdom, wrote from Rome to her children, husband and uncle while they were spending time in the countryside, whether walking and hunting or supervising agricultural and building work.[15] Even as late as early October exposure to the sun is regarded as harmful and Maria repeatedly warns her sons (aged 37, 29 and 28), on a hunting trip, 'not to get too much sun, which I understand is very hot', nor 'to wear themselves out', nor live a disorderly life, all things that may give rise to the overheating of the blood.[16]

When evaluating different forms of physical activity and making recommendations to readers as to how they should exercise, doctors were clearly faced with an onerous task. No one body was identical to another, but even when grouping people together by body type, constitution (hot, cold, dry or humid), age, gender and even class, there were still endless possible permutations in the advice. When reading the medical literature these subtleties must be taken into consideration, since they explain why very few authors agreed entirely on any single issue. The advice for women, for example, was very specific. They were believed to have fundamentally cold humid bodies and Paschetti explained that since exercise consumed superfluous humidity and rid the body of the excrements such bodies generated, the healthiest women and those who live the longest lives were those who exercised the most and tired themselves the most. He adds that exercise also helped women carry a pregnancy better, and give birth more easily,

---

[13] Bartolomeo Traffichetti, *L'arte di conservar la salute tutta intiera ...* (Pesaro, 1565), p. 55. Moreover, the author warns that excess heat 'liquefies' the mucus and catarrh 'excrements' in the head, making them descend to the chest, whilst also pulling evaporations up from the body, thus creating more catarrh (p. 174).

[14] Traffichetti, *L'arte*, p. 58.

[15] Maria Spada's advice to avoid overheating can, for example, be found in the letter to her uncle, the cardinal Bernardino, Archivio di Stato di Roma [ASR], Fondo Spada Veralli, [FSV], B. 619, 15 September 1642; and in the letter from her husband in which he reassures her that he is not exposing himself to too much sun, ASR, FSV, B. 607, 23 April 1658.

[16] ASR, FSV, B. 410, 5 October 1680: 'Si guardino di non pigliar sole che sento sia molto caldo'; 12 October 1680: 'di non si strapazzare e far disordini e soprattutto non pigliar sole e non dare occasione di scaldarsi il sangue'; see also the letters of 9 October 1680 and 30 October 1680.

thus it was of great importance. Indeed, he attacked those 'lazy women who lie around the house or in bed' and warns that both fat and pregnant women should take exercise every day for their health.[17] Pregnant women were advocated to take temperate daily exercise, whilst avoiding all 'excesses' and violent movements; these included dancing, jumping, running, going in carriages, falling, going up and down stairs quickly. In tracts devoted to midwifery and the health of women specifically there were more detailed instructions – although these were always focussed on women's ability to conceive and carry a foetus safely to term. Thus for example women whose failure to conceive was explained by an overly dry complexion and womb were ordered to 'rest most of the time' – since as we have seen, exercise would only dry them up even more. 'Tiring exercises' might also have created an overheated womb, which could dry up the menses. On the other hand, a woman whose menses had stopped because of excessive cold within the body should certainly 'move about'.[18]

Advice also differed considerably according to age. Children of both sexes were understood as having hot damp bodies, and their 'natural' youthful heat and vigour ensured the continual transport of nourishment around the body, which coupled with fresh air was sufficient for the removal of waste products from the body.[19] This meant that they did not need a great deal of exercise. Nor, according to the physician Petronio, did children in particular need any special exercise forms to be devised for them – the implication being that this was common practice. He notes this in a passage where he criticises those – he is presumably alluding to Mercuriale – who having 'rediscovered' different kinds of antique exercise, expect them to be put into practice 'with great care and diligence and consider the slightest mistake to be ... very damaging'. He believed that children naturally took sufficient exercise, with all the 'running and jumping' that they do as a matter of course.[20] Physicians were also concerned about damaging the limbs through overexertion, and were generally quite cautious about the levels of vigour which the child's body could sustain, so some authors specified the appropriate age at which children could safely start certain physical activities. They recommended starting to ride at around age four, moderate running and ball games at seven, and only allowed a significant increase in exercise at around age 12 to 14. This extended to activities such as jumping, *gioco della palla* (a

---

[17]   Paschetti, *Del conservar*, pp. 171–2: 'Donne otiose, le quali nel letto, o in casa giacciono.'

[18]   Scipione Mercurii, *La commare o raccoglitrice* (Venice, 1713, first edn 1596), pp. 80–82. See similar advice in Rannutio Arragoni, *Della Cura singolare del Parto Settimestre...* (Verona, 1663), pp. 18–20, and Petronio, *Del viver*, pp. 260–63.

[19]   Petronio, *Del viver*, pp. 276, 305.

[20]   Petronio, *Del viver*, p. 276.

precursor of tennis), hunting with a cross-bow and dancing galliards, so long as they were done in moderation.[21]

The male body was finally considered fully robust and assumed to be capable of a range of vigorous exercise only at around age 21, a state which lasted until about age 35 or 40.[22] The kinds of activities recommended for men in their prime included jumping, dancing, discus throwing, fighting, running, *palla corda*, fencing, hunting, chivalric games and swimming.[23] After this men entered 'early old age' when they could carry on any activities they had previously undertaken, so long as they did so more gently, following the Hippocratic notion that it was always best for the body to continue any long-standing habits.[24] Once men reached old age, sometime around 65, they were advised to exercise far more gently and slowly. However, stopping altogether was dangerous, since they had to stimulate their inner heat and keep nourishment circulating round the body to counteract the natural tendency of old bodies to cool down, dry out and become blocked by excrements.[25] At this point the kinds of activities recommended included travelling in a litter, boat or carriage, riding only mules, or having massages.[26]

Despite these passages showing that some doctors permitted relatively energetic exercise for the strong and the fit, there is nonetheless a striking, if gradual, shift in medical advice over the sixteenth century, away from hearty recommendations for strenuous exercise and towards an increasingly cautious approach to the matter, particularly for all those who were young, weak or suffering from almost any form of physical disorder. This meant that even in discussions of exercise for adult males, most physicians reiterated the importance of moderation, and some focussed their attention exclusively on mild forms of physical activity.[27]

Key to this cautious approach was the increasing emphasis being placed on the importance of performing all these activities, whatever they were, with due 'decorum' and in such a way as to convey a gentleman's 'honour'. As Traffichetti

---

[21]   Rodrigo Fonseca, *Del Conservare la sanitá* (Florence, 1603), pp. 16–17. Traffichetti, *L'arte*, pp. 145, 153–4.

[22]   Traffichetti, *L'arte*, pp. 154–5, 156, 161; Fonseca, *Del Conservare*, pp. 15–16; Petronio, *Del viver*, p. 274.

[23]   Traffichetti, *L'arte*, p. 161; Bartolomeo Boldo, *Libro della natura et virtú delle cose, che nutriscono ...* (Venice, 1575), p. 213; Giovanni Bertaldi, *Regole della sanità et della natura de cibi ...* (Turin, 1618), p. 22.

[24]   Petronio, *Del viver*, p. 280; Paschetti, *Del conservar,* pp. 156–7: Fonseca, *Del Conservare*, p. 18. Traffichetti, *L'arte*, p. 165.

[25]   On this see Paschetti, *Del conservar*, p. 168; Petronio, *Del viver*, p. 276.

[26]   Petronio, *Del viver*, pp. 276, 282–3; Fonseca, *Del Conservare*, p. 18; Traffichetti, *L'arte*, p. 25.

[27]   We discuss this process at length in our *Healthy Living*, ch. 5.

put it, a man in the prime of life should seek continually to 'acquire honour through all his actions', and this included when exercising, whether riding, jousting, fighting or otherwise 'exercising the military arts, with that decorum and honesty which are expected of a wise and sensible man so that it will bring him honour'.[28] Thus, this caution about the dangers of exertion and overheating from exercise were inextricably linked to changing concepts and expectations of the 'elite' body. Class was coming to form a separate, additional category according to which the human body could be medically described. This was particularly convenient when it came to explaining why it was dangerous for gentlemen to exert themselves in certain activities, but not for peasants or labourers. Not only was the working man's body inherently more resilient but it was already 'used' to exertion and indeed to give up his hard labour would be as damaging to him as doing it would be to the nobleman.[29]

The increased social differentiation in medical definitions of healthy exercise shows how profoundly medical discourse was affected by the changes that were re-shaping the lifestyles, values and aspirations associated with aristocratic culture. The development of princely and cardinal courts in Northern and Central Italy, combined with the early demilitarisation and urbanisation of elite Italian society and the ennoblement of many elite families during the sixteenth century, had led to an 'anthropological mutation' of these groups. This radically transformed the conduct and gestures associated with gentility, making them more attuned to the requirements of courtly and urban life. As numerous scholars have observed, what changes at this time is the aesthetic of the elite male body. The image articulated by countless conduct manuals for the gentleman produced in the second half of the sixteenth century, is no longer the stocky, robust body of a warrior, but a graceful and slender instrument which effortlessly communicates his social distinction through his command of physical movements and gesture.

The imperative for the gentleman to distinguish himself from the lower ranks dictated not just how he moved, but the kind of exercise he might undertake. Scaino in his treatise on ball games explained which games were particularly suitable for them: These included games of *scanno*, *palla corda* (hitting a small ball over a rope) and, even better, *palla racchetta* (using a racquet) and *palla piccola da pugno* (small hand ball). In contrast, soldiers could play *pallon da pugno* (large hand ball) and *calico* (a rough team ball game), both of which were extremely energetic, fast and even somewhat violent.[30] Indeed various authors

---

[28] Traffichetti, *L'arte*, p. 161: 'L'huomo in tutte la attioni sue si debbe forzare acquistarsi honore ... esercitando l'arte militare, con tutto quel decoro, e honesta che ad un huomo savio, e accorto, si richiede, onde ne possi riportare honore.'

[29] Paschetti, *Del conservar*, p. 173. On this point see the more extended discussion in our *Healthy Living*, pp. 155–7, 163–5.

[30] On *ballon* as violent exercise see Graham David Kew, *Shakespeare's Europe Revisited: The Unpublished 'Itinerary' of Fynes Moryson, (1566 –1630)* (Birmingham, 1995), p. 1624.

have documented the popularity and spread amongst courtiers, gentlemen, students and scholars of these new ball games – which also included *pallamaglio* (pall mall – a precursor of golf) and the mounted version of it (a form of polo), and of *trucco* (billiards) and *pallamaglio a tavola* (ping-pong). We also observe the concomitant appearance across Italy, in the palaces and villas of the elite, as well as academic institutions, of new ball courts and areas for playing pall mall.[31]

These recreational exercises were regarded as suited to the refined body of the gentleman. There was, however, mounting criticism even about how impetuous and excessive some ball games could be. Initially praised for the way they exercised the whole body, and recommended for older children (upwards of age 14) and young men (up to 40), ball games were increasingly condemned for inducing much sweat, being played non-stop for many hours, and sometimes in the heat of the day.[32] It was not only doctors who perceived these dangers. Towards the end of the sixteenth century a separate strand of advice manual appeared, often penned by men of the church, which articulated the new counter-reformation models of decorum by stressing the potentially damaging effects of vigorous exercise. They admonished the naturally vivacious behaviour of children, advising that they should be controlled, their actions regulated and rendered decorous. Bishop Antoniano, writing in 1584, is one of those against even playing small ball: 'it seems to me one moves too much, making respiration heavy, so that I recommend billiards and other similar games in which movement and rest are balanced, so that too much exercise doesn't dissolve their strength and expose them to other health risks.'[33] A few decades later the nobleman and art collector Vincenzo Giustiniani also describes the *giuoco della palla* as dangerously violent and tiring, especially for mature men. He had greatly enjoyed it as a young lad

---

On *calcio* see Pietro di Lorenzo Bini, *Memorie del calcio fiorentino* (Florence, 1688).

[31]   Cees De Bondt, *Royal Tennis in Renaissance Italy* (Turnhout, 2006), p. 131; Paul Grendler, 'Fencing, Playing Ball, and Dancing in Italian Renaissance Universities', in John McClelland and Brian Merrilees (eds), *Sport and Culture in Early Modern Europe, Le sport et la civilisation de l'Europe pré–moderne* (Toronto, 2010), pp. 295–319; Patricia Waddy, *Seventeenth-Century Roman Palaces: Use and the Art of the Plan* (Cambridge, MA and London, 1990), pp. 54–5.

[32]   Scipione Mercurio, *De gli errori popolari d'Italia* (Padua, 1645), p. 451.

[33]   Silvio Antoniano, *Dell'educazione christiana e politica de' figlioli libri tre* [1584] (Turin, 1926), pp. 399–400: 'anche se il gioco della palla é molto commendato dai medici a me sembra che vi si faccia un moto troppo continuato che presto commuove il traspiro, onde quello che si chiama il trucco mi par il migliore, ed altri simili che sono temperati di moto e di quiete, dovendo aver riguardo per il troppo esercizio le forze non si dissolvano e non si incorra in altra guisa in alcun pericolo della salute'.

but on one occasion he played it until he was overheated: he then developed a fever which led to an abscess in the groin, and after that he never played again![34]

Giustiniani's arguments partly echo the views expressed by Mercuriale in his encyclopaedic account of exercise in both classical antiquity and sixteenth-century Italy. Here he praises a group of ball games which bear a strong resemblance to contemporary games of boules, croquet and billiards and require less exertion on the part of the player than *piccola palla/palla corda*.[35] They are altogether more sedate and appropriate for men who have passed their prime, but he recommends them particularly for convalescents, the weak and the old. Other than the gentle movement they provide, they specifically exercise one's sight, one's back and stimulate the belly. Certainly, judging from their appearance in the inventories of noble families, by the mid-seventeenth century playing *trucco* appears to have become a common entertainment in Roman noble residences.[36] Moreover Eugenia Maldachini (née Spada) was caught playing *trucco* with the wet-nurse by her father when he paid an unexpected visit, suggesting it was also common for women to play it.[37]

Yet, even these games have drawbacks, potentially harming the head and kidneys because of the constant bending.[38] In fact, as Mercuriale announced, more popular and better known and more often played was the recently invented game of *pallamaglio*. Played by either pairs or teams of men, it required them to hit a ball long distances with a strong 'stick' which had a mallet shaped head attached. The ball could fly through the air, or roll over the ground, and the first to reach a designated finishing point was the winner. Clearly, this was not quite as gentle as the other games, for it necessitated much walking, and Mercuriale considered that it could 'easily' be classed amongst the 'lengthy, vigorous exercises' since it often resulted in perspiration and heavy breathing. He noted also that the legs, arms and back specifically were all strengthened, whilst the whole body benefited from all the virtues of walking.[39]

To these qualities Vincenzo Giustiniani added the intellectual benefits of the game, which, combined with certain physical practicalities, made it 'absolutely

---

[34]   Vincenzo Giustiniani, 'Discorso sopra il giuoco del pallamaglio' [1626], in Bascetta, *Sport e giochi*, p. 329.

[35]   Mercuriale discusses them in relation to a game known as 'trochus' in antiquity which seems to be a hoop and stick game: Girolamo Mercuriale, *De arte gymnastica*, trans. Vivian Nutton (Florence, 2008), p. 379, 381.

[36]   See the inventories of Cardinal Bernardino Spada: ASR, Notai del Tribunale del AC, vol. 5933, c.727; the goods in the Giustiniani villa outside Rome, in Silvia Danesi Squarzina, *La collezione Giustiniani* (Turin, 2003), vol. I, p. 200.

[37]   ASR, FSV, B. 410, 13 April 1658.

[38]   Mercuriale, *De arte*, pp. 649, 653.

[39]   Mercuriale, *De arte*, p. 653.

suited for gentlemen'.[40] He pointed out for example that boules, billiards and croquet required the player to remain more or less fixed on the spot with his eyes cast downwards. He also had to bend down and pick up the ball, neither of which were acts proper to the demeanour of gentlemen. Moreover, it was particularly distasteful that the player might thereby 'dirty his hands', whereas *pallamaglio* 'is played with clean hands'. This was because one end of the mallet was shaped with a depression which could be used to scoop up the ball whilst in a standing position. Being allowed a certain freedom of movement also appears to have counted a great deal in matters of status. He stresses that the players of *pallamaglio* could vary the type of strokes, change balls, even agree on different objectives for the game. They were allowed to walk about as they wished whilst playing, and 'in between one shot and another one is given great liberty not only to converse and conduct business, but to joke and even to break into a run if they so desire'.[41]

Another characteristic of the game which contributed to make it especially suited to gentlemen was the exercise it afforded the intellectual faculties and soul, thereby providing them with 'delight and recreation'. Indeed, what made *pallamaglio* distinctive was the fact that it relied neither just on luck, nor on pure practice and repetition as other games did, but required *industria*, judgement and thought in the choice of clubs, balls and strokes appropriate for the player's abilities and the conditions during the game.[42]

Various considerations therefore, alongside health, determined the appeal of specific forms of exercise. For 'lovers of the muses, patricians, and scholars', their attraction lay both in their moderation and the appropriately 'genteel' manner in which they were played. Moreover, expectations of restraint and composure increased with age as well as with social standing. As doctor Lennio explained, 'there are various kinds of exercise, none of which is appropriate or decorous for every age'.[43]

[40]   Giustiniani, 'Discorso', p. 329: 'È proprio da gentiluomini.'

[41]   Giustiniani, 'Discorso', pp. 329–30: 'Non tiene collegata la persona sempre in un luogo, ma dà libertà grande non solo di discorrere e negoziare ma di burlare e anche di ar una carriera quando vi piace, poi che da tempo dà una botta all'altra.'

[42]   Giustiniani, 'Discorso', p. 330.

[43]   Levinio Lemnio, *Della complessione del corpo humano libri tre* (Venice, 1564), p. 36: 'Io voglio che siano ammoniti tutti e specialmente gli amici delle muse, gli uomini patrici e quelli che continuamente sono applicati alle lettere', 'ma essendo vari generi di esercitazioni, nè ciascuno ne sia atto o decoro ad ogni età ciascuno riconoschi sè stesso'.

Walking and Pleasant Exercise

Given these premises it comes as no surprise to see, by the end of the sixteenth century, a clear consensus emerging amongst physicians that walking was the safest and most laudable physical activity, since it neither involved sweating or overheating. Clerical writers could also find no fault with this view. In their regimens doctors discussed how walking could be varied in terms of speed, direction, duration and place (whether going up or down hill for example, or just pottering about the house), in order to adapt it to all sorts of constitutional needs. By now moreover, the idea that regular exercise was necessary to health had penetrated all sorts of advice literature and walking could be performed almost daily. At the turn of the century for example the clerical author of a conduct book for young pupils recommends that they exercise twice a day. Although permitted to play small ball and even sometimes to go riding for the benefit it confers on the stomach, the emphasis is on gentle exercise, mainly walking in lovely green meadows.[44] A few years later Lombardelli's detailed tract for university students shows how they could fit their exercise into their daily routine. They were advised to walk 150 steps before lunch, or read aloud from Petrarch in the event of bad weather. They should then spend up to an hour playing ball or *pioli* in the courtyard after the first lessons and take another hour of exercise (by which he seems to imply walking) in the evening. In the summer they should also walk slowly after dinner for half an hour. On Sundays the routine is varied, and they may take some 'moderate exercise' by walking to and from holy places, so as to listen to different preachers.[45]

Meanwhile walking was also being facilitated in the public and the private sphere. In Rome the principal streets were increasingly being cobbled and planted on both sides with trees which would provide shade so as to make walking easier and safer.[46] Palaces and villas incorporated porticoes into their designs, and long galleries could be lined with citrus trees in vases, 'so wide that more than four people can stroll comfortably up and down' when the weather did not permit exercise outdoors.[47] Moreover, both the formal gardens and wilder parkland

---

[44] Bartolomeo Meduna, *Lo scolare …* (Venezia, 1588), p. 281.

[45] Orazio Lombardelli, *Il Giovane Studente* (Venice, 1594), pp. 23–4, 29, 31–2, 39.

[46] On paving see Jean Delumeau, *Vita Economica e sociale di Roma nel Cinquecento* (Florence, 1979), p. 69. On trees see Richard Krautheimer, 'Roma verde nel Seicento', in *Studi in onore di Giulio Carlo Argan II* (Rome, 1984), pp. 71–82.

[47] See Maria Spada's description of the gallery in a villa near Viterbo she visited: ASR, FSV, B. 618, 26 November 1678: '[vi é] la galleria larga, e longa, dove ripongono due filari per parte di vasi grandissimi d'agrumi e resto in mezzo campo, capace da poter passeggiare più di quattro persone commodamente. Vi sono fenestre da tutti dui i lati, et un gran finestrone a capo.'

surrounding country villas were equipped with wide tree-lined avenues which provided ample space for walks or even gentle carriage rides for the weak.

To judge from the letters exchanged between members of the noble Spada family who resided in and around Rome, Viterbo and Castelviscardo in the mid-seventeenth century, walking had become the prime form of physical activity performed by (or at least encouraged for) gentlefolk of all ages. Hence Eugenia Spada proudly describes her vivacious three-year-old son Alessandro as 'Our delight; he dances and sings as much as he can, makes us all laugh and it is God's grace that he is very well, has good colour in his cheeks and eats well, but he also takes exercise as he always wants to go walking about outside'.[48] Eugenia's brother, Bernardino, aged 23, takes walks every evening while visiting her in Viterbo[49] and her father Orazio who manages the family estate in Castelviscardo finds having to walk 'for a good part of the day' rejuvenating.[50] Moreover walking was one activity which women could enjoy as well as men, particularly when they were not limited by the severe restrictions on movement imposed upon them during pregnancy, and mature gentlewomen enthusiastically embraced it. Eugenia Spada, aged 46, congratulates herself on taking daily walks at her husband's estate in Giove, even in winter, and in one letter she boasts how she has become a more expert walker, having learned how to walk 'over the cobblestones and through mud' so that she would 'no longer resent walking in Rome, as she used to'.[51] Orazio Spada reminds his wife Maria that she should 'do a bit of exercise' every day at their villa in Tivoli, in the morning and the evening 'if she wants to feel the benefits of the air';[52] but she generally did not need reminding, since even much later in life, when she was in her sixties, she took her doctor's instructions to go out every day 'to take some air and do a bit of exercise' very seriously, even though she had recently fallen and her legs were swollen and sore.[53]

Indeed, it was especially the frequent and often long stays at the family villa which provided the ideal scenario for exercise that stimulated the mind and spirits as well as the body. Here a range of physical activities was an aspect of the recreational programme of *villeggiatura*, which was inextricably linked with the

---

[48]   ASR, FSV, B. 624, 26 October 1672: 'Alessandro é il nostro spasso, che balla e canta quanto puó e fa ridere tutti e per grazia di Dio sta benissimo, é di bon colore e mangia bene ma fa anco esercizio, che sempre vorrebbe andar fuori a piedi'; see also 1 September 1673.

[49]   ASR, FSV, B. 1115, 7 September 1662.

[50]   ASR, FSV B. 607, no date but May 1658: 'Per buona parte del giorno.'

[51]   ASR, FSV, B. 623, 19 December 1685: 'E adesso ho imparato a camminare per li selci e per la fanga che non mi daria piú fastidio il caminare per Roma, come dicevo una volta.'

[52]   ASR, FSV, 24 July 1661: '... ma se non fa un po' di esercizio la mattina e la sera VS non sentirá il beneficio di questa aria'; see also 15 March 1659.

[53]   ASR, FSV, B. 410, 30 October 1680: 'procuro di andare a pigliar aria e fare un poco di esercitio [...] ogni giorno'; for another example ASR, FSV, B. 618, 28 September 1678.

enjoyment of beautiful views, inhaling pure air, enjoying the pleasant company of visitors and the light-hearted atmosphere of villa life. It was a total experience which was encapsulated by the recurrent expression *'godersi la campagna'*, 'enjoying the countryside'. As we move into the seventeenth century we also notice that walking during the *villeggiatura* increasingly takes place in closer contact with nature as people leave their formal gardens for the open countryside, to avail themselves of the long tree-lined avenues (*viali*) that punctuate the rural landscape, or go into the woods where they delight in picking mushrooms or trapping birds – a leisurely form of hunting which we will discuss below.[54] As stressed by medical and lay authors alike, to be beneficial exercise was meant to be pleasurable and environmental factors were crucial in making it so.

Hunting

Given that Mercuriale was an ardent advocate of walking and very cautious about the merits of violent exercise, it comes as some surprise that he considered hunting, which was generally regarded as vigorous exercise, to be an ideal form of exercise. Indeed, it was not often mentioned in regimens. Benzi, writing in the late fifteenth century, had observed that if one has the opportunity to hunt, one must take care not to tire oneself or overdo it. In the following century it is discussed in only two other regimens, both published after the 1560s, where it is included as a 'vigorous' sport for the healthy male in the prime of life.[55] So Mercuriale's eagerness was quite a novelty at the time, presumably thanks to Galen's enthusiastic support for it. According to Mercuriale one reason for its excellence were the many different kinds of exercise it gave the entire body, involving running, jumping, throwing and riding, exercising the voice through shouting and exercising the sight by looking for the quarry. Chief amongst its benefits was the fact – also stressed by Galen – that it combined 'mental and physical pleasure' without exhausting the body. Both these advantages bring us back to those qualities which made certain exercise forms more appropriate for the gentleman.[56]

Hunting was already considered as the ideal exercise for young men by fifteenth-century humanists. They were basing themselves on Greek sources which by the 1440s had started to appear in Latin.[57] Particularly influential were the treatises attributed to Xenophon, which included sections on the health

---

[54]   See for example ASR, FSV, B. 624, 21 September 1674; B. 410, 2 October 1680, 19 October 1680.

[55]   Boldo, *Libro della natura*, p. 213; Traffichetti, *L'arte*, p. 110.

[56]   Mercuriale, *De arte*, pp. 421, 423.

[57]   Giuliano Innamorati, *Arte della Caccia: Testi di Falconeria, Uccellagione e Altre Cacce* (Milan, 1965), p. xxiii.

benefits of this practice while stressing its utility for preparing youths for the rigours of war: it gets them used to rising early, missing sleep, to being tired, hot, cold and hungry. These themes received new impetus in the following two centuries, when the declining identity of the noble-warrior and the growing uncertainty surrounding the acquisition of nobility stimulated a massive debate on what constitutes noble behaviour. In these texts hunting was a prominent feature.[58] In a period in which the Italian nobleman was less and less likely to actually ride off to fight in wars, hunting offered him the opportunity to exercise the traditional noble virtues and achieve honour.

The renewed interest in this practice inevitably affected medical writers. In 1544 the physician Michelangelo Biondo dedicates a work to hunting and in 1626 Doctor Bertaldi praises the activity in the comments he interpolates into a much older regimen.[59] However, those factors which made it ideal for future soldiers were at the same time the reasons why hunting was seen as potentially damaging! Even Mercuriale pointed out that it generally required a complete overturning of one's daily regimen, forcing one to exercise directly after eating, to skip meals completely, to miss sleep in order to rise very early and so on, all of which was definitely undesirable for those who were not in excellent health. Moreover, it was so vigorous that one risked serious damage to the head or breaking veins in the chest and, of course, falling off the horse. These contradictions penetrate a number of other texts: it is 'wonderful exercise', particularly for kings and princes, notes one late seventeenth-century author, but he warns, it should not be overdone, since 'too much exercise damages the body'.[60]

So in spite of the renewed interest in hunting, we cannot assume that the kind of arduous hunting on horseback which was envisaged by these texts was actually the norm for all young nobles. Instead, hunting appears to have become a 'node' around which different ideals of masculinity clustered and conflicted.

The cultural tensions embedded in the topic emerge clearly from the dialogue on hunting published in 1616 by Simoncelli, a nobleman who held several military offices under the Medici.[61] Simoncelli's key argument is indeed that hunting is a 'noble' and virtuous sport, and he is clearly seeking to defend

---

[58]   On tracts specifically in praise of hunting see Giovanni Barberi-Squarotti, *Selvaggia Dilettanza. La Caccia nella letteratura Italiana dalle Origini a Marino* (Venice, 2000).

[59]   Michelangelo Biondo, *De canibus et venatione* (Rome, 1544); Bertaldi, *Regole*, p. 22; see also above fn. 54.

[60]   Gregorio Leti, *La lode Della Caccia ...* (Geneva, 1664), pp. 18–19: 'Gran'esercitio in vero è la caccia', but 'il troppo esercitio danneggia tutto il corpo'.

[61]   Baldovino di Monte Simoncelli, 'Il Simoncello: o Vero della Caccia. Dialogo di Baldovino di Monte Simoncelli', in Giuliano Innamorati (ed.), *Arte della Caccia: Testi di Faconeria, Uccellagione e Altre Cacce* (Florence, 1616 (original edn); 2 vols, Milan, 1965). On Simoncelli, born 1570, see pp. 391–2.

it against a 'few' city dwellers who, he says, disdain it for 'political' reasons.[62] By this he was presumably referring to the urban elites, occupied with government and political office, who would have been adherents of the counter-reformation model of decorous and restrained masculinity. They had distanced themselves from a more rustic ideal of masculinity, dependent on strength, vigour and fearlessness, as exemplified in the courageous hunting of wild beasts. The main interlocutor is an 80-year-old man, Sig. Belisario, who despite his great age still hunts regularly. He is clearly intended to be a living example of the health benefits of the practice, which, he notes, is taken up by 'many people who have no intention of ever fighting' but practice it for its secondary aim of 'recreating the soul and for the health of the body'.[63] We see here also how notions of 'recreation' and pleasure were deployed in support of hunting as an activity which was particularly appropriate for the elite male. By improving the health of the intellectual faculties, located in the noblest region of the body, the sport was seen as being inherently more suitable for the nobility.[64]

Also, as part of this clash of cultural ideals, the long-standing battle between '*lettere ed armi*' (scholarship and military life) makes an appearance. The dialogue is constructed around a conversation between Belisario and two young noblemen from the city, who were students at a college and had never hunted. Anxious not to characterise himself as an uncivilised countryman, he praises the honourable study of literature, but ironically concedes that these 'soft and delicate' noble youths may have been too busy 'sweating' over their studies to appreciate the pleasures of hunting.[65] He then however attacks the inadequate riding skills of those youths who try to hunt, or indeed, go to war, despite being familiar only with the elegant equestrianism and dressage skills which had become so popular at the time.[66]

Indeed, the Spada-Veralli letters seem to endorse this sense that noblemen were becoming less skilled as horsemen. Although as youths they participated in ritualised chivalric tournaments they rarely rode in everyday life and by the 1630s people of this social standing travelled by coach, not on horseback. While at the turn of the century male members of the Spada-Veralli family (Paolo Spada and Giovan Battista Veralli) still rode, and carriages or coaches (*cocchi* or

---

[62]   See also Simoncelli, 'Il Simoncello', p. xxix on Simoncelli's as a rather antiquated text harking back to these traditional themes whilst eminently practical in the technical sections.

[63]   Simoncelli, 'Il Simoncello', p. 401: 'Adoperandosi in essa molte persone, le quali ne hanno in animo di guerreggiar già mai'. And 'Ordinata alla ricreazione dell'animo o alla sanità del corpo'.

[64]   On the relationship between exercise and the intellect and soul see our *Healthy Living*, ch. 6.

[65]   Simoncelli, 'Il Simoncello', p. 398.

[66]   Simoncelli, 'Il Simoncello', pp. 409–17.

carrozze) were a means of transport specifically for women and children,[67] three decades later we find that no man of the family ever travelled on horseback, this being reserved for the male servants who accompany them. Only in emergencies, such as when the carriage or litter breaks down and it is impossible to wait for repair, did male travellers resume their old riding skills and cover the distance on horseback.[68]

Hunting tracts from the period also point to other practical changes which were taking place in Italy. It appears that by the middle to the end of the sixteenth century many different forms of hunting were practised that could cater for different levels of physical fitness and riding ability. These were to some extent also linked to the social hierarchy: references are made to the suitability of different types of hunting for different classes of men, as regards both the nature of the prey hunted, the hunting methods and the weapons used at the kill. First in this hierarchy came the chasing of large wild animals; whether deer, which were considered the most 'noble' of beasts, or the more dangerous and difficult wild boar, or bears. These animals had long been the preserve of kings, princes and the nobility since this kind of hunting required the stamina and strength associated with rulers, but also for the simple reason that they had the territory and financial resources to mount such hunts, in terms of supplying horses, dogs and servants.[69] Smaller game, and particularly hares, were considered appropriate for the lesser nobility and people of more lowly condition who could enjoy the sport with relatively little expense.[70]

The link between the ruling elite and the vigorous hunting of dangerous animals had its origins in antiquity. Physical vigour and bravery were indispensable to the exercise of power and were therefore a political virtue that was often remarked upon, hence ideals which were increasingly out of vogue for the nobility at large, remained unchanged for rulers as late as the end of the seventeenth century. In this vein we find many accounts of the robust, healthy lifestyles of the rulers of the courts of the Este at Ferrara or the Medici in Tuscany, which always included their love of hunting. Moreover, well into the seventeenth century there is evidence that young men raised in such ruling families were out hunting by the age of 12 or 13.[71] This also seems to have been true for some of the women. Isabella de' Medici, and her sisters, born in the 1540s, were riding by the age of three or four, and the Princess Isabella was frequently out hunting with her brothers as a teenager.[72] By her early twenties,

[67] See Daria Albicini's letters to husband Paolo Spada (1594–1612) and Giulia Benzoni's to Giovan Battista Veralli (1590–1610), in ASR, FSV, B. 589 and B. 449.

[68] We trace this shift from horse to coach in our *Healthy Living*, pp. 168–70.

[69] Eugenio Raimondi, *Delle Caccie* (Naples, 1626), p. 8.

[70] Carlo di Stefano, *L'Agricoltura e Casa di villa* (Venice, 1623), p. 384.

[71] Gaetano Pieraccini, *La Stirpe de' Medici di Cafaggiolo* (Florence, 1924), pp. 463, 485.

[72] Caroline Murphy, *Murder of a Medici Princess* (Oxford, 2008), pp. 39, 80.

she enjoyed hunting wild boar, stags and was particularly keen on hare coursing.[73] Moreover, her letters show that she was well aware of the beneficial effects of riding and hunting as exercise, as on the occasion when she writes to her husband that she was 'waiting to be able to take some exercise, to see if I can finally shake off this feeling of biliousness', and then went out hunting.[74] For women rulers (regents in particular) hunting was a symbol of their integration into power positions that were normally regarded as male, hence their involvement in hunts is often celebrated in encomiastic texts and portraits such as those representing members of the late seventeenth-century Savoy family.[75]

Leaving aside exemplary women like Isabella de' Medici, by about 1600 it is unclear how many noblewomen learned to ride well enough to actually follow the hunt, as opposed to showing up for the final kill (see Figure 8.1). Shortly after the marriage of 15-year-old Margherita Gonzaga to the Duke of Ferrara, in 1579, one of her ladies-in-waiting wrote to her father, the Duke of Mantova, describing how she, Margherita, and a lady of honour had 'started to go riding'. Her account gives a clear impression that none of them were particularly skilled riders. For example, the Duchess had fallen off once and the lady-in-waiting twice, though neither had hurt themselves. The writer herself – 'because I am braver (*più animosa*)' – was given a more difficult horse, a *corsiero*, which kept on rearing, though she 'clung on so tightly' that they all laughed at her.[76] Judging from a 1589 account by a court secretary, within 10 years the Duchess had in fact become a skilled huntswoman, whose weapon of choice was a gun made especially for her, 'with which she shoots many wild animals', so, presumably, her riding had improved, too.[77] However, this relative unfamiliarity with riding is also documented for us at the turn of the century near Faenza, amongst the Spada family, which had not yet been ennobled. Amongst the women riding appears to have been exceptional and done reluctantly when, due to the weather conditions, no other means of transport was available.[78]

[73]   Murphy, *Murder of a Medici Princess*, pp. 89, 94, 160.

[74]   Cited in Murphy, *Murder of a Medici Princess*, p. 88.

[75]   See the many accounts and images in Conte Amedeo di Castellamonte, *Venaria reale palazzo di piacere, e di caccia ...* (Turin, 1674).

[76]   Angelo Solerti, *Ferrara e La corte Estense nella seconda metà del secolo decimosesesto* (Venice, 1898), pp. 49, 50.

[77]   Solerti, *Ferrara*, p. 50.

[78]   ASR, FSV, B. 410, 21 January 1612, 25 January 1612.

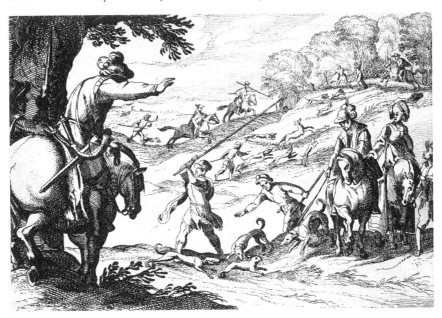

Figure 8.1 Women of the elite riding to a hunt

Note: Women of the elite did ride to hunts, as illustrated in many of the engravings by Antonio Tempesta. However, the presence of grooms holding the harness of the women's mounts, as in this image, suggests they were not viewed as particularly skilled riders. Moreover, women are usually positioned at the side of the frame, looking on at the action, suggesting that their participation was restricted to following at a safe distance.

Source: Antonio Tempesta, *Men and Dogs Hunting Hares and Deer*, 1624. © Harvard Art Museums/Fogg Museum, Gift of Eric A. von Raits in memory of Helen van C. de Peyster von Raits, M22312.37.

In Italy, hunting large wild game appears to have become the preserve of the few by 1600. High levels of urbanisation and intense deforestation around cities and towns in the later Middle Ages followed by the vogue for suburban villas had resulted in ever greater tracts of productive land being put under cultivation, resulting in the loss of hunting territory and game. The ruling elites, such as the Medici, who owned feudal hunting rights, reacted to this loss by passing legislation which banned anybody from hunting, even from carrying weapons on huge areas around the city.[79] Around Rome, the newly rich papal families bought the highly prestigious hunting rights from the declining older feudal

---

[79] See Hervé Brunon, 'La chasse et l'organisation du paysage dans la Toscane des Medicis', in Claude d'Anthenaise and Monique Chatenet (eds), *Chasses princières dans l'Europe de la renaissance* (Arles, 2007), pp. 219–47, 224–5.

families – essentially exchanging cash for status – and by the early seventeenth century had transformed their lands to include a stocked and walled game park, known as a *barco*.[80]

So, although we have evidence that the early seventeenth century saw the creation of new hunting parks for those at the apex of Italian society and that rulers were still often portrayed visually and verbally with reference to vigorous hunting, the extent to which this kind of hunting was actually practised throughout the upper echelons of society needs to be questioned. Following a tradition which had been established in the late Middle Ages, princely hunts were often used in an almost theatrical way to impress foreign dignitaries and other rulers. Or amongst the nobility themselves, guests and allies could be entertained with small hunting parties often held within the confines of their *barco*.[81] In Florence in the 1590s, there were even hunting competitions between rival groups of hunters, which could call on as many as a 3,500 men.[82] Such events were not only described in contemporary accounts, but illustrated in engravings of hunts by artists such as Giovanni Stradano and his pupil Antonio Tempesta. From this variety of sources it appears that there would have been a core of elite, relatively young, noblemen who participated actively on horseback in most stages of the hunt, and would also have given orders to other members. There would also have been professional huntsmen who performed the rather more arduous tasks of reconnoitring for the hunt in the run-up to the event, locating the animals and, if necessary, luring or chasing them to a place where they could then be pursued and killed by their lords. Other noblemen could have accompanied the hunt on foot, with highly prized hunting dogs.[83] Generally, the beaters who were on foot would have been peasants or other local men, paid to help with the event. At the bigger more 'staged' events, animals had already been hunted, rounded up and 'trapped' in a large open space in the forest by means of a series of large 'tele', cloths which were attached between the trees. Shady pavilions or raised platforms might even be erected in advance to provide a comfortable viewing point for the crowds of onlookers, courtiers and dignitaries, male and female, who simply watched the kill.[84] Although some noblemen and even noblewomen

[80] For an account of this process Tracy L. Erlich, *Landscape and Identity in Early Modern Rome: Villa Culture at Frascati in the Borghese Era* (Cambridge, 2002), pp. 218–19, 232.

[81] Erlich, *Landscape and Identity*, pp. 180, 218–19, 227.

[82] Giulio Dati, 'Disfida di Caccia tra I Piacevoli e I Piattelli descritta da Giulio Dati', in Giuliano Innamorati, *Arte della Caccia: Testi di Falconeria, Uccellagione e Altre Cacce* (Milan, 1965), pp. 343–68, 365.

[83] On these different roles see Dati, 'Disfida di Caccia', pp. 352–55.

[84] For accounts of such hunts see Giancarlo Malacarne, 'Les chasses des Gonzagues a Mantoue au temps de la renaissance', in Claude d' Anthenaise and Monique Chatenet (eds), *Chasses princières dans l'Europe de la Rénaissance* (Arles, 2007), pp. 137–54.

apparently did accompany the hunt on horseback, as we can see from the many pictures by Tempesta, it is clear from other illustrations and written accounts that courtiers were also simply carried to the entertainment by carriage: and in one account from Ferrara, by boat, since some of the women were pregnant.[85] It appears then that there were vastly different degrees of participation in hunts, as well as many different kinds of hunting party and that for the majority of participants it could be a relatively moderate form of exercise.

There were however many forms of hunting which were less physically and financially demanding, particularly hunting only with dogs, and hunting small game with guns, or nets, and going birding. Although already known and practised by 1500, the fashion for birding spread through the sixteenth century and by 1600 many owners of villas had planted special thickets (*paretaio*, or *frascato*) or small groves of evergreens (*boschetti* or *uccellatoi*), which were designed to attract large numbers of small birds.[86] Indeed, one of the main drives behind the fashion for birding in Italy is thought to have been the loss of forests, and pressure on land around the cities. By the seventeenth century, this seems to have become the most widespread form of hunting in Italy. Yet its popularity reveals once again a clash in ideals and practices of masculinity. In hunting tracts and even in Mercuriale, the authors dismiss it as not worthy of the name 'hunting', and not appropriate to 'real men'.[87] However, more than anything these comments actually document the extent to which birding had become hugely popular across the Italian peninsula.

The practice was disdained, partly because of the devious methods employed, since it merely required the hunters to lay traps, whether using nets or spikes, or even putting glue on the boughs of small trees to catch their prey. Yet, in contrast to Scipione Mercurio's description of it as being 'of medium vigour', offering the perfect balance of exercise and moderation, Simoncello considers it unworthy of being called hunting because it does not harden the body and soul to withstand the ordeal of war.[88] Certainly, the engravings by Tempesta suggest that it was

---

[85]   Richard Almond has suggested that Tempesta's images show adult women actually being instructed in how to hunt. Our interpretation is that they show women following the hunt and certain events being pointed out to them. Richard Almond, *Daughters of Artemis: The Huntress in the Middle Ages and Renaissance* (Cambridge, 2009), p. 62. See for example the 'Ladies watching hunters chase animals into a pit' or 'Men and Dogs hunting hares' in Tempesta's *Hunting Scenes, I* (Vienna, 1595) and *Hunting Scenes, II* (Vienna, 1598), reproduced in *The Illustrated Bartsch*, vol. 36 (New York, 1983), p. 261. For images of people travelling by carriage, see the last engraving in 'La Curea' in Castellamonte, *Venaria* (no page number); for the account of going to the kill by boat, see Solerti, *Ferrara*, p. 194.

[86]   For a comprehensive account of this see Brunon, 'La chasse', pp. 229–39.

[87]   Mercuriale, *De arte*, p. 421; Simoncelli, 'Il Simoncello', p. 403.

[88]   Mercurio, *De gli errori*, p. 309 and Simoncelli, 'Il Simoncello', pp. 403–4.

above all peaceful recreation, requiring participants to sit still for long periods, even in hiding, waiting for their prey to fly into the trap (see Figure 8.2).[89]

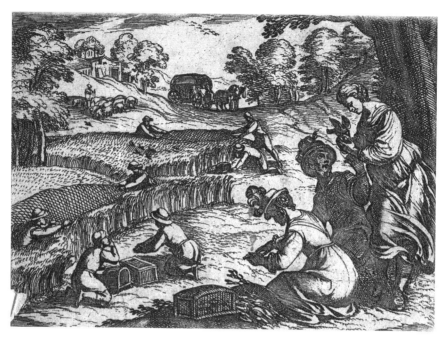

Figure 8.2   This image shows one of the ways in which small birds were hunted and it was evidently a leisurely pursuit. The actual trapping is done by servants whilst the ladies and gentlemen stay in the shade having been brought by carriage

Source: Antonio Tempesta, *Hunters Trapping Small Birds in the Brush*, sixteenth century, Etching, Harvard Art Museums/Fogg Museum, Gift of Herrman L. Blumgart, by exchange, S9.85.5. © President and Fellows of Harvard College.

Despite disdain for the practice in some didactic sources, it would seem from contemporary accounts that gentlefolk felt perfectly at ease enjoying this kind of small-scale leisurely hunting of birds and smaller game. In part this may well have been because birding fitted very well into the pastimes which livened up the extended periods that the urban elites spent at their country villas, in the spring, early summer and autumn. Activities like birding were ideal because they were gentle enough to be enjoyed by groups of people of both sexes and all ages, and could also be undertaken quite simply, without the need for horses.

---

[89]   'Bird Hunters with Different Traps and Snares', in *The Illustrated Bartsch*, p. 306.

Count Fabroni, a nobleman from Pistoia, kept a diary of his hunting *villeggiature* for more than 20 years in the second half of the seventeenth century which records his activities and shows how the prey was mostly represented by very small birds which were perhaps not all even edible (larks, thrushes, titmouses, robins, partridges, quails, blackbirds, jay birds, sparrows). Hares were the second most common prey, while only very rarely they caught a fox and even more exceptionally a roe deer. As illustrated also by the nice drawings included in the diary (see Figure 8.3), hunting was done on foot, with dogs, and using 'the arquebus' (musket) which was the only weapon employed.[90]

Birds were also the kind of game most frequently given to the Spadas as a gift during the hunting season. Receipt of a hare, roe deer or even of partridges was a treat.[91]

Some members of the Spada family also enjoyed hunting although participation appears to have been related to age. From numerous letters we learn that only men in their late teens, twenties or thirties appear to have gone hunting.[92] Their father, on the contrary, felt compassion for the roe deer that were ruining his olive groves and couldn't bring himself to do away with them – a sentiment more akin to the attitude of the church, which depicted hunting as cruel and barbaric.[93] The women might occasionally participate in birding at the *paretaio* but mostly bombarded their dear ones with recommendations to be careful not to wear themselves out while running after hares, wild beasts (*fiere selvaggie*) or domestic boars (*cinghiali domestici*).[94] As suggested by the mocking tone in these phrases women do not seem to have taken their younger brothers' or sons' hunting ambitions too seriously and disrespectfully teased them about their abilities as hunters.[95]

Overall, by the early seventeenth century, a preference for gentle or moderate exercise had been established, thanks particularly to a dramatisation of the dangers of overheating the body and the head present in the medical discourse about exercise. This condemnation of vigorous exercise was also reinforced by new constructions of nobility which identified civility with bodily restraint and decorum. Whilst walking was the ideal exercise form, also because of the simplicity and ease with which it could be practised, *Pallamaglio*, *trucco* and birding came a close second for nobility and gentlefolk. These were all 'exercises' which could be enjoyed in the open air, at one's country villa – or even in the

---

[90]   Biblioteca Nazionale Centrale di Firenze, Rossi Cassigoli ms. 380: 'Ricordi di villeggiatura, di caccia e altro'.

[91]   See for example ASR, FSV, B. 624, 6 September 1674; B. 410, 23 October 1680.

[92]   See ASR, FSV, B. 1115, 7 November 1664; B. 618, 4 May 1678, 24 September 1678, B. 607, 1 October 1663 and 4 May 1664 and 13 May 1664: see also fn. 16.

[93]   ASR, FSV, B. 607, 1 April 1659.

[94]   ASR, FSV, B. 1115, 16 October 1669; B. 410, 19 October 1680, 30 October 1680.

[95]   See also ASR, FSV, B. 624, 6 September 1674.

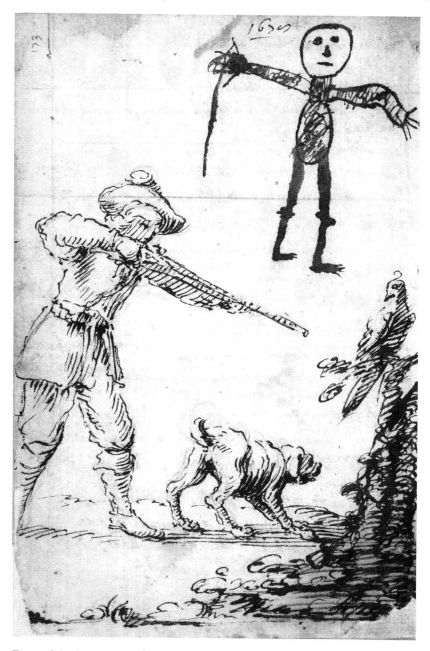

Figure 8.3 An amateur drawing showing a man hunting birds with his dog and arquebus from the hunting diary of Count Fabroni

Source: Biblioteca Nazionale Centrale di Firenze, Rossi Cassigoli 380, c.12v., 'Ricordi di villeggiatura, di caccia e altro', 1664–90.

great villas on the edge of the city, with minimal sweating, overheating and other dangerous or unpleasant effects. Meanwhile, given the many different forms of hunting which existed, according to the quarry and methods used, hunting could still combine new notions of gentility and moderate exercise with traditional expressions of 'noble' identity.

Chapter 9

Exercise, Health and Gender: Normative Discourses and Practices in Eighteenth- and Nineteenth-Century German-Speaking Countries*

Martin Dinges

Jean-Jacques Rousseau is always good for a snappy dictum. In *Emile*, published in 1762, he maintained that 'the only useful branch of medicine is health theory, and this is less a science than a theory of virtue'.[1] In a quite modern way Rousseau points out that maintaining health should be the main priority. Nowadays we would talk of what the health sociologist Aaron Antonovsky called 'salutogenesis'. This approach examines how health can be maintained despite all the challenges presented to both body and soul.[2] Antonovsky, whose ideas emerged in the context of stress research, comes to the conclusion that an individual who sees his life in the world as meaningful, understandable and manageable has better general health resources by which to overcome everyday stress. He calls this attitude *Kohärenzgefühl* (sense of coherence). Stress, he says, can even play a part in strengthening health resources.

In today's debate about health in post-industrial service societies a healthy lifestyle is becoming increasingly important.[3] There are two reasons for this: The (infectious) nation-wide diseases have largely disappeared and other acute

---

*   This chapter was translated by Jane Rafferty.

[1]   Jean-Jacques Rousseau, *Émile ou De l'éducation* (Paris, 1961; original edition 1762), p. 28: 'La seule partie utile de la médecine est l'hygiène; encore l'hygiène est-elle moins une science qu'une vertu.'

[2]   Aaron Antonovsky, *Salutogenese: zur Entmystifizierung der Gesundheit* (Tübingen, 1997), esp. pp. 33–5; Jürgen Bengel and Regine Strittmatter, *Was erhält Menschen gesund? Antonovskys Modell der Salutogenese – Diskussionsstand und Stellenwert; eine Expertise* (Cologne, 2003), pp. 93–5.

[3]   David Armstrong, 'The Origins of the Problem of Health-Related Behaviours: A Genealogical Study', *Social Studies of Science*, 39 (2009): pp. 909–26, esp. 918. See also Thomas Altgeld, 'Mehr Bewegung im Alltag statt Run auf Risikosportarten? Gesundheits- und Sportverhalten von Männern', in Ilse Hartmann-Tews and Britt Dahmen (eds),

illnesses can be treated better than ever. But ever-increasing life expectancy has led to a growing number of chronic illnesses. These can be prevented at least to some extent by a lifestyle that promotes health. So in this chapter exercise should be understood as one of the health resources that individuals can tap into. It is initially of little importance whether they tap into them with the intention of promoting health or not.

The idea of exercise as a health resource is not as modern, let alone anachronistic, as it first appears. For exercise as a health resource one can easily draw a line from ancient dietetics, that is, the doctrine of a healthy life, via the older dietetics of the Renaissance, right up to present-day fitness sport.[4] With reference to Antiquity Renaissance dietetics also recommended robust sporting activities. Apart from that, exercise in the fresh air was the main recommendation. So it was not entirely surprising to historians of medicine that Wolfgang Behringer recently re-assessed the importance of sport in the Early Modern period, giving it greater significance than previous research had done.[5] I shall now, as examples, assess German-speaking theories of health during the eighteenth and nineteenth centuries in terms of how they thematise exercise in general. The focus on this period results from the significantly growing interest in health issues indicated by the increasing number of publications in this field from the 1750s. This new interest in health can be explained partly by contemporary demographic policies and partly by individual re-orientations as a phenomenon of secularisation.

Rousseau, as cited earlier, remarked that health doctrine should be seen not so much as a science but as a doctrine of virtue. He points here to the strong normative character of these doctrines that always involve value judgements. So to start with I shall look at normative discourses as presented by health advisors, and then give examples of exercise as mentioned in personal testimonies. This dual approach means that it is not only the upper and upper-middle classes (as is largely the case with bourgeois sport) who are taken into account.

Gesundheit in Bewegung: Impulse aus Geschlechterperspektive (Sankt Augustin, 2010), pp. 99–105.

[4]   For an overview see Heikki Mikkeli, *Hygiene in the Early Modern Medical Tradition* (Helsinki, 1999), esp. pp. 60–64.

[5]   Wolfgang Behringer, 'Arena und Pall Mall: Sport in the Early Modern Period', *German History*, 27 (2009): pp. 331–57. He basically offers information on the princely courts and the sporting practices of the upper and middle classes; his focus is on the sixteenth and seventeenth centuries.

Normative Discourses of the Health Advisors

Exercise as one of the six 'res non naturales' is a classification that has become a convention since Galen.[6] What is designated as unnatural here are those external influences that do not already exist in a healthy body, these being the elements, the parts of the body, or particular abilities. Depending on circumstances the individual external conditions that promoted health, in other words the 'res non naturales', were discussed to varying degrees of intensity. So it is not possible to generalise as to whether exercise, compared for instance to nourishment, sleep or digestion, was a particularly important or less significant aspect.[7] But in any case exercise appears in the very first regimes or in the first Greek Diaita from the fourth century BC. As with the other 'res non naturales' a pair-concept is used, 'motus et quies' or 'exercitium et otium', that is movement and rest, like for instance filling the body and emptying it. In the teleological concept of health of that time it is assumed that by its nature the body strives for a healthy balance. So this dialectic concept of 'motus et quies' refers to the vitally important balance between rest and body movement.

So perhaps we should ask briefly why exercise should be important for health at all. For the answer I shall now leap into the eighteenth century.[8] The doctor of the Hallenser Reformuniversität, Friedrich Hoffmann (1660–1742), argued in 1715 in a thoroughly classical way. In his theory of health, written in the vernacular, he says:

> Every indisposition, illness and unhealthy movement consists directly in the fact that the fluid parts are moving too slowly or too quickly, which causes the circulation to become irregular and the necessary elimination of unused parts cannot take place. [What is good is] everything that brings about gentle, calm and moderate movement in the blood, which contributes a great deal to health and the prolongation of life.[9]

---

    [6]   There were also discussions about the number (six).
    [7]   Mikkeli, *Hygiene*, p. 16: 'aer, cibus et potus, motus et quies' or 'exercitium et otium, somnus et vigilia, repletio et evacuatio' and 'secreta et excreta, accidentia animae' or 'affectus animi' or 'passiones'.
    [8]   I will not go into the convolutions of how this has been received in the meantime since these are of more interest in terms of intellectual history.
    [9]   Friedrich Hoffmann, *Herrn Friedrich Hoffmanns, weitberühmten Medici gründliche Anweisung, wie ein Mensch vor dem frühzeitigen Tod und allerhand Krankheiten durch ordentliche Lebens-Art sich verwahren könne*, Theil 1 (Halle, 1715), cited from Günter Henner, *Quellen zur Geschichte der Gesundheitspädagogik* (Würzburg, 1998), pp. 127–8: 'Alle Unpässlichkeit, Kranckheit und ungesunde Bewegung bestehet unmittelbahr darin, dass die flüssigen Theile entweder in einer gar zu langsamen oder gar zu schnellen Bewegung sind, welches verursacht, dass die Circulation ungleich wird und die gehörige Absonderung

So Hoffmann accepts the body image canonised since late Antiquity, according to which the fluids in the body must be kept in balance.[10] As we know, this was regarded as health. The precondition for this is that the fluids must be kept moving, and unwanted materials eliminated from the body. The end of the quotation refers to this.[11] Another condition for health is that the fluids should not flow too quickly or too slowly – the 'golden mean'. Too much movement is just as bad as too little. And it is noticeable that the dangers of too much movement are quite clearly addressed. So Hoffmann is by no means putting forward one-sided pro-exercise propaganda here.

The regimes of Antiquity already had different recommendations for men and women, for particular ages – in particular for children and old people – and also sometimes for athletes.[12] So let's have a closer look now at who was recommended to take exercise at the end of the eighteenth century. Instead of compiling pieces of advice from numerous writings,[13] it is heuristically more fruitful to assess the sum of these recommendations as put together by Doctor Johann Peter Frank in his nine-volume 'System einer vollständigen medicinischen Polizey' between 1779 and 1819. Frank had a great many international contacts because he himself was a leading light in the health administration of several European countries.[14] What is more, in the second volume he devoted a whole chapter to the 'Wiederherstellung der Gymnastick' (restoration of gymnastics) (section 3,3, pp. 607–92), but he also discussed the issue of health and exercise in other chapters, for instance in a chapter 'on excessive strain put too early onto the juvenile bodily strength and animal spirits'[15] or in the section on 'public physical education for adolescent daughters to become future mothers'[16] in the

---

der unnützen Theile wohl nicht geschehen kann ... alles dasjenige, was eine sanffte, ruhige und gemäßigte Bewegung in dem Geblüth erweckt, zu der Gesundheit und Verlängerung des Lebens sehr zuträglich sey.'

[10]   Karl Eduard Rothschuh, *Konzepte der Medizin in Vergangenheit und Gegenwart* (Stuttgart, 1978), esp. p. 195.

[11]   Michael Stolberg, *Homo patiens. Krankheits- und Körpererfahrung in der Frühen Neuzeit* (Cologne, 2003).

[12]   Mikkeli, *Hygiene*, p. 15.

[13]   Such a compilation could easily be made using for example Georg Friedrich Müller, *Das Turnen als Schutz- und Heilmittel für körperliche Leiden beider Geschlechter* (Reutlingen, 1847), pp. 229–31 for masturbation; pp. 239–40 for early menstruation; pp. 263–5 for women.

[14]   See the most recent study of Frank: Markus Pieper, 'Der Körper des Volkes und der gesunde Volkskörper. Johann Peter Franks "System einer vollständigen medicinischen Polizey"', *Zeitschrift für Geschichtswissenschaft*, 46 (1998): pp. 101–19.

[15]   'zu frühe Anspannung der jugendlichen Seelen- und Leibeskräfte'.

[16]   'öffentlichen physischen Bildung erwachsender Töchter zu künftigen Müttern'.

first volume (pp. 473–98).[17] These chapters have so far not been systematically assessed from the point of view of exercise, health and gender.

Frank, like other doctors of the Enlightenment, positioned himself as a general health advisor who wants to reform the whole of public life, so ultimately he discussed just about everything. This kind of general discourse on health created a need for expert advice discussing problems created by society – as for example in Frank's case the people's dramatically declining health.[18] His assertion that the German people had generally become soft is the central theme in our context. It is a topos he repeatedly takes up. In his criticism of coach driving, for instance, he maintains:

> What a difference between one and the same nation in a period of not even three and a half hundred years! ... then still kings, princes and women on horseback ... A strong manly body, the honour and pride of the German youth ... the praiseworthy object of the blue-eyed girl straight as a cedar tree with toned arms and swift feet! ... today everyone who wants to distinguish himself from the common people, pulled along in cradles by horses ... today Germany's sons of heroes with the features of women, their feet in shiny white silk ... hardly strong enough even to raise the silk parasol against the sun which dares to shine on the face of this wimpish doll of a man if he ever leaves the shining coach to stagger across the road like a puppet! ... the future mother of the defenders of Germany's honour and name, the pale cheeks and withered breast thickly painted in white and red ... tied all day long, unmoving, to a plush sofa surrounded by faded upstarts ... A declared enemy of all housework and one-time uncompassionate half-mother of ailing sons.[19]

---

[17]   References to Peter Frank, *System einer vollständigen medicinischen Polizey*, vol. 1: *Von der Fortpflanzung der Menschen und Ehe-Anstalten ...* (Mannheim, 1784); vol. 2: *Von der außerehelichen Zeugung, dem geflissentlichen Mißgebähren ...*(Mannheim, 1780). For Frank's significance in sport history see Joachim K. Rühl, 'Die Bedeutung der Leibesübungen in Johann Peter Franks "System einer vollständigen medicinischen Polizey" (1779–1817)', in Thierry Terret (ed.), *Sport et santé dans l'histoire* (Sankt Augustin, 1999), pp. 453–64.

[18]   Martin Dinges, 'Medizinische Aufklärung bei Johann Georg Zimmermann. Zum Verhältnis von Macht und Wissen bei einem Arzt der Aufklärung', in Martin Fontius and Helmut Holzhey (eds), *Schweizer im Berlin des 18. Jahrhunderts* (Berlin, 1996), pp. 137–50.

[19]   Frank, *System*, vol. 2, pp. 684–5: 'Welch ein Unterschied zwischen einer und der nemlichen Nazion, in Zeit von nicht gar dritthalb hundert Jahren! ... dort noch Könige, Fürsten und Frauen zu Pferde ... ein starker mannbarer Körper, die Ehre und Zierde des deutschen Jünglings ... der rühmlichste Gegenstand des blauäugichten Mädchens von Zeder-geradem Wuchse, mit nervigtem Arme und flinkem Fuße! ... heute alles, was sich nur vom Pöbel unterscheiden will, in Wiegen von Pferden gezogen ... heute Deutschlands Heldensöhne mit Weiberzügen, die Füße in weißglänzender Seide ... kaum noch kräftig genug, den seidenen Schirm der Sonne entgegen zu halten, die es wagen darf, der zierlichen

So decadence was caused by becoming soft, which was particularly evident in the ruling classes, and this since 1430! Frank polemicised against the notion that physical fitness endangered young people:

> if health never was endangered by sudden changes in weather and occurring accidents; what then! ... then the young weakling will stay in his mother's lap, where he will never twist his ankle ... But what is the point of cushioning the boy against the impression of foreign objects, if not to see over the years the man or rather the manly woman die of the snuffles or break his neck when jumping a span-high hedge?[20]

So toughening up through exercise is recommended – and at the same time this proves to be a way of becoming a man, of literally moving away from the mother's lap instead of degenerating into the effeminate man already mentioned.

The same basic pattern also applies to young women. Admiringly quoting Lykurg, one of the well-established authorising references to Antiquity as a role model at the time, he describes how Lykurg had

> tried to keep young girls' bodies in constant motion by running-races, wrestling, javelin throwing and archery so that the seed of future generations would grow stronger roots and would flourish better but also so that, through their bodily strength, they would be better equipped to bear the pain of childbirth.[21]

Mannspuppe ins Angesicht zu scheinen, wenn sie je den glänzenden Wagen verlässt, um Gliedermännchenmäßig über die Strassen hinzuhüpfen! ... die künftige Mutter der Verfechter der deutschen Ehre und Nahmens, die blassen Wangen und welke Brust weiß und roth dick überfirneist ... den ganzen Tag im Kreise fader Kleinmeister unbeweglich auf dem wohllüstigen Sofa hingefesselt ... eine erklärte Feindin aller häuslichen Beschäftigungen und dereinst unbarmherzige Halbmutter siechender Söhne.'

[20]   Frank, *System*, vol. 2, pp. 646–7: 'wenn die Gesundheit bei einer unthätigen, nichts wagenden Lebensart, von dem öfteren Wechsel der Witterung und der aufstossenden ohngefähren Zufällen nie etwas zu ahnden hätte; wohl dann! ... so bleib' der junge Weichling im Mutterschose, wo er seinen Fuß nie verrenken wird ... allein was nützet es, den Knaben, mit Federdecken vor dem Eindrucke fremder Gegenstände zu verwahren, um mit der Zeit den Mann oder vielmehr das männliche Weib von einem Schnuppen töden, und über einer Spannehohen Hecke den Hals einstürzen zu sehen?'

[21]   Frank, *System*, vol. 2, pp. 611–12: 'die Körper der Mädchen, durch Wettlaufen, Ringen, Spiesswerfen und Bogenschiessen in immerwährender Bewegung zu erhalten gesucht: damit der Keim zukünftiger Geschlechter festere Wurzeln schlagen und in ihrem Schosse besser gedeihen könnte, besonders aber damit sie, durch die Stärke des Körpers, gegen die Schmerzen der Geburt, abgehärtet würden.'

It is not surprising for an author of this time that the role of the woman is primarily defined by her ability to bear children.[22] But in any case a precondition for this is behaviour that promotes health, in other words appropriate exercise instead of slovenliness and sensuality.

Frank summed this up in the formula: 'Physical exercise in the fresh air is equally necessary to both genders: it promotes the circulation of the fluids and the life-giving fire of the nerves, without which children are born only half-alive.'[23] It is highly relevant for our context that Frank is not just thinking about free movement without any relation to work. In fact he calculates the normal exertions of everyday life into the individual exercise account. Here he argues in a thoroughly class-orientated way: 'Is not the fate of the common peasant girl's bodily condition much better the more her laborious work differs from the lethargic upbringing of the urban beauty?'[24] Being active, working, and moving about in the process, this reinforces the health of the young woman on the land far better – and is of course an argument criticising the nobility.[25]

Frank also compares bourgeois daughters who, as adolescents, were 'locked up in good Turkish fashion' and then become 'useless weaklings', with peasant girls.[26] According to him, everyone who considered themselves to be socially superior to the rank of the peasants and lower burgesses locked up their girls from the age of 10 until puberty, so that through 'endless sitting and never using their exercise muscles' weak circulation occurred. He says, 'circulation only takes place in those arteries whereto the powers of the faint heart can barely carry the humours themselves, but there is barely a trace of inner movement of the blood in such parts'.[27] This 'semi-constricted circulation' stands in contrast to

---

[22] Rudolf Helmstetter, 'Popularisierungen. Wissen für Frauen zwischen "Fortpflanzungszwecken und Schönheitsidealen"', in Renate Lachmann and Stefan Rieger (eds), *Text und Wissen* (Tübingen, 2003), pp. 181–95, at 189–90; Helga Glantschnig, 'Der fortschrittliche Umgang mit dem Körper. Zur Entstehungsgeschichte der Leibesübungen im 18. Jahrhundert', *Das achtzehnte Jahrhundert und Österreich*, 10 (1995): pp. 45–54, at 53–4, see also Claudia Honegger, *Die Ordnung der Geschlechter. Die Wissenschaft vom Menschen und das Weib 1750–1850* (Frankfurt M., 1991).

[23] Frank, *System*, vol. 1, p. 483: 'Die Bewegung des Körpers in freier Luft ist beiden Geschlechtern auch gleichnothwendig: sie unterhält den Kreislauf der Säfte und das beseelende Feuer der Nerven, ohne welches nur halb lebendige Kinder geboren werden.'

[24] Frank, *System*, vol. 1, p. 484: 'Ist nicht das Schicksal der gemeinen Bauerndirnen, in Rücksicht ihrer körperlichen Beschaffenheit, um soviel besser, je weiter ihre geschäftige Lebensart, von der schläferigen Auferziehung der Stadtschönen abstehet.'

[25] Frank clearly recognises the dangers of heavy work, especially during the last months of pregnancy, Frank, *System*, vol. 1, pp. 540–42.

[26] Frank, *System*, vol. 1, p. 477: 'auf gut Türkisch eingeschlossen', 'unbrauchbaren Weichlingen'.

[27] Frank, *System*, vol. 1, p. 474: 'ewige Sitzen und die nie unterbrochene Ruhe ihrer Bewegungsmuskel', 'Kreislauf findet dann nur in denjenigen Gefäßen statt, wohin die

the 'healthy blood of the robust peasant girl', which 'floods the firm cheeks all over, and proclaims a happy excess of the balsamic fluids from which future solid citizens will be created'.[28]

The business of fluids applies in much the same way to birth and its consequences. Due to lack of exercise the town-dwelling woman, when giving birth, must 'get much hotter and strain her nerves much more than the hardened peasant woman'. This leads to 'childbirth fever from fluids stuck in worn-out or narrow arteries, which right from the first day after the birth turns into gangrene and putrefaction or leaves blockages in the internal birth parts'.[29]

This brings us to Frank's notions about the connection between health and exercise. As in the quotation above his argumentation repeatedly involves the state of the bodily fluids. Thus gymnastic exercises or dancing should never be stopped abruptly so that 'nature has time to moderate the flow of the fluids without endangering health and of re-closing the expulsion channels that had been opened'.[30] Abrupt transitions between motus and quies are undesirable.

However, Frank's hopes for the positive effects of exercise on health went further than this. According to his image of the human anatomy exercise in children increases the firmness of brain cells and muscle fibres.[31] He goes on: 'Thus we can see in people who work hard how much diligent exercise increases the size and strength of the muscles.'[32] Here again exercise as part of work is a way of continually strengthening the body.

Furthermore he mentions at least once the strengthening of individual organs, specifically the innards, by playing skittles. This, he said, promoted health and should therefore not be looked down on as a peasants' game.[33] He also reports

---

Kräften [*sic*] des matten Herzens für sich allein, die Säfte noch wohl bringen können; aber es ist kaum ein Verdacht von innerer Bewegung des Bluts, in solchen Theilen'.

[28]   Frank, *System*, vol. 1, p. 475: 'das überall zu den festen Backen heraus will, und den glücklichen Überfluss balsamischer Säfte ankündigt, aus welchen der zukünftige kernhafte Bürger erschaffen werden wird.'

[29]   Frank, *System*, vol. 1, p. 477: 'weit mehr erhitzen und ihre Nerven anspannen als das abgehärtete Bauernweib'; 'Kindbetterfieber, von ausgetrettenen oder in feinen Gefäßen stockenden Säften, welche gleich in den ersten Tagen nach der Geburt, in Brand und Fäulung übergehen, oder in den inneren Geburtstheilen Verstopfungen zurücklassen'.

[30]   Frank, *System*, vol. 2, p. 677; Frank, *System*, vol. 1, p. 487, zu Tanzvergnügen: 'damit so die Natur Zeit gewinne, ohne Nachtheil für die Gesundheit, den Lauf der Säfte zu mäßigen und die geöffneten Absonderungswege wieder zu schliessen.'

[31]   Frank, *System*, vol. 2, p. 526.

[32]   Frank, *System*, vol. 2, p. 528: 'So sehen wir deutlich an arbeitsamen Menschen, wie sehr eine fleißige Bewegung selbsten die Größe und Stärke der Muskel erhöhe.'

[33]   Frank, *System*, vol. 2, p. 635.

without comment that in northern countries bathing has reduced the incidence of scurvy.[34] So here exercise is supposed to prevent individual illnesses.

If we accept Frank's positive assessments of exercise, then we might perhaps expect recommendations for specific types of exercise with details of the anticipated health benefits. But this is not the case. Instead, the high number of warnings in relation to exercise is striking: in the chapters analysed, health warnings are issued 23 out of the 46 times exercise is mentioned (exactly a half).[35] It is generally easier to talk about dangers to health and the risk of accidents than about positive health benefits.[36] In a work about the medical police that was to be set up this obviously applies even more. Nonetheless, let us start with his positive statements.

Recreation days are recommended for schoolchildren (vol. 2, p. 605) where they can play outside, and apart from that, exercise in very general terms instead of scribbling in the schoolroom (p. 614). In addition Frank encourages instructive walks for boys as the Jesuits used to do (p. 629). The body formation of French peasants by their corporals in the army is stated to be exemplary (p. 630); Frank advises scholars to alternate between exercise and intellectual activity (p. 631); also exemplary are the Swiss territorial reserve soldiers who exercise in the hills (p. 632), as well as their running races, wrestling and archery (p. 634). Boys should do long-distance running and throwing (p. 634), and also play skittles. The 'female' gender is advised for the first time to do skating – though Dutch women are held up as examples to their German counterparts (p. 635). Youngsters are urged to play ball games (p. 635), do fencing (p. 637) and riding (p. 639).[37] Obviously dancing is recommended for both genders (p. 637). Young people should swim (p. 641); boys should climb up trees and walls – incidentally, to train themselves not to become dizzy. Boys are also advised not to go out of their way to avoid the dangers of exercise (p. 646). An exercise room is mentioned in connection with priests/seminarists, soldiers and young students (pp. 648f.). And now comes the only positive recommendation that applies solely to women: The shepherdesses in Bretten (today Baden) turn their run into a race – though in light clothes (p. 654). Apart from that there is only one other example from abroad for German women; these are the West

---

[34]   Frank, *System*, vol. 2, p. 642.

[35]   In this count double references particularly to dancing are included which occur in several passages in the text.

[36]   Oliver Stenzel, *Medikale Differenzierung: der Konflikt zwischen akademischer Medizin und Laienheilkunde im 18. Jahrhundert* (Heidelberg, 2005), p. 11.

[37]   See also August Nitschke, 'Gymnastik, Fechten und Tanz im 18. Jahrhundert. Die Ausbildung des Körpers auf den Schulen von August Hermann Francke', in Josef N. Neumann and Udo Sträter (eds), *Das Kind in Pietismus und Aufklärung* (Tübingen, 2000), pp. 333–47.

Mongolian Kalmück horsewomen, who apparently did the same sort of exercise as the men (vol. 1, p. 482).

So here we have quite a long list of recommended types of exercise for recreation which significantly does not contain any references to desirable movement while at work or its usefulness to health. This sphere only reappears again when it comes to the warnings, when he is talking about apprentices being over-taxed (vol. 2, p. 556), which the 'father of labour medicine', Ramazzini, had completely failed to notice (p. 559).[38] So Frank offers us a positive list of exercise types, almost all of which are intended for children, adolescents and young adults.

Apart from the scholars already mentioned, adults are referred to entirely unspecifically. Frank remarks as an example that 'old and young' walk on stilts, albeit in the Biscay area (presumably in Aquitainia) (vol. 2, p. 646). And his praise of going for walks is directed at all 'classes of people' (p. 682). Since weaker people are also mentioned, for whom benches should be set up, we can assume that the elderly are also included here, though Frank's whole exercise propaganda clearly applies almost exclusively to those under the age of 25. This makes a certain sense from the point of view of his medical police project: from the perspective of increasing the population for the purposes of the state, young subjects are particularly relevant – they should become useful as child-bearers and soldiers. So here the discourse on exercise turns out to be biopolitics. Individual health brought about by exercise is a means of improving the nation's body.[39]

We have already established that Frank recommends exercise to both genders. As far as women are concerned, he always argues from the point of view of their ability to bear children. If we look more closely the gender-specific inequalities become even more obvious. The addressees were almost exclusively lads, boys, schoolboys, male youngsters, soldiers, priests, male students, male artisans, in other words, men, or those who would and should become men. The same applies to the term 'youth', which in the broader context always has male connotations. If swimming is supposed to be good for many people and of interest to youngsters (p. 641), the implied reference later turns out to be to 'lads and young men' (p. 672). When Frank writes about 'children' swinging on ropes in the barn (p. 671), elsewhere the reference is again to lads (p. 627). So the recommended exercise for children is by no means gender-neutral. On the contrary, whenever concrete examples are given this discourse on exercise is directed almost exclusively towards the physical development of men.

---

[38] This applies despite his references to unhealthy work materials and dangerous workplaces. Bernardino Ramazzini, *Die Krankheiten der Handwerker* (Würzburg, 1998 [1700]), in the case of work-related illnesses distinguishes between men, women and Jews.

[39] Pieper, 'Körper'.

Again, for girls and young women there is just the extremely unspecific instruction that in running races the demands should be differentiated according to age and gender (p. 654). On the other hand, girls are mentioned rather more often when it comes to the numerous warnings, Frank's second major theme. They are accused of sitting too much (p. 611), but like the boys they should desist from 'Burzelbaum- und Radeschlagen' (doing somersaults and cartwheels) because of the danger of accidents (p. 628). Jumping over the bonfires on St John's eve (Johannisfeuer) was particularly dangerous for girls because they jumped a shorter distance and wore skirts that could catch in the fire (p. 657). Finally, the dangers of dancing for women who have their 'monthly' are stressed (p. 664), pregnant women should be forbidden to do it altogether (p. 667) and the 'dance heroines' are warned once again about getting over-hot (vol. 1, p. 486). So while on the one hand the girls, pampered town-dwellers and young women are constantly criticised for their lack of exercise, Frank makes no constructive suggestions beyond going for walks and vague ideals of skating Dutch women and West Mongolian Kalmück horsewomen.

Apart from all this, the doctor, eager for reform, seeks to regulate exercise in many ways. Thus when playing cards people should not sit hunched up (vol. 2, p. 622), and the 'less-supple boys' in particular should avoid games that are too dangerous (p. 627). Peasants' swings should be secured in case the ropes broke and the children fell off (pp. 627, 671); youngsters in the countryside should take care when climbing trees (p. 628). On the other hand, organised tree-climbing and competitions to climb up a greasy pole are praised. According to this Swabian custom, prizes were attached to the top such as shoes, stockings, bodices, aprons and scarves, which 'the victor would then throw down to his anxiously thrilled girl with a pubescent cheer' (p. 645).[40] We can see here how Frank imagines restricting such practices – and at the same time gives them erotic connotations.

Hence 'little daredevils' should not jump headfirst from the bridges (p. 628). When playing skittles the ball should be thrown precisely (p. 660), the common lads, when ice-skating, should be protected by the medical police from parts of the pond that had thawed out; the police should also forbid skating parties of little 'daredevils' if these blocked public pathways (p. 661). He is adamantly against 'fencing games', which, he maintained, did not lead to toughening up, but to brutality (p. 667). It could, however, be taught by an expert instructor who should proceed step by step, and not over-tax his pupils, thereby endangering their health (p. 628). When riding, no unsuitable horses should be used and above all no children should be allowed to sit on them or take the horses to the drinking trough (p. 669). Young people should not imitate the tricks performed

---

[40] '[wirft] der Sieger endlich seinem ängstigfrohen Mädchen das eroberte mit mannbarem Jauchzen zu'.

by English acrobats on horseback (p. 672). Lads and male adolescents should have swimming lessons, where they should be instructed by 'skilled and cautious men' (p. 672).

What is surprising is that in this dietetics so little reference is made to the other circumstances of exercise activities. Frank does at least advise against dancing, especially in the heat of the summer (p. 663), warns against taking cold drinks after getting hot (p. 676) and criticises the 'dusty air in the schoolroom', which should be avoided at all costs (vol. 1, p. 485). Apart from that, he says, the public exercise area should be set up 'in an open space on slightly raised ground where healthy air can blow unrestricted', and should be covered in grass or sand (vol. 2, p. 649). Johann Bernhard Basedow is more precise about this when in 1774 he warns, for instance, against exercising to the point of exhaustion, 'especially just before and after a meal'.[41]

So on the one hand exercise is considered to be a generally good thing for specific classes of people, that is, when it concerns the work of peasants and artisans. On the other hand, in practical terms, exercise is only recommended in combination with various precautionary measures. Frank systematically imposes restrictions on exercise. Gender is clearly the most important dividing line, next comes age, since for 'children' in particular, mainly boys, age-specific precautions are recommended. In the case of young women above all additional dangers are pointed out. Adults beyond their mid-twenties are of virtually no interest at all. Nor do the times of day (after meals) or of the year (summer/winter) play a significant role. So this is a sort of 'light' dietetics.

Samples from Witness Statements

For a better assessment of how the ideas articulated by Frank were disseminated I should like to present some random samples from the digitalised corpus of the 'Deutsche Autobiographien 1690–1930'.[42] The subtitle of the collection announces texts by 'workers, scholars, engineers, artists, politicians and writers'. Consequently, the literate higher classes are also over-represented here. By using various relevant search terms I have looked at almost 60 per cent of the corpus (up to 'Lehmann'); if the number of hits was not much more than 500, I have looked at the entire corpus of about 70,000 pages. This assessment should also point the way to other research possibilities.

---

[41]   Johann Bernhard Basedow, *Elementarwerk mit den Kupfertafeln Chodowieckis et al.* (1774), ed. T. Fritzsch (3 vols, Leipzig, 1909), vol. 1, p. 185, quoted from Henner, *Quellen*, p. 136.

[42]   Oliver Simons (ed.), *Deutsche Autobiographien 1690–1930, Digitale Bibliothek* (Berlin, 2004).

The first result is a certain disillusionment about the semantic scope of some of the concepts: basically every conceivable thing is 'practised': attraction, friendship, jurisdiction or rights, deadly seriousness, hospitality, devilment – and apart from that, generally an instrument or a language – but exercise, by contrast, far less often. The earliest use of the term in connection with climbing trees is by Amalia Schoppe, born in 1791 – a girl! – and with sporting activity in the present-day sense by Kügelgen, born in 1802.[43]

The search term 'ball' mostly leads to the sort of ball where you dance. Verbs in the past tense prove to give quite good access, although people ran and rode constantly – like we drive cars – without any obvious reference to our topic. Of course, members of the lower classes run a good deal – specifically alongside the coaches, which is at least an indication that exercise was integrated into their daily lives, something that would please any preventative medical practitioner today. Otherwise people occasionally jumped up from a chair, or from something else, but none of the 865 cases give any reference to long jump.

Naturally the search term 'horizontal bar' gives fewer, though more precise results, the first, incidentally, from Immermann, born in 1796, who during his youth reports on gymnastics instructor Jahn.[44] Quite some time later comes a medically interesting reference to horizontal bar exercises as a cure for masturbation, given by the labourer Bromme, born in 1873.[45] Apart from that, we learn that in the gardens of some bourgeois houses in the second half of the nineteenth century horizontal bars were erected; sometimes they had already been set up between the doors of the rooms inside.[46] While Hufeland (1762–1838), later to become a famous dietician, was still in his youth 'the young people of the family ... met in the garden or for walks on Sunday afternoons'. And there they would 'do gymnastics, play ball, have war games, and in winter especially would stage comedies in small theatres with self-made figures'.[47] So in the 1770s people largely managed without equipment, but still enjoyed exercise.

---

[43] Simons, *Deutsche Autobiographien*, p. 61247 (Amalia Schoppe, *Erinnerungen aus meinem Leben in kleinen Bildern* (2 vols, Altona, 1838), vol. 2, p. 122). Simons, *Deutsche Autobiographien*, pp. 41159, 41295 (Wilhelm von Kügelgen, *Jugenderinnerungen eines alten Mannes* (6th edn, Leipzig, 1959), pp. 306, 374.

[44] Simons, *Deutsche Autobiographien*, p. 37724 (Karl Immermann, *Memorabilien* (München, 1966), p. 159).

[45] Gudrun Piller, *Private Körper. Spuren des Leibes in Selbstzeugnissen des 18. Jahrhunderts* (Cologne, 2007), p. 60.

[46] Simons, *Deutsche Autobiographien*, p. 18760 (Karl Deussen, *Mein Leben* (Leipzig, 1922), p. 54).

[47] Simons, *Deutsche Autobiographien*, p. 35180 (Christoph Wilhelm Hufeland, *Selbstbiographie* (Berlin, 1863), pp. 30–31: 'sonntags nachmittags ... die jungen Leute der Familien, welche auch Hofmeister hatten ... im Sommer im Garten oder auf Spaziergängen',

In the first third of the nineteenth century Immermann (1796–1840) criticised the supposed ability of gymnastics to make boys into men, and in this he strongly opposed Frank's view: 'Why tell the young boys of proud things from which those immature human beings will only receive the illusion that they will become men of sterling qualities by doing exercise at jungle gym and vaulting horse and that self-reliance will only be accomplished at the *Ger* and horizontal bar.'[48] How many other criticisms of this sort are to be found later is something that still needs to be investigated. In any case Kügelgen tells us about a certain outcry caused by gymnastic activities amongst the citizens of Bernburg because the young men went about it all too forcefully and too obviously.[49]

We could also give ourselves the dubious pleasure of investigating whether or not all Johann Peter Frank's good advice was actually followed. What emerges, of course, is that the wildest and most dangerous tobogganing was still undertaken and that six-year-old boys, like the future painter Karl Blaas (1815–1894) continued to be put on horses, thereby experiencing their greatest childhood pleasure, while the strict doctor would have complained about the dangers on public thoroughfares.[50] This otherwise rather questionable methodology would nonetheless remind us that the normative texts should not be taken too seriously.

For the 1830s Gustav Freytag (1816–1895) tells us about the confidence-building from his time in the army and the value of exercise: 'In bayonet fencing

---

'[da wurde] geturnt, Ball geschlagen, Krieg gespielt, im Winter besonders auf kleinen Theatern mit selbstverfertigten Figuren Komödien aufgeführt').

His recommendations for physical exercise in the chapter of the same name in Christoph Wilhelm Hufeland, *Makrobiotik* (Stuttgart, 1958; original edn 1796), pp. 205–6, aim at one hour a day in the fresh air – though not shortly before a meal and up to three to four hours after it – and never 'to the point of heavy sweating'. For an example of the public 'infrastructure' for exercise see Gerhard Grasmann, 'Körperübungen im Lebensvollzug von Kindern und Jugendlichen im 19. Jahrhundert. Dargestellt am Beispiel der Hansestadt Stralsund', in Werner Buchholz (ed.), *Kindheit und Jugend in der Neuzeit 1500–1900* (Stuttgart, 2000), pp. 281–94.

⁴⁸   Simons, *Deutsche Autobiographien*, p. 37724 (Immermann, *Memorabilien*, p. 159): 'Warum dem jungen Stolze Dinge sagen, aus denen unreife Menschen abnehmen mußten, sie würden zwischen Kletterbaum und Springpferd Kerle von ganz besonderem Korn und Schrot, aus denen sie die Einbildung schöpften, nur an Ger und Reck werde die echte Selbstständigkeit herangepflegt?'

⁴⁹   Simons, *Deutsche Autobiographien*, p. 41181 (Kügelgen, *Jugenderinnerungen*, p. 317).

⁵⁰   Simons, *Deutsche Autobiographien*, p. 8948 (Karl Blaas, *Selbstbiographie des Malers Karl Blaas. 1815–1875* (Vienna, 1876), pp. 5–6): 'The house was no longer the same one in which I was born, and in 1821 we moved again. When we moved in my older brother Franz put the horse in front of the furniture van, I rode for the first time and left the house in jubilation, something that I will always remember.' For leg-breaking while skiing see Simons, *Deutsche Autobiographien*, p. 8958 (Blaas, *Selbstbiographie*, p. 13).

I charged and jumped around every opponent and noticed that this gymnastic exercise could be of lasting use to me.'[51] Admittedly we know that such insights are often ignored in later practice, but still the positive connection between military drill and gymnastics is posited here, something I have never noticed in earlier soldiers' sources.[52] Otherwise, as one would expect, gymnasia and student clubs are mentioned as institutions in which gymnastics, fencing and training took place.

Until motorisation, riding was a banal practice. Nonetheless in the 1840s Theodor Fontane (1819–1898) makes an attempt to find riding therapeutic. He writes of an acquaintance: 'He rode a lot, for the sake of his health, and when I met him in the *Tiergarten* I rode along with him for a while and let him tell me about it.'[53] In retrospect, during the last third of the nineteenth century riding was also a suitable means of self-stylisation for emancipated women. Thus the Prussian general's daughter and future socialist Lily Braun (1865–1916) reports how correctly she and the coachman sat up straight on the horse in the afternoons. For in actual fact the coachman was only supposed to be with 'the lady' when she came to the stable in the mornings and – without paternal supervision! – rode through the village, admired by all the peasant children.[54] And behind this successful woman too was an encouraging father: 'Mama thought I was at work, my father was riding through the woods with my little sister as he once did with me.'[55] As today, more strenuous or dangerous forms of exercise were facilitated by the fathers, behind the backs of the somewhat more cautious mothers.[56]

---

[51] Simons, *Deutsche Autobiographien*, p. 24077 (Gustav Freytag, *Erinnerungen aus meinem Leben*, Gesammelte Werke (16 vols, 2. Reihe, Leipzig, n.d.), vol. 8, p. 518): 'Ich chargierte und sprang im Bajonettfechten jedem Feinde verderblich umher, und merkte, daß diese Turnübung für mich von dauerndem Nutzen sein könne.'

[52] See also Martin Dinges, 'Soldatenkörper in der Frühen Neuzeit – Erfahrungen mit einem unzureichend geschützten, formierten und verletzten Körper in Selbstzeugnissen', in Richard van Dülmen (ed.), *Körpergeschichten* (Frankfurt M., 1996), pp. 71–98. A later example in Nicole Schweig, *Gesundheitsverhalten von Männern: Gesundheit und Krankheit in Briefen 1800–1950* (Stuttgart, 2009), p. 75.

[53] Simons, *Deutsche Autobiographien*, p. 22932 (Theodor Fontane, *Von Zwanzig bis Dreißig* (new edn, 25 vols, Munich, 1967), vol. 15, p. 268): 'Er ritt viel, von Kur wegen, und wenn ich ihn im Tiergarten traf, ging ich eine Strecke neben ihm her und ließ mir von ihm erzählen.'

[54] Simons, *Deutsche Autobiographien*, p. 11829 (Lily Braun, *Memoiren einer Sozialistin*, Gesammelte Werke (5 vols, Berlin, 1922), vol. 2, p. 43).

[55] Simons, *Deutsche Autobiographien*, p. 12351 (Braun, *Memoiren*, p. 409): 'Mama glaubte mich bei der Arbeit, der Vater ritt mit dem Schwesterchen durch die Wälder, wie einst mit mir.'

[56] Horst Petri, *Väter sind anders. Die Bedeutung der Vaterrolle für den Mann* (Stuttgart, 2004), pp. 74–6.

Karl Friedrich Burdach (1776–1847), future professor of medicine, points us to another agent of socialisation, namely the peer group. As we know, in today's sociology of boys, 'serious competitive games', not without their dangers, very much attract the attention of research.[57] The future professor of medicine Burdach says of his time as a student: 'I was no swot: I fenced, rode and danced, admittedly only moderately well, but adequately, in order to have fun and not to be left behind entirely by my peers.'[58] On the other hand, little girls were put off dangerous games as early as possible, as the laddish socialist Braun reports: 'If I played nicely with a ball and hoop without crawling into the bushes, then Mademoiselle praised me: "Comme elle devient raisonnable!", she said.'[59]

Dietetics of everyday life can be written most easily about going for walks, something that appears almost 1,800 times: times of the year and day, seasonal regularities, expectations of the effect on digestion and many other things can easily be put together from the source corpus.[60] And for the time around 1700 too there are already differentiated findings, so that the previously preferred view of going for walks as a bourgeois practice can be put aside. Indeed, the most explicit reference to salutogenesis comes from a very early testimony. The Leipzig Pietist Adam Bernd (1676–1748) who also reflected theoretically about body and soul, said: 'I was so happy that I no longer had to go walking in this village or the other for the sake of my health, but could do it in one place.'[61]

---

[57]   Gabriele Klein and Michael Meuser, 'It's a Men's World: ernste Spiele männlicher Vergemeinschaftung', in Michael Meuser (ed.), *Ernste Spiele: zur politischen Soziologie des Fußballs* (Bielefeld, 2008), pp. 113–34.

[58]   Simons, *Deutsche Autobiographien*, p. 14669 (Karl-Friedrich Burdach, *Rückblick auf mein Leben* (Leipzig, 1848), p. 56): 'Dabei war ich kein Stubenhocker: ich focht, ritt und tanzte, zwar Alles nur mittelmäßig, aber hinreichend, um mir Vergnügen zu machen und hinter meinen Commilitonen nicht ganz zurück zu bleiben.'

[59]   Simons, *Deutsche Autobiographien*, p. 11796 (Braun, *Memoiren*, p. 20): 'Spielte ich dann artig mit Ball und Reifen, ohne in die Büsche zu kriechen, dann lobte mich Mademoiselle: "Comme elle devient raisonnable!" sagte sie.' See also Jürgen Baur, Ulrike Burrmann and Katharina Krysmanski, *Sportpartizipation von Mädchen und jungen Frauen in ländlichen Regionen* (Cologne, 2002), p. 41: Girls are taught to practise reserved, 'sensible' physical activities while boys are encouraged to practise 'vigorous' physical activities which involve lots of movement and spatial exploration. So girls are prepared to practise moderate exercise while boys are encouraged to practise competitive sports. These embedded preferences are backed by the example of the peers and society in general. This statement is relativised on p. 42. Similar historical evidence in personal testimonies can be found in Susanne Hoffmann, *Gesunder Alltag im 20. Jahrhundert? Geschlechterspezifische Diskurse und gesundheitsrelevante Verhaltensstile in deutschsprachigen Ländern* (Stuttgart, 2010), pp. 217–18, 229.

[60]   See also Gudrun M. König, *Eine Kulturgeschichte des Spazierganges* (Vienna, 1996).

[61]   Simons, *Deutsche Autobiographien*, p. 6064 (Adam Bernd, *Eigene Lebens-Beschreibung* (Munich, 1973), pp. 362, 61: 'Ich hatte eine rechte Freude, daß ich nun nicht

Previously he had described his daily speed-walks as a 16-year-old, which in 1692 were certainly supposed to promote religious self-discovery. Later he also supported medical opinions and advised melancholics:

> to do moderate exercise and go for walks, and to keep going until you work up an adequate sweat, by sweating them away the evil and superfluous fluids in the body and the thick blood are thinned, the dark and weak thoughts made strong, so that it will seem to you as if you were new-born, have been given hope, heart and happiness, and will wonder where the horrible thoughts disappeared which plagued you just a short time before.[62]

And do we really have to read Johann Wolfgang Goethe (1749–1832) to get the impression that nurses and maids liked to go for walks?[63]

Unfortunately, as far as swimming goes we only hear about record-breaking, like crossing Lake Constance at its widest point, or Leopold von Sacher-Masoch's (1836–1895) complacent assertion: 'That I, as a young Gentleman, did a lot of swimming, riding fencing and gymnastics goes without saying.'[64]

Summary

The testimonies about types of exercise have led us from the pietist self-doubter to the person who gave masochism its name. Nonetheless, we cannot seriously imagine that between 1700 and 1870 exercise mutated from a religiously

---

immer bald auf dieses, bald auf jenes Dorf Gesundheits halber spazieren gehen, oder fahren durfte, sondern nur bei einem Ort allein es bewenden lassen könnte.'

[62] Simons, *Deutsche Autobiographien*, p. 5727 (Bernd, *Lebens-Beschreibung*, p. 198): ' mäßige Bewegung und Spazier-Gang vornehmen, und so lange damit anhalten, bis ein zulänglicher Schweiß erfolget, so wird durch das Wegschwitzen der bösen und überflüssigen Feuchtigkeiten im Leibe gleichwie das dicke Blut verdünnet, also das finstere, und schwache Haupt heiter und stark gemacht, daß es ihnen auf eine Zeit ist, als wären sie neu geboren, Hoffnung, Herze, und frohen Mut bekommen, und sich wundern müssen, wo die schrecklichen Gedanken hin verschwunden, die sie nur kurz zuvor noch geplaget'.

[63] Simons, *Deutsche Autobiographien*, p. 26749 (Johann Wolfgang Goethe, *Aus meinem Leben. Dichtung und Wahrheit*, Hamburger Ausgabe (14 vols, Hamburg, 1948ff.), vol. 9, p. 27).

[64] Simons, *Deutsche Autobiographien*, p. 57506 (Leopold von Sacher-Masoch, 'Eine Autobiographie', *Deutsche Monatsblätter. Centralorgan für das literarische Leben der Gegenwart*, 2/3 (Bremen, June 1879): pp. 259–69, here p. 262): 'Daß ich viel schwamm, ritt, focht und turnte, versteht sich bei einem jungen Gentleman von selbst.'

motivated activity to a purely physical one.[65] In fact, the testimonies illustrate very well the diffusion process of gymnastic exercises, while references to earlier practices are sadly rather few and far between if one is looking for a connection with health, at least an implicit one. And the positive assessment of exercise seems to prevail over other dietetic constraints. On the other hand it is far more difficult to designate statements about exercise in everyday life in terms of their relevance to health since motus is generally mentioned without comment.[66]

Before the nineteenth century the gender-specific aspects of certain types of exercise seem to me to be less explicit. Nonetheless, the student practice of a nightly 'walk', which served, amongst other things, to mark the public space, would illustrate very well, of course, the context of gender-specific socialisation and exercise – but for this other sources would have to be used.[67]

Otherwise the autobiographies also demonstrate that types of exercise are only recorded up to about the age of 25 – with the exception of a few references to riding out, though health factors are mentioned less and less here.[68] On the other hand, a representative corpus of correspondence by men examined by Schweig shows that middle-aged married men in particular valued going for walks as a health measure very highly in the mid-nineteenth century.[69] And even for young singles going for a walk was still the quintessence of exercise and balance until 1900, whether labourer or industrial worker. By contrast gymnastics and speed-walking are not mentioned until after 1900, sporting activities not until the Weimar period.[70] This warns us once again not to over-estimate physical exercise.

In order to learn more about the role of exercise and its significance in the lives of certain people a detailed analysis of individual autobiographies would be needed. But in any case the normative and autobiographical discourses complement and relativise one another to such a high degree that the possibilities of both types of source should be used to the full.

---

[65]   See Jacques Gleyse, 'Gymnastik als Gestaltung des Körpers in der Frühen Neuzeit: Diskurse, Praktiken oder Transgressionen?', in Rebekka v. Mallinckrodt (ed.), *Bewegtes Leben, Körpertechniken in der Frühen Neuzeit* (Wolfenbüttel, 2008), pp. 125–42. See also Werner Körbs, *Vom Sinn der Leibesübungen zur Zeit der italienischen Renaissance* (2nd edn, Munich, 1988; original edn Berlin, 1938), pp. 137–40.

[66]   See the views of Ulrich Bräker in Susanne Hoffmann, *Gesundheit und Krankheit bei Ulrich Bräker (1735–1798)* (Dietikon, 2005), S. 84–5.

[67]   Barbara Krug-Richter, '"Gassatum gehen". Der Spaziergang in der studentischen Kultur der Frühen Neuzeit', *Jahrbuch für Universitätsgeschichte*, 9 (2006): pp. 35–50.

[68]   Jens Lachmund and Gunnar Stollberg, *Patientenwelten: Krankheit und Medizin vom späten 18. bis zum frühen 20. Jahrhundert im Spiegel von Autobiographien* (Opladen, 1995), p. 224.

[69]   Schweig, *Gesundheitsverhalten*, pp. 129–30.

[70]   Schweig, *Gesundheitsverhalten*, p. 132. For the sporting generations see Hoffmann, *Alltag*, p. 189.

PART IV
Enhancing or Endangering Status and Identity?

Chapter 10

Masculine and Political Identity in German Martial Sports

B. Ann Tlusty

Introduction

In his sixteenth-century narrative poem *The Lucky Ship from Zurich*, Johann Fischart described the triumphant arrival of a group of 54 Swiss marksmen at a shooting match in Strasbourg after managing to sail from their home in Zurich in only 19 hours. In order to prove their feat, the Swiss shooters, dressed in their hometown livery, brought with them a great pot of porridge cooked in Zurich that they kept warm until their arrival in Strasbourg. Fischart, who himself claimed to have attended the 1576 match, characterized this display of perseverance and masculine skill in the pursuit of friendly intercity competition as an illustration of civic virtue. In fact, the political overtones of the poem (which in its full version includes hints at bitter rivalry as well as expressions of friendship and good neighbourly relations) completely eclipse the match itself, which Fischart does not actually describe.[1]

As suggested by Fischart's poem, shooting matches and other martial sports competitions served a variety of political functions. Not only did they help to cement diplomatic ties between friendly states, but they could also diffuse political tension between rivals by providing an opportunity for non-threatening competition and displays of hospitable goodwill. Large shooting matches were often organized specifically with an aim of normalizing relations after periods of tension or as a backdrop for courting allies. Conversely, misunderstandings or social slights at these events could also lead to diplomatic breakdowns and even feuds.[2]

At the same time, by encouraging ownership of firearms and skilled swordplay, martial sports contributed to early modern associations of weapons with masculine values such as physical competence, financial strength and fair play, all understood as elements of civic virtue. This chapter will trace the rise

---

[1]   Johann Fischart, *Das glückhafft Schiff von Zürich* (Strasbourg, 1576).
[2]   August Edelmann, *Schützenwesen und Schützenfeste der deutschen Städte vom 13. bis zum 18. Jahrhundert* (Munich, 1890), pp. 67, 112–18.

and fall of state-sponsored martial sporting events over the course of the early modern period, concentrating on their relationship to masculine and political identity in the German cities.

A cornerstone of the performance of masculinity was readiness to face risk in the public arena. This included not only being willing to defend and protect oneself, one's household, and one's neighbourhood and city when threatened, but also risking defeat in contests of skill and chance. Martial sports provided opportunities to elevate individual and communal reputations through peaceful competition in the arts considered necessary for war without actually risking life and limb. Aside from serving as collective training camps for wartime skills,[3] martial competitions also encouraged the purchase of weaponry needed to bolster local defence systems. In a world in which those in control often viewed leisure activities as suspect, representing idleness, frivolity and disorder, martial sports were thus an exception, supported by local authorities as a form of political leisure.

Men, Arms and the Martial Ethic

The weapons culture that flourished throughout the German-speaking lands during the early modern period was embedded in the layered power structures characterizing the Holy Roman Empire. In theory, the community of independent households that made up a neighbourhood, a village or a town also equated to a military unit that represented the power and autonomy of the individual entities making up the Empire. Each of these political bodies, or estates (i.e. princely and ducal territories, free imperial cities, etc.) understood their right to protect themselves from incursion by outside powers in terms of the right to resist (*Widerstandsrecht*), which also embodied the right of resort to arms.

In order to protect this right, city and town governments throughout the empire required all male householders to keep arms and stand ready to bear them if required to do so by their government. Socialization to the martial role thus began at the level of the household, itself a kind of defence unit with its own chain of command under the governance of the householder. The householders were in turn subject to the command of local guard captains. Rulers naturally understood these local militias not as a counter to local power, but as an expression of it. To put it in Hobbesian terms, armed citizens embodied the

---

³   As did nearly all early modern sports, if not always as directly. Gregory M. Colón Semenza, 'Sport, War, and Contest in Shakespeare's Henry VI', *Renaissance Quarterly*, 54/4 (Winter, 2001): pp. 1251–72, here p. 1251.

arms of the body politic. As such, they were subject to rule by the 'head' (ruler) that they had taken an oath to serve and protect.

Tension arose out of the fact that the freedom to keep and bear arms in defence of one's community, in the name of authority, also implied freedom to defend oneself. According to custom, defending oneself included defending one's name and one's honour, a principle that also made it into some early modern law codes.[4] These rights, however, could easily come into conflict with the authority of lawmaking bodies, whose decrees repeatedly demanded that men turn to the courts to handle disputes rather than settling them privately through resort to arms in personal duels.[5] But even among lawmakers, a conflict of interest was inevitable, since concern with protecting the right of resistance was not limited to free citizens claiming the right to self-justice. This goal was also shared by the town leaders responsible for enforcing laws, who themselves struggled to protect their own sovereignty against the growing power of territorial princes. The princes, in turn, manoeuvred to defend their autonomy from the Emperor. Facing death in a duel thus became more than a matter of personal honour. It was an expression of the German ideal of a free citizen and a microcosm of the right of the estates to resist tyranny by force of arms.

For this reason, resort to arms in defence of honour was widely tolerated by the courts in spite of the many laws against duelling that appeared throughout the early modern period. This was as true of private duels among townspeople as it was of swordplay among the nobility. After all, good fighters made good soldiers, and as any student of Machiavelli knew, good soldiers made good townsmen. Military virtues such as martial courage, respect for the rules of honour and fraternal identity, militia theorists argued, would naturally translate into the civic virtues necessary to good citizenship.[6]

Good townsmen, then, were armed, some of them heavily.[7] So in turn were the towns they were bound to protect. By the fifteenth century, towns were

---

[4] E.g. the *Carolina*: Charles V, *Constitutio Criminalis Carolina (Peinliche Halßgerichts Ordnung)* (Frankfurt, 1565), 40r.
[5] Stefan Brüdermann, *Göttinger Studenten und akademische Gerichtsbarkeit im 18. Jahrhundert* (Göttingen, 1990), p. 170; Roger Manning, *Swordsmen: The Martial Ethos in the Three Kingdoms* (Oxford, 2003), p. 218.
[6] Niccolò Machiavelli, *The Art of War*, trans., ed. and with a commentary by Christopher Lynch (Chicago, 2003), pp. 19–25, 243–57; John Pocock, *The Machiavellian Moment: Florentine Political Thought and the Atlantic Republican Tradition* (Princeton, 2003), pp. 201–2.
[7] One Augsburg household in 1645 reported possession of 300 muskets: Jürgen Kraus, *Das Militärwesen der Reichsstadt Augsburg 1548 bis 1806* (Augsburg, 1980), p. 85; other wealthier citizens kept enough weapons to outfit a company of men, some maintaining their own armoury rooms filled with finely decorated suits of armour and gilded and jewelled swords and knives: Hauptstaatsarchiv Stuttgart (HSAS), C3 RKG Bü 418, 423, 675, 3557;

stockpiling weapons in civic armouries in order to ensure sufficient capability for defence, with both citizenship and guild membership sometimes linked to providing weapons and armour for the armoury. The armoury provided a means of arming the poorer members of the citizenry in case of emergencies, while also ensuring that the government was at least as well armed as its people.[8] At the same time, armouries could serve a representative function as symbols of local power and prestige. This was also true of ceremonial events such as military musters, receptions for visiting dignitaries, and even processions attending elite weddings and holiday celebrations, all of which provided an opportunity for local householders to appear in force and dressed up in their required arms and armour.

These public displays of wealth and military commitment, town leaders believed, enhanced the reputations of local governments, fostered community pride, and encouraged a martial identity among their citizens. This was equally true of participation in martial sports. Especially during the sixteenth century, towns and courts throughout Germany competed with one another not only to produce the best swordsmen and marksmen, but also to provide the most elaborate forms of hospitality in hosting martial sports competitions. The largest of these also provided opportunities for full military musters and parades of citizens displaying their martial readiness.

Sword Fighting and the Culture of the Sword

The most enduring symbol of martial identity in the European tradition was the sword. Associated during the late Middle Ages primarily with the nobility, whose role in theory was to protect and defend, wearing a sword by the sixteenth century had come to represent masculine autonomy and civic freedom for German men. But a sword at a man's side was more than a symbol of his status as a free citizen. It also functioned as a public marker of his willingness to face risk in the name of honour and reputation, since it implied that the bearer was willing to use it to protect his name. This, if done honourably, also meant facing the point of the sword of an adversary. Because this public expression

---

Stadtarchiv Memmingen (STAM), A 086/07; A 134/14; Stadtarchiv Augsburg (StAA), Spreng'sches Notariatsarchiv 1568–1594.

[8]   Karl Saur, *Die Wehrverfassung in schwäbischen Städten des Mittelalters (Strassburg, Basel, Augsburg, Ulm, Rottweil, Überlingen, Villingen)* (Bühl, 1911), pp. 7–8, 79; Otto Mörtzsch, 'Das wehrhafte Freiberg im Mittelalter', *Zeitschrift für historische Waffenkunde* (*ZHW*), 7 (1915–17): pp. 216–24, here p. 217; Michael Kaiser, 'Bürgermilitär', in Michael Diefenbacher and Rudolf Endres (eds), *Stadtlexikon Nürnberg* (Nürnberg, 2000), p. 170; Hartwig Neumann, *Das Zeughaus. Die Entwicklung eines Bautyps von der spätmittelalterlichen Rüstkammer zum Arsenal im deutschsprachigen Bereich* (Koblenz, 1991), p. 13.

of individual martial courage was so crucial to the performance of masculine identity, the side arm was an indispensable fashion accessory for early modern German townsmen, especially those of middling status and above. According to military musters, nearly all early modern German householders kept one or more swords in their homes, and countless sources including court testimony, illustrated broadsheets, chronicle illuminations, and other works of art provide overwhelming evidence that few adult townsmen except those at the very lowest ranks were willing to walk the streets without at least some kind of a blade at their sides.

Among artisans as well as aristocrats, then, swords were ready at hand. For this reason, swords were the weapon of choice for most men during the early modern period for fighting duels of honour, whether they occurred spontaneously in the streets or in accordance with formal military and aristocratic tradition. During the sixteenth century, when the concept of the duel was still influenced by late medieval traditions of judicial duelling, honour was best restored by winning the fight. Skill with a sword was thus understood as a masculine virtue, creating a market for training in the form of competitive sports.

Studies of the German sword-fighting tradition normally begin with the techniques of the fourteenth-century sword master Johann Liechtenauer, whose style was preserved in 1389 in an illustrated text attributed to Hanko Döbringer. Liechtenauer's school formed the basis for most of the fencing manuals of the next two centuries, in Italy as well as Germany.[9] Although the richly illustrated sword-fighting manuals of the fourteenth and fifteenth centuries were often produced as a form of representational courtly art, the sword masters themselves came primarily from the burgher classes. Thus the art of sword-fighting was influenced early on by the strong guild culture of the German cities. Sword fighters in German towns began by the fifteenth century to organize as guild-like 'brotherhoods' in which men studied the sport under the hand of an established master sword-fighter. Like journeymen craftsmen, sword-fighting masters typically spent two to three years traveling both to learn and to teach their art in so-called 'Fencing schools' (*Fechtschulen*). These 'schools' were not permanent institutions, but public competitions or training sessions offered by a traveling swordsman.

---

[9]   Heidemarie Bodemer, *Das Fechtbuch. Untersuchungen zur Entwicklungsgeschichte der bildkünstlerischen Darstellung der Fechtkunst in den Fechtbüchern des mediterranen und westeuropäischen Raumes vom Mittelalter bis Ende des 18. Jahrhunderts* (PhD dissertation, University of Stuttgart, 2008), pp. 66, 102–9.

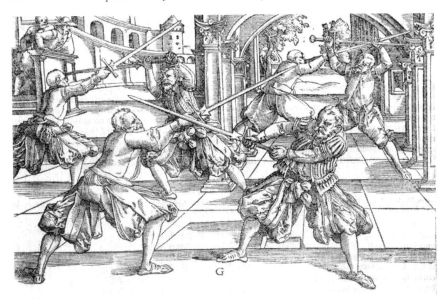

G

Figure 10.1 Long-sword fighting school. From Joachim Meyer's illustrated
fencing manual *Gründtliche Beschreibung der freyen Ritterlichen
vnnd Adelichen kunst des Fechtens*, Strassbourg, 1570, 32v

Source: By permission of the Bayerische Staatsbibliothek München, Res/4 Gymn. 26 t.

During the sixteenth century, two major fencing guilds came to dominate the
sword-fighting landscape in Germany. The older of these organizations was
generally known as the 'Marcus brothers' (*Marxbrüder*), a name that derived
from their traditional veneration of Saint Marcus. The *Marxbrüder* were centred
in Frankfurt and held their yearly master's examinations at Frankfurt's large
annual fair. A rival organization alternately known as 'free fencers' (*Freifechter*)
or 'feather fencers' (*Federfechter*) established their own fencing guild during the
1570s around a school that originated in Prague.[10] The masters of these two
schools spent the next century disputing both organizational points and sword-
fighting methods, regularly competing with one another to prove the superiority
of their respective approaches. At the same time, they also held joint fencing
schools and exhibitions, cooperated on requirements for achieving the status of

---

[10]   The origin of the name *Federfechter* is not clear: G. Liebe, 'Die Ausgänge des deutschen
Fechterwesens', *ZHW*, 6 (1912–14): pp. 134–7, here p. 134; Karl Wassmannsdorf, *Sechs
Fechtschulen der Marxbrüder und Federfechter aus den Jahren 1573 bis 1614* (Heidelberg,
1870), p. 8; Karl Lochner, *Die Entwicklungsphasen der europäischen Fechtkunst* (Vienna,
1953), p. 16.

master sword-fighter, and shared experts to act as examiners.[11] The rivalry was generally good-natured, but sometimes led to fights breaking out between fans of the rival schools. In this they were very much like modern sports clubs.

As guild-like associations, early modern sword-fighting schools were closer to sport clubs than to military organizations. In fact, critics of the sport argued that the continued emphasis on fighting with heavy long swords made them irrelevant to wartime readiness. By the sixteenth century, long swords were already on the decline as weapons of war, being replaced by lighter side arms that did not get in the way of the soldiers' primary functions as gunners or pikemen.[12] Increasingly, heavy fighting swords were replaced in local weapons inventories by light dress swords and rapiers introduced from Italy and France. German fencing masters initially condemned the new swords both due to their foreign origins and the style of fighting they introduced, which was based on cuts and jabs rather than 'manly' swings. But the new style persisted both in military and civilian life, for the long swords, pikes and shields that were standard equipment for the early fencing masters were also not practical for wearing on one's person as demanded by current fashion. By the later sixteenth century, fencing masters typically provided training in both older and newer sword-fighting styles.[13]

City leaders supported sword-fighting schools regardless of whether the styles they taught were directly applicable to war. In theory, fencing was a martial art, and as regularly argued by fencing masters, this most 'chivalrous' (*ritterlich*) of arts instilled men with all of the virtues of the martial ethic, including courage, strength and respect for fair fighting.[14] For this reason town councils provided space for the training sessions, sometimes also contributing funds to pay fencing masters' fees, wages for guards and musicians, and other expenses.[15]

Sword-fighting schools could be festive affairs, opening with parades and displays of weapons, accompanied by music and other entertainments, and concluding with hearty drinking bouts.[16] Larger competitions were sometimes arranged as part of wedding festivities or other celebrations, while more modest schools took place fairly regularly, in some years as often as every two to four

---

[11]   Lochner, *Die Entwicklungsphasen*, pp. 16–18; Stadtarchiv Nördlingen (StANö), R39F5/10, Fechtschule 1534–1618, c. 1600; Liebe, 'Die Ausgänge', p. 135.

[12]   Hans-Peter Hils, *Meister Johann Liechtenauers Kunst des langen Schwertes* (Frankfurt, 1985), pp. 9–11.

[13]   Joachim Meyer, *Gründliche Beschreibung / der freyen Ritterlichen vnd Adelichen Kunst des Fechtens* (Augsburg, 1600), 50r; Markku Peltonen, *The Duel in Early Modern England: Civility, Politeness, and Honour* (Cambridge, 2003), pp. 61–4.

[14]   For numerous expressions by sword-fighting masters of the chivalric and military virtues of sword fighting see StANö, R39F5/10, Fechtschule 1534–1618.

[15]   Staats- und Stadtbibliothek Augsburg, 2°Cod.Aug.246, p. 53.

[16]   Fürstlich Oettingen-Wallersteinische Bibliothek an der Universitätsbibliothek Augsburg, Hs.I.6.2°5; Wassmannsdorf, *Sechs Fechtschulen*, pp. 9, 13–31.

weeks.[17] In the tradition of the late medieval masters whose methods were recorded in lavishly illustrated fencing manuals, expert sportsmen demonstrated their martial skills at these events not only by fighting with swords, but also with pikes, halberds, daggers and knives. To draw attention to the school and increase its entertainment value, larger sword-fighting competitions not only featured music and parades, but were sometimes also accompanied by theatrical sword dances.

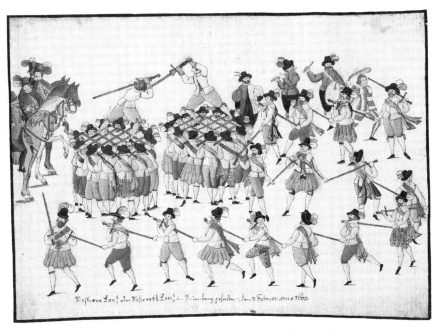

Figure 10.2 Sword dance in Nuremberg at Shrovetide, c. 1600

Source: By permission of the Germanisches Nationalmuseum, HB 3361 Kaps 1379.

Like sword-fighting schools, sword dances were a guild art, performed mainly by journeymen and the sons of local citizens.[18] Wearing bells on their clothes

[17] StANö, R39F5/10, Fechtschule 1534–1618, 1598; Dieter Meyer, *Literarische Hausbücher des 16. Jahrhunderts* (2 vols, Königshausen, 1989), vol. 1, pp. 435–49.

[18] Jean-Pierre Bodmer, *Aus Zürichs Bibliotheksgeschichte. Beiträge von 1964 bis 2007* (Zurich, 2007), p. 39; Walter Schaufelberger, *Der Wettkampf in der alten Eidgenossenschaft: Zur Kulturgeschichte des Sports vom 13. bis in das 18. Jahrhundert* (Bern, 1972), pp. 107–8; Stephen Corrsin, *Sword Dancing in Europe: A History* (Enfield Lock, 2005), pp. 10–11, 31–8; G. Liebe, 'Der Schwerttanz der deutschen Handwerker', *ZHW*, 3 (1902–5):

that jingled in time to the recurring sound of striking blades, sword dancers performed complicated synchronized steps that often included jumping or dancing over rows of swords to the rhythmic accompaniment of drums and fifes.

Although neither sword dancing nor, at least by the sixteenth century, long-sword fighting translated directly into military skills, both provided opportunities for public displays of masculine agility as well as martial identity and risk-taking. Long-sword fighting was a dangerous blood sport, so much so that it eventually drew criticism from theologians who accused fencers of fighting for the sake of spectacle and exploiting blood lust for income.[19] Sword dancing also played with themes of danger, including jumping over or handling sharp blades, fighting mock battles, and acting out stories of death and rebirth. Injuries were common in both sports, and sword-fighting schools could be deadly. Both of these artisan-dominated pursuits began to be attacked from elite quarters by the end of the sixteenth century as inappropriate, even 'uncivilized', entertainments.

All martial sports suffered during the difficult seventeenth century, especially during the decades of the Thirty Years War, which was fought by professional soldiers, not civic militias. As civic support for militias declined, the culture of the sword among the burgher and artisan classes also came under the scrutiny of town and territorial rulers, who launched a campaign during the latter seventeenth century to get swords out of the hands of commoners. Ostensibly, safety was their major concern, for particularly among the young journeymen, wearing swords led to 'all kinds of dangerous altercations, fights and swordplay in the streets', and at times even to homicide.[20] But the fact that restrictions on wearing swords ultimately appeared in sumptuary laws, which regulated appropriate clothing for persons of different social rank, rather than in police ordinances concerned with safety and violence suggest different motives among lawmakers. Sumptuary laws limited the wearing of dress swords first only to master craftsmen, then to those in upper-level trades, and finally only to men of the highest social ranks.

Meanwhile, as elite men took up the 'civilized' and less dangerous French sport of fencing with foils, the artisan-dominated sport of fighting with heavy swords declined into a shabby sideshow event taking place at markets, fairs and shooting matches. The contrast of foil fencing provided elites with an additional context for condemning common sword-fighting contests as coarse and

---

pp. 252–5, here p. 253; Hanns Bächtold-Stäubli, *Handwörterbuch des deutschen Aberglaubens* (10 vols, Berlin, 1927–42), vol. 7, pp. 1548–50; Eugen Mogk, 'Volkstümliche Bräuche der Vorfrühlingszeit im Wandel der Zeiten', *Niederdeutsche Zeitschrift für Volkskunde*, 7 (1929): pp. 143–52, here pp. 147–8.

[19] Zachäus Faber, *Antimonomachia* (Leipzig, 1625), F4r–v; Matthäus Krägelius, *Duellum & Bellum von Kampff vnd Krieg* (1644), pp. 49–51; Liebe, 'Die Ausgänge', p. 136.

[20] StAA, Polizeiwesen 54, Ordnungen, Degen tragen, Regensburg 1658; Nuremberg, 1709.

dangerous. Eventually the reputation of the traditional travelling masters of the long sword became so questionable that the German word *fechten* itself (which can be translated as 'fighting', but is most often understood as 'fencing' or 'sword fighting') came to be associated with vagrancy.[21] Sword dancing, meanwhile, re-emerged briefly after the Thirty Years War, but with more participation by military men than by journeymen. Then it, too, went into a permanent decline.[22]

It is no coincidence that the decline of sword sports among urban artisans neatly parallels the campaign by elites to monopolize the sword as fashion. By the mid-eighteenth century, wearing a sword had become a privilege only of military men, students and members of the patrician and noble classes. These shifts paralleled a general process of increasing segregation between civilian and military life.

Shooting Matches, Sportsmanship and Civic Identity

Although the sword was the natural choice for personal defence, military strength increasingly depended on projectile weaponry. The most elaborate of martial competitions during the early modern period were thus centred on the sport of shooting. By the fifteenth and especially the sixteenth centuries, both gun and crossbow shooting societies or clubs (*Schützengesellschaften*) were well-established in all the German towns, leading to a culture of peaceful martial competition that was played out at elaborate shooting matches. Nobles and patricians also hosted shooting matches at their private estates. At their zenith in the sixteenth century, these matches were among the grandest entertainments available to those of common status.

Shooting societies pre-dated guns, beginning as cross-bowmen's guilds in the twelfth or thirteenth centuries. From the beginning, they had no direct relationship to military institutions, but were created on the model of religious confraternities or brotherhoods, and later organized on the guild model. During the fourteenth and fifteenth centuries, as the political power of the artisans grew and guild masters gained seats in local councils, one city after another established permanent shooting grounds, maintained at civic expense, where townsmen could practice and compete.[23]

The competitions hosted by local shooting societies were of several different types. Most were limited to either crossbows or guns, although double matches

---

[21] Bodemer, *Das Fechtbuch*, p. 58; Liebe, 'Die Ausgänge', pp. 136–7; Jakob and Wilhelm Grimm, *Der Digitale Grimm: Deutsches Wörterbuch von Jakob und Wilhelm Grimm*, ed. Hans-Werner Bartz et al. (33 vols, Frankfurt, 2004), vol. 3, col.1387, 1.

[22] Corrsin, *Sword Dancing*, pp. 50–54; Liebe, 'Der Schwerttanz', pp. 252–3.

[23] Edelmann, *Schützenwesen*, p. 4.

including both kinds of competition were possible. Strictly local competitions for a few guldens' worth of prizes that served as training for the local shooting society could occur several times a year, even every weekend during the summer months. Some matches pitted only two neighbouring towns against one another in the spirit of friendly rivalry. At the other end of the scale were the large festive matches for which invitations could be sent to dozens of shooting clubs located throughout the empire and beyond. Open shoots (*Freischießen*) welcomed all comers, whereas Lord's matches (*Herrenschießen*) limited participation to those of privileged status. In Tyrol, only those with at least the status of master craftsmen could belong to a shooting society by the end of the seventeenth century.[24] Elite gun enthusiasts occasionally held private matches on their noble estates, inviting a closed circle of friends, although even these sometimes included invitations to civic councilmen to bring along a small group of talented marksmen from their local society, apparently without respect to rank.[25]

Preparations for the great shooting matches that dominated the early modern entertainment scene began months before the shoot, with the painting of targets, the construction of decorations in town colours, and the engagement of pewter-, silver- and goldsmiths to craft prizes and souvenirs.[26] The most impressive matches were lauded in verse in richly illustrated pamphlets and chronicles, providing both a literary and a visual record of the events. Some of these were created by artisan poets in the tradition of the Paddle-Master (*Pritschenmeister*). Paddle-Masters served the larger martial competitions as combination jesters, disciplinarians and poets, entertaining the crowd with clever rhymes and paddling those who broke minor rules or performed extremely badly with a special paddle called a *Pritsche*.[27] Afterwards, they celebrated the matches and their own antics in verse.[28]

Augmenting these literary descriptions are details provided in the hundreds of shooting competition invitations (*Schützenbriefe*) held in archives throughout Germany. Together, these sources describe lavish processions and great banquets

---

[24]   Max Radlkofer, 'Die Schützengesellschaften und Schützenfeste Augsburgs im 15. u. 16. Jahrhundert', *Zeitschrift des historischen Vereins für Schwaben*, 21 (1894): pp. 87–138, here 112–13; Otto Stolz, *Wehrverfassung und Schützenwesen in Tirol von den Anfängen bis 1918* (Innsbruck, 1960), p. 164.

[25]   StANö, R29F4 Schützengesellschaften, Schützenbriefe 1437–1802, Ansbach 1495.

[26]   Radlkofer, 'Die Schützengesellschaften': p. 99; StAA, Schützenakten, Fasc V, Schießgraben und Rosenau, Silber-, Zinn-, Kegel- u. andere Spiele, 1559–1807.

[27]   The *Pritsche* was made of two or more hinged boards designed to make a loud clap, which could serve to exaggerate the paddling or otherwise draw attention to the Paddle-Master's antics.

[28]   Some *Pritschenmeister* made a name for themselves as literary figures: Hans Rupprich, *Die deutsche Literatur vom späten Mittelalter bis zum Barock* (2 vols, Munich, 1973), vol. 2, pp. 245–7.

along with dances, music, lotteries, fireworks and other entertainments. For a small fee, participants and spectators at the matches could compete in a variety of sports and games of chance in addition to shooting, including races both on foot and on horseback, jumping and stone-throwing contests, bowling, jousting, wrestling and, of course, sword fights. The entrance fees for these events paid for prizes and helped offset the cost of other entertainments. The inevitable raffle or lottery, forerunners of later state-sponsored lotteries, could be an especially lucrative commercial enterprise.[29] According to Peter Opel's description of the daily raffle at a Regensburg match in 1586, a six-*kreuzer* ticket provided players a chance to win one of 244 prizes, the most valuable of them a serving dish worth 100 gulden. Lesser prizes ranged from swords and daggers decorated with silver to items more appropriate for women, such as pairs of scissors or a woman's belt. By selling a total of 32,290 tickets, the lottery took in 3,229 gulden, while the total cost of the prizes was only 1,494 gulden.[30]

While games, lotteries and other entertainments were open to spectators as well as shooters, only competing marksmen and local shooting society members took part in the banquets and drinking bouts that took place inside the Shooting House, a kind of private clubhouse located at the shooting grounds that catered to shooting society members and their guests. This privilege, too, came at a price. In order to compete in any public shooting match or belong to a local shooting society, one had to own a gun or a crossbow as well as to pay entrance fees. Entrance fees for shooting matches ranged from one to two gulden during the sixteenth century and rose to four gulden in the eighteenth. A good crossbow or a newly made gun was also not cheap, although the two- to four-gulden price of a simple musket during the first decades of the seventeenth century would not have been beyond the means of an average craftsman willing to sacrifice a week or two of his wages.[31] These expenses, then, would have been

---

[29] Ernst Freys, *Gedruckte Schützenbriefe des 15. Jahrhunderts* (Munich, 1912), p. 7; Gustav Freytag, *Bilder aus der deutschen Vergangenheit* (5 vols, Leipzig, 1891), vol. 4, 1700–1848, p. 343.

[30] Edelmann, *Schützenwesen*, pp. 128–54 (1 gulden = 60 kreuzer).

[31] Johann Schultze, 'Verteilung von Waffen unter die Untertanen des Stifts Fulda 1619/1620', *ZHW*, 7 (1915–17): pp. 22–5; P. Uhlig, 'Rüstungssorgen einer mittelalterlichen Stadt', *Zeitschrift für historische Waffen- und Kostümkunde*, 15 (1937–9): pp. 246–7; HSAS, C3 Bü 425, Q8. For context, see incomes for carpenters and day-labourers employed by the city of Augsburg in 1595 (about a gulden per week) and journeymen working for Nördlingen during the early seventeenth century (one to two gulden per week). Independent master craftsmen earned somewhat more: B. Ann Tlusty, *Augsburg during the Reformation Era: An Anthology of Sources* (Indianapolis, 2012), pp. 154–6; StANö, R29F4 Schützenmaister, Rechnung; UB 1612–40, 132. Joyce Malcolm came to a similar conclusion for seventeenth-century England: *To Keep and Bear Arms: The Origins of an Anglo-American Right* (Cambridge, MA, 1994), pp. 83–4.

affordable to most artisans of middling status or above, but discouraging to those lower on the economic scale. Because fiscal health was also a masculine value, participation in a shooting match could therefore serve a representative function. The chance to mix public displays of martial skills with conspicuous consumption undoubtedly upped the social capital to be gained by gun and crossbow ownership among townsmen.

As gun technology improved, gunpowder weapons began to replace crossbows in the hands of city guards, in the homes of artisan householders, and in the plans of military theorists. This also affected the choices of marksmen at sporting contests. To be sure, during the fifteenth century and at least the first decades of the sixteenth, crossbows were still at least as useful in battle as the primitive hand guns then available. But gunpowder weapons were already appearing in civic muster lists by the late fourteenth century and they caught on quickly, outnumbering crossbows among ordinary citizens a century later.[32] During the sixteenth century, between about 10 per cent and 35 per cent of German households kept one or more firearms in their homes; this increased to 50 per cent or more during the early decades of the seventeenth century. By this time crossbows were no longer of interest to town captains, who did not include them on muster lists.[33]

Nonetheless, crossbows remained popular for sport shooting throughout the early modern period. Dedicated crossbow aficionados even argued that theirs was the more chivalrous sport, branding guns as cowardly and inferior for competition.[34] It is perhaps for this reason that crossbow matches gradually came to be dominated by a more privileged class of shooters. Competition with guns remained primarily a burgher sport throughout this period, while crossbow matches, viewed increasingly as purely for entertainment and less and less as military training, wound up as an elite amusement.

Despite some setbacks in weapons ownership caused by the fortunes of war (i.e. disarmament by rival powers, plunder by marauding soldiers and economic hardship), gun ownership among ordinary townsmen continued to rise over the course of the seventeenth century, while the numbers of swords and pole arms

---

[32]   Kraus, *Das Militärwesen*, p. 88; Wendelin Boeheim, *Handbuch der Waffenkunde. Das Waffenwesen in seiner historischen Entwicklung vom Beginn des Mittelalters bis zum Ende des 18. Jahrhunderts* (Leipzig, 1890), p. 445; Rolf Kießling, *Die Stadt und ihr Land. Umlandpolitik, Bürgerbesitz und Wirtschaftsgefüge in Ostschwaben vom 14. bis ins 16. Jahrhundert* (Cologne, 1989), pp. 26, 627; STAM, II L a1; StANö, Verzeichnisse des Kriegsvolks, Rottirung Register, 1488.

[33]   B. Ann Tlusty, *The Martial Ethic in Early Modern Germany: Civic Duty and the Right of Arms* (Houndmills, 2011), pp. 135–45.

[34]   Stolz, *Wehrverfassung*, p. 159.

dropped.[35] In some towns, gun ownership became a requirement of citizenship during the first decades of the Thirty Years War. Nearly all cities were also encouraging local men to participate in regular target practice by this time, in some cases making it obligatory for at least a portion of the male population.[36]

Because prevailing notions of civic republicanism assumed a natural relationship between martial skill, defence duties and the civic virtues that bred good citizens, city governors who encouraged participation in shooting had greater goals in mind than merely training men to be good marksmen. Competitive shooting, they believed, could also serve as a school of masculine values by fostering martial honour and fair play. The goal of any public confrontation between men was to establish one's superiority over the adversary without resort to an unfair advantage. The peaceful world of martial sports was no exception to this nearly universal code of honour, for as is the case in other sports, carefully prescribed and standardized rules enhanced the value of winning.

Rules governing shooting matches thus emphasized sportsmanship and friendly competition, and sought to limit any form of antagonism among shooters. Fights and insults of all kinds were forbidden during the matches. Aiming a gun or a crossbow at a fellow shooter was considered an especially serious offence, not only due to the danger it posed to life and limb, but even more because such an action violated the atmosphere of brotherhood and mutual respect that shooting competitions were supposed to foster. Other angry gestures, such as throwing down a gun or drawing a knife, could result in expulsion from the shooting grounds and even forfeiture of one's gun. In some cities, men were asked to remove their swords before entering the shooting stand, a symbolic gesture of peace that had more in common with guild custom than with military tradition.[37]

---

[35] Tlusty, *Martial Ethic*, pp. 137–45; StANö, Kriminalakten, Melchior Aufschlager, 9 June 1581; StANö, Verzeichnisse des Kriegsvolks, Musterung 1615; StANö, Specificatio aller Lierhaimischen Vnderthanen vnd Haußgenoßen; Stadtarchiv Rothenburg, A164 (1583, copy from 1786).

[36] Cipriano Gaedechens, *Hamburgs Bürgerbewaffnung: Ein geschichtlicher Rückblick* (Leipzig, 1872), pp. 13–14; Herzog August Bibliothek (Wolfenbüttel), M: Gm 3920 (1), A1v; Universitätsbibliothek Johann Christian Senckenberg (Frankfurt), Ffm W 112 No. 3, Wachtordnung 1621, 7; Tlusty, *Martial Ethic*, pp. 204–5.

[37] StAA, Schützen-Akten VII, Frevel 1551–1804, Jörg Halbritter, 1560–3; StANö, R2F3 /1 Statuten vnnd Ordnungen 1553–1567, Schützen Ordnung 1557–87; R29F4 Schützengesellschaften, Schützenmaister 1675. Craftsmen were often expected to lay aside their swords during craft and guild meetings: Wolfgang Maria Schmid, 'Passauer Waffenwesen', *ZHW*, 8/10–11 (1918–1920): pp. 317–42, here p. 322; StAA, Zünfte 2, 304r–9v; Zünfte 3, 517r, 702r–4r; Zünfte 5, 16v–17r.

Other rules were simply aimed at levelling the playing field. Shooting was to be done standing, for example, without any kind of support. Each shooter had to fire his own gun, and to shoot alone, without help. Shooters also had the right to concentrate while in the stand without interference from spectators or taunting from other men. To ensure that each shooter had an opportunity to properly prepare for the match, invitations also typically described in detail the distance of the shooting stand from the target, the size of the target, the limit placed on the numbers of shots, etc.[38]

Punishment for cheating, fighting or other inappropriate behaviour was usually immediate and could be humiliating. Rather than referring such incidents to the local courts, as would have been the case if they occurred in the streets or in public houses, witnesses to bad behaviour at the shooting grounds needed only to inform the acting Shooting Master, who passed judgement on the spot. Shooting Masters received authority from city leaders to levy fines, confiscate guns and crossbows, and ban troublemakers from the shooting grounds. Minor infractions could lead to a public paddling from the Paddle-Master, a ritual gesture aimed at diffusing anger through jest. These rules served to promote communal identity and solidarity among the shooters by playing down social and economic difference and ensuring equal treatment.

Ordinances also forbade technological experiments that could give one shooter an advantage, such as firing with multiple or split bullets or using a nail in the stock to stabilize the trigger finger. Such rules became especially controversial with the introduction during the sixteenth century of rifled barrels. Initially, this new technology seemed simply unfair, for no shooter with a smooth-bore musket could compete with the more accurate rifle. As a result, many towns initially forbade rifles at shooting matches entirely.[39] Thus city leaders sometimes found themselves in the unusual position of discouraging use of the latest military technology in order to promote good sportsmanship. Because the rifled guns were expensive, making the decision to allow rifled barrels meant that the price of equal competition in a shooting match went up. Some towns experimented with separate competitions for those with rifled and

---

[38] Because no standard existed for units of measure, invitations often included real-size images of the target, as well as lines or even attached pieces of string to demonstrate local standards for measuring distance. Freys, *Gedruckte Schützenbriefe*; StAA, Schützen-Akten 1/3, 1567.

[39] Anne Braun, *Historische Zielscheiben: Kulturgeschichte europäischer Schützenvereine* (Gütersloh, 1981), p. 38; StAA, Ordnungen und Statuten, K18, no. 391, Ordnung vnd Gesatz der Erbarn Gesellschafft vonn Zil vnd Birsch Schutzenn 1562, 1570; Schützen-Akten VIII, Artikel und Ordnungen 1540–1832, 20 March 1574; STAM, A 296/02, 1562.

those with straight barrels; the result, of course, was the segregation of shooters based on their economic status.[40]

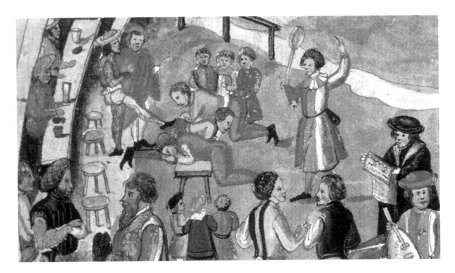

Figure 10.3 Paddle-Master paddling errant shooters, Augsburg, c. 1570–7. This detail from an illuminated manuscript commemorates a shooting match that took place a century before, in 1470

Source: By permission of the University Erlangen-Nürnberg Library, Ms. B 213, fol. 180v, probably commissioned by Landsknechtführer Sebastian Schertlin von Burtenbach.

As this example makes clear, although shooting match rules were aimed at promoting social levelling, brotherhood and fair play, both society membership and the right of participation in individual matches could be exclusive. Shooters had to be male and wealthy enough to own the right kind of gun or crossbow. Many smaller matches were limited to local residents, and some were restricted to those of elite status. Shooting matches could also be divided by religious confession by the later seventeenth century, although this was the exception rather than the rule.[41] The majority of shooting societies remained confessionally mixed throughout the early modern period, and invitations to larger matches

[40]   Anton Diemand, 'Zur Geschichte des Schützenwesens der Stadt Oettingen', *Historischer Verein für Nördlingen und Umgebung*, 6 (1917): pp. 1–18, here 11. Due to their expense, rifled barrels did not become standard military equipment until the nineteenth century.

[41]   Diemand, 'Zur Geschichte des Schützenwesens': p. 10. In bi-confessional cities, Catholics and Protestants shared power and were bound by law to tolerate one another's religious practice.

did not distinguish between Catholics and Protestants.[42] The general paucity of confessional issues arising in the records suggests that religious identity usually took a back seat to martial skill.

Larger matches in most cases also pit men of very different social status against one another in the spirit of fair competition. Shooting masters in taking their oath swore to preside without distinction over rich and poor as well as over both local and visiting marksmen. Rules also ensured that the presiding shooting masters came from a mixed social background, and were not dominated by elite members.[43] Although lords and nobles were undoubtedly given their due in terms of social respect, their status did not enter into the rules of play, for in theory, the only thing that mattered was who was the best shot. Nobles and craftsmen regularly competed against each other without preference. During a 1565 match in Prague, for example, Archduke Ferdinand of Austria, son of Emperor Ferdinand I, made a point of insisting on competing fairly against any and all comers, 'rich or poor'.[44] At a crossbow match in 1518, Emperor Maximilian was bested by a miller's son from the Swabian village of Gisslingen. And at the halfway mark during Augsburg's double crossbow and harquebus match of 1509, the young Duke of Bavaria Wilhelm IV, as one of 15 shooters who had not yet managed to hit the target at all, took a public paddling from the Paddle-Master apparently with goodwill, while the top prize for the competition went to a cabinet maker.[45]

Women, too, were a regular presence at shooting matches, as is evident by their inevitable appearance in images of shooting grounds, but their role was carefully proscribed. Women had joined men in shooting brotherhoods from their inception in the late Middle Ages as passive 'sisters' rather than active members, and prior to the Reformation, they occasionally joined in athletic events such as footraces.[46] Local girls from good families sometimes honoured the best marksmen by handing out prizes and dancing with the winners. Women

---

[42]   Greater segregation is evident at smaller matches, most likely due to regional confessional dominance more than any intentional efforts at religious isolation. Schaufelberger, *Der Wettkampf, pp.* 38–44; StAA, Schützen-Akten I, Augsburger Schießen 1554–1833; on mixed confessions at matches see also Wolfgang Behringer, 'Arena and Pall Mall: Sport in the Early Modern Period', *German History*, 27/3 (2009): pp. 331–57, here 345–6.

[43]   StANö, R2F3/2, Ayd Buch der Statt Nördlingen 1572; StAA, Schützen-Akten I (Stuttgart, 1560); Schützen-Akten VIII, Püchsenschützen wahl, 1570–1658.

[44]   'Er sey Reich oder Arm': Edelmann, *Schützenwesen*, p. 122.

[45]   Radlkofer, 'Die Schützengesellschaften': pp. 105–7, 110; see also Behringer, 'Arena', pp. 345–6.

[46]   Stadtbibliothek Nuremberg, Ms B213, 175r, 176v–7r; as the early modern period progressed, women's fashions increasingly restricted physical activity, which both hindered their participation in athletic events and reflected social condemnation of such behaviour:

of status also occasionally enjoyed shooting in private matches, but these events belonged strictly to the world of elite amusement.[47] Among the burgher classes, civic republicanism rested upon an assumption of masculine identity that did not allow for martial competition against women, so that target shooting remained entirely a male preserve. Despite the often fair-like atmosphere of the larger shoots, practice with guns was a serious business, and just as was the case with other defence-related activities, women were supposed to stay out of the way.[48]

As suggested by Fischart's story of the Strasbourg match with which we began, the reputations forged and maintained at large shooting matches were important for collective as well as individual identity. Public displays of weaponry, town colours, expensive hospitality and collective martial skill combined to enhance town status. In fact, as local shooting societies often argued in their petitions for council support, letting too much time lapse without hosting a match could even bring the entire town into disrepute. Invoking images of the greenery that traditionally decorated the winner's wreath, shooting masters warned against letting the local wreath 'wilt' (*verdorren*). In order for their home town to bear the fruit of goodwill among its neighbours, the shooter's wreath had to be 'refreshed' and made green again on a regular basis, which could only happen with the council's generous support for a new invitation.[49]

The goal of these marksmen, of course, was not only to compete, but to win, and whichever shooter took first place also conferred honour and status upon his home town. With support from sponsors, the best marksmen travelled from match to match, some attaining the status of semi-professional sportsmen. Since it was traditional practice for the town who took home the wreath to host a match the following year, winners not only found themselves the centre of attention at the prize ceremony and had their names recorded in chronicle entries, but they were celebrated again at the home match, sometimes even

---

See Geoffrey Squire, *Dress and Society 1560–1970* (New York, 1974), p. 54. On prostitutes in foot races see also Schaufelberger, *Der Wettkampf*, p. 90.

[47]   Lady Mary Wortley Montagu, *The Complete Letters of Lady Mary Wortley Montagu*, ed. Robert Halband (3 vols, Oxford, 1965–67), vol. I, 1708–20, pp. 268–9; Richard Froning (ed.), *Frankfurter Chroniken und annalistische Aufzeichnungen des Mittelalters* (Frankfurt, 1884), pp. 268–9. For other examples of private women's shooting matches see Theo Reintges, *Ursprung und Wesen der spätmittelalterlichen Schützengilden* (Bonn, 1963), pp. 298–9.

[48]   Tlusty, *Martial Ethic*, p. 25.

[49]   StANö, R29F4 Schützengesellschaften, 6 May 1577; 20 April 1580; Edelmann, *Schützenwesen*, p. 65; *Festschrift zum Jubiläumsschießen aus Anlaß des 550-jährigen Bestehens des königlich privilegierten Schützenvereins Augsburg vom 16. bis 26. Mai 1980* (Augsburg, 1980), p. 41.

appearing in commemorative broadsheets as celebrities comparable to modern sports heroes.[50]

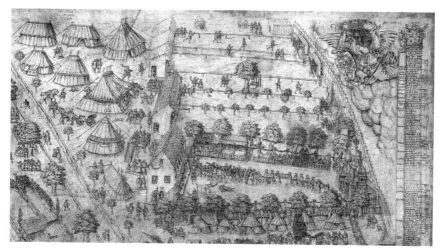

Figure 10.4   Broadsheet commemorating a large shooting match held in Regensburg in 1586 by engraver and gunsmith Peter Opel. Note the list of participants along the side of the print with flags denoting winners

Source: By permission of the Bayerische Staatsbibliothek München, Cod.icon. 399 a.

Military Professionalization and Commercialization of Sports

As the art of war came to depend less on individual fighting skills and more on technology and collective drill, martial sports began to lose the backing of local governments and moved increasingly into the private sector. Like most entertainments, expensive shooting festivals experienced a decline during the Thirty Years War. Target practice continued as both a sport and a form of military training throughout the early modern period, but shooting competitions never recovered their place of honour as a focus of civic pride and popular entertainment.

Pressure for shooting clubs to privatize came primarily from their government sponsors. City governments that were increasingly strapped for cash began in the later seventeenth century to resist supporting shooting grounds and buildings. First crossbow clubs and then gun clubs gradually had to take over the expense of

---

[50]   Wolfgang Harms, *Deutsche illustrierte Flugblätter des 16. und 17. Jahrhunderts* (7 vols, Berlin, 1985–97), vol. 7, p. 162.

maintaining their own buildings, sometimes engaging in decades-long struggles over financial responsibility while the facilities fell into disrepair. The decline in official support for shooting societies did nothing to dampen the interest of those who remained dedicated to the sport, however – it only forced them to become self-sufficient. Monetary support increasingly came from sponsors, often innkeepers who provided space and grounds in return for the lucrative business of putting up large numbers of guests and serving drinks and meals.[51]

Commercialization was also accompanied by a resurgence of the play function of the competitions, which had declined during the economic downturn of the seventeenth century. Eighteenth-century shooting matches thus began to take on the character of folk festivals that catered to the general public. The secondary entertainments at these events, which included beer and wine tents, food stands, puppet shows, and trained animal acts along with games, music and dances, eventually came to overshadow the shooting competitions entirely. Target shooting continued to provide a context, but was no longer the focus of the festivals.[52] Meanwhile, state-sponsored shooting matches moved in the direction of official military training, combining the mandatory target practice with military drill and introducing requirements for standardized firearms.[53] The result was a sharp division between shooting sports, which pitted individual men and guns against each other in the spirit of competition, and military exercise, in which the individual was subordinated to collective discipline and the audience had disappeared.

In the mountainous regions of Tyrol and Switzerland, where travel was dependent on narrow passes that could effectively be defended by a few riflemen, shooting societies were eventually militarized and professionalized, developing during the seventeenth and eighteenth centuries into modern defence organizations. Despite efforts in this direction by some territorial rulers, this development did not take place in other German-speaking lands, where the split between privatized sport and military drill reflected the new division between civilian and military identity.[54] With the advent of universal conscription into a professional army, military service became a phase of life for most men rather

---

[51]   *Festschrift*, p. 44; StANö, R29F4, Schützengesellschaften; StAA, Schützen-Akten I, 16 April 1695; Schützengesellschaften IV, Schüzenwirt 1562–1791.

[52]   Ulrich Rosseaux, *Freiräume: Unterhaltung, Vergnügen und Erholung in Dresden (1694–1830)* (Cologne, 2007), pp. 160–72.

[53]   A[ugust] L[udwig] Reyscher, *Vollständige, historisch und kritisch bearbeitete Sammlung der württembergischen Gesetze* (19 vols, Stuttgart and Tübingen, 1828–49), vol. 19, pp. 487–9; Gaedechens, *Hamburgs Bürgerbewaffnung*, pp. 13–14; Kraus, *Das Militärwesen*, pp. 80–81, 89.

[54]   Stolz, *Wehrverfassung*, pp. 57–8, 68; Walter Schaufelberger, 'Krieg und Kriegertum im eidgenössischen Spätmittelalter', in Walter Schaufelberger, *Spurensuche. Siebzehn Aufsätze zur Militärgeschichte der Schweiz* (Effingerhof, 2008), pp. 141–74, at pp. 172–3; Martin

than a lifelong commitment to local defence. Martial identity moved out of the household, neighbourhood, and community, and was transferred to the State.

Conclusion

The sixteenth and early seventeenth centuries in Germany marked a zenith in the celebration of the burgher-dominated sports of sword fighting, sword dancing and target shooting. At the heart of the love affair with martial sports was a nearly universal commitment on the part of early modern civic institutions to encourage in their townsmen an identity with the martial ethic. During this age of urban militias, martial skill and martial identity were linked to layered notions of individual, local and political sovereignty. Thus to early modern theorists, martial sports were schools of civic republicanism. The fact that martial sporting competitions included elements of play did not diminish their political role. In fact, because the entertainment aspect of these events increased their visibility, it also enhanced their value as a public performance of masculine and civic values.

Although they were associated with martial skill, shooting societies and sword-fighting schools were never military organizations. Their club-like atmospheres were intended to emphasize individual rather than collective ability and social levelling rather than military hierarchy. Like modern sports events, the competitions also strengthened communal identity and cultivated local pride, occasionally even creating heroes analogous to modern sports idols. In fact, in both shooting and fencing matches, the rules of good sportsmanship and male sociability could take priority over military effectiveness. Even technical innovations could be hindered in the interest of fair play.

This changed with the rise of absolutist models and the triumph of standing armies. The process of military professionalization with its emphasis on drill, uniforms and disciplined subordination required a different kind of martial training, one that was not reconcilable with the play elements of early modern shooting and fencing matches. German shooting societies declined in importance and size during the later seventeenth century and were already taking on the character of modern sports clubs by the eighteenth, with their entertainment value eventually eclipsing military interest entirely. Meanwhile, sword fighting, which was an artisanal skill in the sixteenth and seventeenth centuries, almost completely disappeared, replaced by the less dangerous and more elite sport of fencing with foils.

The fact that the weapons culture of the German towns was being redefined and redirected just as the militia model was gaining ground both in England and

---

Schennach, *Tiroler Landesverteidigung 1600–1650: Landmiliz und Söldnertum* (Innsbruck, 2003), pp. 267–70.

the United States is not coincidental. The role of an armed citizenry as a check on unbridled government power, viewed positively by the drafters of the American Bill of Rights and its English antecedent, clearly ran counter to the interests of the increasingly absolutist rulers of the Empire. The German-speaking world was thus characterized by an increasingly clear demarcation between military and civilian life. As military training was disengaged from the world of sports and entertainment, masculine fashion also lost its martial element. By the later eighteenth century, swords were ubiquitous only at the sides of soldiers, students and aristocrats, while fashionable German townsmen carried walking sticks.

Chapter 11
French Enlightenment Swimming*

Rebekka v. Mallinckrodt

During the Enlightenment swimming became both one of many areas for world improvement and a topic for authors to make a name for themselves. Like other efforts to promote public health, publications about how to swim were aimed at keeping potential readers from deadly perils and helping them toughen up physically. Whereas only 15 publications that deal specifically with swimming are documented for the years between 1587 and 1771 in all of Europe, the number had already climbed to 98 between 1772 and 1836, and still increased to 376 in the remainder of the nineteenth century.[1] Swimming became both the topic of independent publications and a component part of the pedagogical, military and natural scientific writings of the time.

Research on the history of swimming often took this as a clue that the practice of swimming only spread from the late eighteenth century on. Still, there are many sixteenth-, seventeenth- and eighteenth-century sources that hint at a practice independent from this textual tradition of swimming manuals. In this chapter I therefore want to disentangle discourses and practices in showing that there was a practice before and independent of these treatises. In taking France in the second half of the eighteenth century as an example, I analyse who published these swimming tracts and why. By specifying the social background and intentions of these authors it is possible to show that their treatises did not stand for the whole epoch and population, but served definite needs and functions for specific social groups. In qualifying the validity of these texts this chapter also opens up the field for new research as many Enlightened authors claimed to introduce new practices (without doing so). It is therefore necessary to look beyond these texts and also contrary to their authors' intentions in order to discover swimming (and also other sportive) practices in the Early Modern period.

Furthermore, Enlightened writers stressed the value of swimming for strengthening the body, but even more as a life-saving skill. Swimming was first and foremost seen in these tracts as an instrumental body technique, only in the

---

* This chapter was translated by Elizabeth Bredeck.

* This chapter was translated by Elizabeth Bredeck.
[1] Thierry Terret, *Naissance et diffusion de la natation sportive* (Paris, 1994), p. 14.

second place as an exercise.[2] These were typical eighteenth-century justifications for swimming that was at the same time practised for pleasure, in the context of sportive activities as well as for practical needs. These different contexts and aims cannot always be disentangled due to the fact that swimming was always also a life-saving technique. But cutting off swimming from these manifold contexts would mean cutting off modern swimming practices from their pre-modern predecessors that were not perceived and practised solely but also as sports and pastimes. Like modern swimming the pre-modern practice was simultaneously a life-saving measure, a sport, an exercise, an instrumental body technique and/ or a leisure activity depending on who performed it in which situation and for what purpose.

A New Practice? A New Science!

Evidence of swimming practices in the pre-modern period is actually widely scattered; what proof does exist is usually little more than a passing reference, i.e. it does not allow for any further interpretation of how swimmers and swimming practices were perceived. It is still not entirely clear if this scant evidence reflects the state of the research, if it is because swimming was such an everyday occurrence that it was not worth mentioning, or if it is for precisely the opposite reason: widespread ignorance about swimming. Actual references to swimming practices may provide only an incomplete picture, but it is still important to view them here for France in the seventeenth and eighteenth centuries, since they place the swimming manuals in a new light, and allow at least a preliminary comparison between the practices they describe and what we find in other written evidence. The practice of swimming was in fact more common than Enlightenment authors would have us believe, since when they labelled their work 'new' and noted the widespread ignorance of a life-saving technique, they were at the same time promoting themselves and legitimizing their own publications,[3] because the most profitable books were 'those that attack prejudices', as one eighteenth-century French writer explained to a publisher.[4]

As early as the seventeenth century we find references to professional divers in France. In 1678 the minister of the navy Seignelay commented that people should avoid diving bells since using them was difficult, and the work done

---

[2]   For Marcel Mauss' term and concept of 'body techniques' see Rebekka v. Mallinckrodt, 'Introduction. Body Techniques in the Early Modern Period', in Rebekka v. Mallinckrodt (ed.), *Bewegtes Leben. Körpertechniken in der Frühen Neuzeit* (Wolfenbüttel, 2008), pp. 1–14, especially pp. 3–4.

[3]   See for instance Nicolas Roger, *Essai sur l'art de nager* (London, 1787), p. 17.

[4]   Robert Darnton, 'A Pamphleteer on the Run', in Robert Darnton, *The Literary Underground of the Old Regime* (Cambridge, MA, 1982), pp. 71–121, here p. 110.

better by divers.[5] A list of divers living along the banks of the Dordogne dating from 1704 contains brief descriptions of individual people and their respective diving abilities. We learn for example that despite his gout and 45 years of age, Bertrand Belot, known as Picard, could dive four-and-a-half meters deep and remain a good 15 minutes under water.[6] Beginning in the seventeenth century such divers were employed permanently by the navy.[7]

Françoise Bayard, who has studied files on incidences of drowning in Lyon between 1624 and 1789, also found numerous swimmers among bathers.[8] The swimming references in the files date from the seventeenth century.[9] In no case is swimming mentioned as an unusual ability. Instead, we learn that while some people were so proficient that they could swim across the river, others were just learning or had a friend show them how it was done. Given her particular research interests, Bayard does not usually differentiate between bathers and swimmers, so from her work on the first group we can only deduce the social background, age and gender of the swimmers. Most were young (85 per cent); more than three-quarters of them were male; and craftsmen (59 per cent) as well as domestic servants (20 per cent) represented the largest social groups.[10]

We find evidence of swimming in other sources, too. In a posthumously published text on swimming (1696), Melchisedech Thévenot (ca. 1620–1692) supported his theory of an innate human ability to swim by referring to contemporary practices.[11] At the same time he noted that while swimming was not widespread, it was nonetheless common among sailors and boatmen as a necessary skill, and among the lower ranks as a form of entertainment.[12] However, his suggestion that swimming practices were concentrated in the lower ranks is relativized by other written evidence. The naturalist Gilles-Augustin Bazin (1681–1754) wrote in 1741 that swimming was so familiar that he need not discuss it in any more detail.[13] The author and dramatist Jean-François

---

[5]   Ministère de la Culture et de la Communication, *Sur l'eau ... Sous l'eau. Imagination et technique dans la Marine 1680–1730*, exhibition catalog Archives Nationales Hôtel de Soubise Mai–Décembre 1986, p. 51.

[6]   *Sur l'eau ... Sous l'eau*, p. 54, catalog number 69b.

[7]   *Sur l'eau ... Sous l'eau*, p. 55.

[8]   Françoise Bayard, 'Nager à Lyon à l'époque moderne (XVIIe–XVIIIe siècles)', in Actes du 116e congrès national des sociétés savantes (Chambéry 1991), Section d'histoire moderne et contemporaine, *Jeux et sports dans l'histoire*, vol. 2, *Pratiques sportives* (Paris, 1992), pp. 229–45.

[9]   Bayard, 'Nager à Lyon', pp. 232–3.

[10]   Bayard, 'Nager à Lyon', p. 233.

[11]   Melchisedech Thévenot, *L'art de nager* (Paris, 1696), p. 2.

[12]   Thévenot, *L'art de nager* (1696), preface, no pagination.

[13]   Gilles-Augustin Bazin, *Observations sur les plantes et leur analogie avec les insectes. Précédées de deux discours. L'un Sur l'accroissement du Corps humain, l'autre Sur la cause pour*

Marmontel (1723–1799) practised it in the early 1740s during his youth at the Collège de Mauriac (Auvergne).[14]

For the late eighteenth century, the reports about accidents on the Seine and its banks that were collected and published by the Paris Lifesaving Association often provide just as much information about people's inability to swim as they do about competent swimmers. For instance, a 25-year-old journeyman baker named René Huault died on 16 June 1772 after swimming twice across the Seine.[15] In contrast, the day labourer Pierre-Maurice Brit fell into the water by accident and was saved by M. Rossignol, a courier on the stagecoach to Lyon who was able to swim.[16] In a dramatic rescue effort, Claude Verdot dived to the bottom of the Seine and saved 14-year-old Jacques Le Blond, who had jumped into the water to retrieve his hat.[17] A woman who apparently wished to commit suicide and was therefore unwilling to give any further personal information was rescued by a journeyman of the dyers' guild who knew how to swim.[18] These are just a few of the many examples documented in the reports. Here, too, the swimmers are predominantly young men from the ranks of craftsmen and servants, but by no means exclusively people who worked on the water or the waterfront. In addition, even before a swimming school was officially established in Paris in 1785, sailors, mariners, ferrymen and harbour workers apparently gave commercial swimming lessons[19] and the founder of the swimming school, Barthélémy Turquin, aimed to suppress this competition by applying for a royal privilege, which was granted in 1787.[20]

Thus, when late eighteenth-century authors of swimming manuals called it a practice of the lower ranks and seamen, this is certainly borne out by the existing evidence, if not always quite so exclusively or pointedly. As a topos this was instead characteristic of Enlightenment writings, and as such, it leads us to ask what purpose this rhetorical device served. Manual authors usually explained that swimming was considered disreputable precisely because it was an amusement of the rabble, and this explanation – like the references to an ostensibly widespread inability to swim – helped justify their own efforts to speak out against such

---

laquelle les Bestes [sic] nâgent naturellement, & que l'Homme est obligé d'en étudier les moyens (Strasbourg, 1741), pp. 46–47.

[14]   Jean-François Marmontel, *Mémoires*, ed. Maurice Tourneux (3 vols, Paris, 1891), vol. 1, pp. 20–21. I am grateful to Ulrike Krampl (Tours) for this reference.

[15]   [Philippe Nicolas] Pia, *Détail des succès de l'établissement que la ville de Paris a fait en faveur des personnes noyées* (7 issues in 5 vols, Paris, 1773–1782), vol. I, 1, pp. 12–14.

[16]   Pia, *Détail des succès*, vol. I, 2, pp. 38–9.

[17]   Pia, *Détail des succès*, vol. I, 2, pp. 47–51.

[18]   Pia, *Détail des succès*, vol. I, 2, pp. 59–60.

[19]   Nicolas Roger, *Méthode sûre pour apprendre à nager en peu de jours* (Paris, 1783), pp. 16–17; see also Roger, *Essai*, p. 38.

[20]   Archives Nationales, Paris, F 17/1350, dossier 2, No. 17.

'prejudices'. Jean-Jacques Rousseau, who defended swimming in his novel *Émile* (1762), explained that it was neglected because it was useless in terms of social distinction:

> An exclusive education, which merely tends to keep those who have received it apart from the mass of mankind, always prefers the most expensive instructions to the most common, even when the latter is of more use. Thus all carefully educated young men learn to ride, because it is costly, but scarcely any of them learn to swim, as it costs nothing, and an artisan can swim as well as any one.[21]

Swimming thus seemed to be not only a useful skill but also an egalitarian one, and as such it was a typical Enlightenment project. It was also usefulness that distinguished the Enlightened 'philosophe' from the 'érudit'. When Poncelin de la Roche-Tilhac, editor of the re-published Thévenot work (1782), likewise spoke of the rural pleasures of 'peasants' and the 'rabble', he combined it with an obvious jibe at the court and its admirers:

> The limpness that comes from false courtliness soon destroyed these salutary institutions ... Most citizens of the other ranks, anxious to imitate domestic paladins, renounced the old customs; rural pastimes and innocent recreation like the art of swimming were left to the peasants and the rest of the rabble. Since the time of this upheaval, the fateful age of the reversal of good manners, our little lords have despised the pleasures that the people might share with them.[22]

The topos of physical (and especially sexual) degeneration was frequently used to delegitimize the noble elite's ruling function,[23] and under the conditions

---

[21] Jean-Jacques Rousseau, *Émile*, trans. by B. Foxley, introduction by P.D. Jimack (London, 1974), p. 96. 'Une éducation exclusive, qui tend seulement à distinguer du peuple ceux qui l'ont reçue, préfère toujours les instructions les plus coûteuses aux plus communes, et par cela même aux plus utiles. Ainsi les jeunes gens élevés avec soin aprennent tous à monter à cheval, parce qu'il en coûte beaucoup pour cela; mais presque aucun d'eux n'apprend à nager, parce qu'il n'en coûte rien, et qu'un artisan peut savoir nager aussi bien que qui que ce soit' (Jean-Jacques Rousseau, *Émile ou de l'éducation* (orig. publ. 1762) (Paris, 1992), p. 137).

[22] Melchisédech Thévenot, *L'art de nager* (Paris, 1782), pp. 14–15: 'La mollesse, à laquelle une fausse urbanité donna naissance, détruisit bientôt ces institutions salutaires ... La plupart des citoyens des autres ordres, jaloux d'imiter ces Paladins Casaniers, abdiquerent les vieux usages; & les récréations champêtres, les délassemens innocens, tels que l'Art de nager, furent livrés aux paysans & au reste de la populace. Depuis cette révolution, époque fatale du renversement des bonnes mœurs, nos petits-maîtres dédaignerent les plaisirs que le peuple pouvoit partager avec eux.'

[23] See for example Antoine de Baecque, *The Body Politic: Corporeal Metaphor in Revolutionary France 1770–1800* (Stanford, 1997), pp. 8, 11, 29–71; Natalie Scholz, *Die*

imposed by the censors, in many cases it was just such apparently non-political topics as swimming that offered the chance for critique.[24]

At the same time these depictions were often ambivalent. On the one hand, 'naturalness' and 'simplicity' had positive connotations, but on the other, repulsion is also evident in these representations of the lower ranks since the authors by no means wished to sink to their level. The same ambivalence and the same political thrust emerged in discussions about those other outstanding swimmers in Enlightenment treatises, namely, 'noble savages'. Whereas early swimming manuals from the sixteenth and seventeenth centuries did not yet differentiate between European and non-European swimmers, the 'noble savage' meandered amphibian-like and equipped with fantastic abilities through the writings of the eighteenth century:

> Today you find good swimmers in climate zones where our luxurious lifestyle and our delicacy have not yet advanced. Asia, Africa, and America contain many people of every gender and age and from varied circumstances who highly value this important form of recreation. All Negroes learn to swim at a tender age. Hence we are often amazed at the long distances they can cover, whether to fish or to return to their hometown. Reliable observers have confirmed that they use astonishing power to swim a distance of forty miles.[25]

Enlightenment defenders of swimming found two solutions to this dilemma of their role models' social ambivalence. First, they frequently invoked traditions from antiquity since doing so was socially safe: in the eyes of both aristocratic and bourgeois readers, such traditions were uncontroversial.[26] This appeal to antiquity might still be coupled with the hope for a revival of the spirit of

---

imaginierte Restauration. Repräsentationen der Monarchie im Frankreich Ludwigs XVIII (Darmstadt, 2006), pp. 32–4.

[24]   See Robert Darnton, *Glänzende Geschäfte. Die Verbreitung von Diderots 'Encyclopedie'* [sic] *oder: Wie verkauft man Wissen mit Gewinn* (Frankfurt/M., 1998) (orig. publ. 1979), pp. 19–20.

[25]   Thévenot, *L'art de nager* (1782), pp. 16–17: 'Les bons Nageurs sont aujourd'hui relégués dans les climats, où notre luxe & notre délicatesse n'ont pas encore pénétré. L'Asie, l'Afrique & l'Amérique, offrent une foule de personnages de tous les sexes, de tous les âges & de toutes les conditions, qui estiment pour beaucoup cette récréation importante. Tous les Negres sur-tout apprennent à nager dès la plus tendre jeunesse. Aussi est-on souvent étonné des trajets immenses qu'ils font, soit pour aller à la pêche, soit pour regagner leur patrie. Des Observateurs dignes de foi attestent les avoir vus nager avec vigueur surprenante pendant l'espace de quarante lieues.'

[26]   See for example Thévenot, *L'art de nager* (1782), pp. 8–12.

the Roman Republic, and thus politicized.[27] The other option was to draw a clear distinction between contemporary (and allegedly) lower-class and non-European practices on the one hand, and a new art of swimming on the other. Swimming for recreation was a practice of the lower ranks, but swimming in order to increase one's physical powers or to save a life was the serious business of the Enlightened elites.[28] 'Unconscious' swimming was something practised by 'savages', the methodical step-by-step learning to move through the water, in contrast, was as much a handicap as it was an expression of European rationality.

Thus, what was new in the eighteenth century was not the introduction of swimming practices, but their increasing textualization. By writing about swimming, authors intended to elevate its status as both an 'art' and a 'science', as the title pages of the manuals clearly show,[29] and thereby aimed at distinguishing this new 'Enlightenment-style swimming' from existing practices. How did they conceptualize swimming in this new context?

Enlightenment-Style Swimming

As publisher and editor of the Thévenot text, Poncelin de la Roche-Tilhac was responsible for three editions of this swimming manual in the 1780s. By including supplementary essays about bathing, swim aids and resuscitation

---

[27] See for instance Chantal Grell, *Le dix-huitième siècle et l'antiquité en France 1680–1789* (2 vols, Oxford, 1995); Claude Mossé, *L'Antiquité dans la Révolution* (Paris, 1989). For references to the Roman Republic, see for instance Thévenot, *L'art de nager* (1782), p. 11 and in particular the ideal described there: 'delà, cette vigueur héroïque, ce tempérament robuste, cette santé parfaite, dont jouissoit le plus grand nombre des soldats Romains'. See also Thévenot, *L'art de nager* (1782), pp. 39–40 ('ces Républicains', 'leur simplicité'); and p. 69: 'Les Anciens, parmi lesquels la vigueur du corps étoit beaucoup plus considérée qu'elle ne l'est de nos jours'.

[28] In the Thévenot edition of 1782, the term 'usefulness' is used three times on the title page alone as a form of advertisement. See also Thévenot, *L'art de nager* (1782), p. 56, note; also pp. 131–2: 'Enfin, c'est en contractant l'habitude de vous remuer ainsi en tout sens, & de subjuguer l'élément impérieux dont vous avez soumis les caprices à vos réflexions, que vous pourrez secourir efficacement ceux qui seront en danger de se noyer.' See also pp. 152–3: 'Ne pensez pas que tous ces rafinemens, toutes ces especes de tours de force, que je vous indique ici, n'aient que le pur agrément pour objet. Chacune de ces manieres de nager offre une utilité particuliere, dans cette foule de pressans dangers auxquels nous pouvons nous trouver exposés.' See also pp. 156–7, 159–61, 165, 167–8.

[29] *L'art de nager, avec des avis pour se baigner utilement*, Précédé d'une Dissertation, où l'on développe la science des Anciens dans l'Art de nager, l'importance de cet exercice & l'utilité du bain, soit en santé, soit en maladie. Ouvrage utile à tout le monde, & destiné particuliérement [sic] à l'éducation des jeunes Militaires du Corps Royal de la Marine, Paris 1782.

methods, he on the one hand placed Thévenot's work in a dietetic-utilitarian framework: in the revised Thévenot text itself he also repeatedly emphasized the usefulness of many swimming techniques. On the other hand, by referring to numerous historical sources, travel reports, medical treatises and scientific writings, Poncelin introduced swimming in an erudite discourse. To most authors who saw themselves in this scientific context, being scientific meant discovering laws or guiding principles.[30] The foundation of 'Enlightened' swimming therefore had to be a study of its prerequisites, namely, the build and weight of human beings. Both topics had long since been discussed, and not just in swimming manuals.

In a detailed essay of 1741, the aforementioned naturalist Gilles-Augustin Bazin explained why animals could swim naturally but humans could not: while quadrupeds retained their natural gait in water, a human being would sink if he tried to walk as if on land.[31] In 1775 the mathematician Jean Baptiste de la Chapelle likewise drew a sharp dividing line between human bipeds and animal quadrupeds who in his view were fundamentally better equipped to swim:

> When swimming, it is important and even essential to hold the head above the surface of the water: a constant effort and fairly tiring for human beings who, unlike many quadrupeds, are not designed by nature to swim, and who – simply because of this 'flawed' build – can suffocate, even if they know how to swim well and are completely healthy.[32]

All other physical requirements aside, swimming was always going to be a dangerous business for human beings in Chapelle's view because of the

---

[30]   See Thévenot, *L'art de nager* (1782), p. 164: 'les bons Nageurs, maîtres de l'élément, dont ils ont étudié les loix, se jouent de ses caprices'. See also Roger, *Méthode sûre*, p. 28: 'elles [the swimming techniques, RvM] portent toutes sur un petit nombre de principes simples & faciles à retenir, savoir: que nos corps sont plus légers que l'eau: que nos corps ne sont pas par-tout également légers: qu'il faut donner aux parties les plus légères un poids capable de les tenir en équilibre avec les plus pesantes: que les différentes parties de notre corps ne peuvent acquérir cette variété de poids que par la diversité de leur position, ou par la résistance de l'eau.' In addition, see Roger, *Essai*, pp. 50–51 and also Thévenot, *L'art de nager* (1782), who first discusses Borelli's views (*De motu animalium*) on pp. 5–8.

[31]   Bazin, *Observations*, pp. 35–6.

[32]   Jean Baptiste de la Chapelle, *Traité de la construction théorique et pratique du Scaphandre, ou du bateau de l'homme* (Paris, 1775), pp. 12–13: 'Ce qu'il y a d'important & même d'essentiel dans l'art de nager, c'est de soutenir toujours sa tête au-dessus de la surface de l'eau: travail perpétuel & bien laborieux pour l'homme, qui n'est point construit pour nager naturellement, comme sont plusieurs quadrupèdes, & qui pourroit, par le seul défaut de conformation, être suffoqué, en nageant parfaitement bien & dans toute la plénitude de ses forces.'

unnatural posture it required. The naturalist Mathurin-Jacques Brisson (1723–1806) likewise wrote in 1781 in his *Dictionnaire raisonné physique* that the human body's centre of gravity was in the chest area, unlike animals whose centre of gravity was near the abdomen. Brisson held that the volume of the brain accounted for the greater weight of the human head compared with that of animals, so holding it up in order to breathe in the water involved more work.[33]

While these authors' arguments were strictly physiological, their emphasis on the upright posture that made horizontal swimming seem laborious, dangerous or even impossible needs to be seen against the background of an extensive religious, philosophical and pedagogical tradition. In this literature the upright walking position – like the capacity for reason (and with it the drawback of the heavy head) – was both a criterion for distinguishing humans from animals and a means of social distinction.[34] We can therefore assume that when the above authors addressed the problem of horizontality, they were also influenced by this tradition.

The conclusions they drew were nevertheless varied. When describing a type of cork 'armour' that he had designed, Chapelle, who rejected swimming, underscored one advantage in particular: wearing this outfit allowed a person to move about while remaining vertical in the water, which corresponded to the 'natural' human posture (see Figure 11.1).[35] Using the same line of argument, other authors proposed that humans should swim in an upright position.[36] Nicolas Roger emphasized that this was a matter of achieving proper balance.[37] Drawing on Borelli's views of human anatomy, Poncelin de la Roche-Tilhac

---

[33]   Mathurin-Jacques Brisson, *Dictionnaire raisonné de physique* (3 vols, Paris, 1781), vol. 2, pp. 201–2, article '*nager*'.

[34]   Georges Vigarello, 'The Upward Training of the Body from the Age of Chivalry to Courtly Civility', in Michael Feher (ed.), *Fragments for a History of the Human Body*, vol. 2 (New York, 1989), pp. 148–99; Ludwig-Uhland-Institut für empirische Kulturwissenschaft der Universität Tübingen (ed.), *Der aufrechte Gang. Zur Symbolik einer Körperhaltung*, exhibition catalogue (Tübingen, 1990); Anselm Schubert, *Das Ende der Sünde. Anthropologie und Erbsünde zwischen Reformation und Aufklärung* (Göttingen, 2002), pp. 108–24; Kirsten O. Frieling, 'Haltung bewahren. Der Körper im Spiegel frühneuzeitlicher Schriften über Umgangsformen', in Rebekka v. Mallinckrodt (ed.), *Bewegtes Leben. Körpertechniken in der Frühen Neuzeit* (Wolfenbüttel, 2008), pp. 39–59.

[35]   Chapelle, *Traité*, pp. 30–34.

[36]   Oronzio de Bernardi, *Vollständiger Lehrbegriff der Schwimmkunst auf neue Versuche über die spezifische Schwere des menschlichen Körpers gegründet. Aus dem Italienischen* übersetzt und mit Anmerkungen begleitet von Friedrich Kries, Professor an dem Gymnasium zu Gotha (2 vols, Weimar, 1797), vol. 2, p. 65.

[37]   Roger, *Méthode sûre*, pp. 11–14, 28.

concluded that by nature people were unable to swim, since human posture was actually opposed to it, but it was possible using an acquired skill.[38]

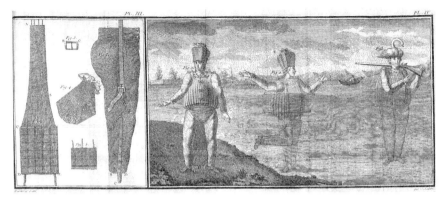

Figure 11.1   Chapelle proposed using a 'cork armour' instead of learning how to swim

Source: Jean Baptiste de la Chapelle, *Traité de la construction théorique et pratique du Scaphandre, ou du bateau de l'homme* (Paris, 1775). By permission of the Württembergische Landesbibliothek Stuttgart (Gew.oct.3398).

In addition to discussing posture, these writers also looked at the specific gravity of humans in relation to water. Bazin came to the conclusion that the specific gravity of human beings corresponded almost exactly to that of water, which was actually conducive to swimming.[39] As long as physicists were not in complete agreement, however, Bazin preferred to be on the safe side and assume that humans had a higher specific gravity than water.[40] He noted that this 'excess weight' could be counteracted easily by taking one deep breath, whereas while exhaling a slight movement of the arms was required.[41]

The unnamed author of the 1765 *Encyclopédie* article '*nager*' shared this working assumption about the specific gravity of the human body. According to this article, it was the weight of the head with its brain mass that particularly distinguished human beings from animals. Drawing on Borelli, the author nonetheless optimistically concluded that because the difference was so slight, a little movement was the only thing needed to stay afloat.[42]

---

[38]   Thévenot, *L'art de nager* (1782), pp. 5–8.

[39]   *Journal des Savants* (1742), p. 617.

[40]   Bazin, *Observations*, p. 39.

[41]   *Journal des Savants* (1742), p. 618. See also Bazin, *Observations*, pp. 47–8.

[42]   Denis Diderot and Jean Le Rond d'Alembert (eds), *Encyclopédie ou Dictionnaire raisonné des sciences, des arts et des métiers* (17 text and 11 illustrated vols, Paris, 1751–1772),

Jean Baptiste de la Chapelle also took human anatomy into account, but the picture he painted of human weightiness was more dramatic. He did this at least in part to help promote the sale of his own cork 'armour'.[43] In eighteenth-century France, however, he was the exception. Brisson wrote in 1781 that although humans were heavier than water, the degree of difference was so small that simply expanding the ribcage and making several slight movements of the arms and legs would suffice to keep a person afloat.[44] Nicolas Roger claimed that humans had to be lighter than water, since otherwise all swimming skills would be futile.[45] Poncelin de la Roche-Tilhac pointed out that it was impossible to sink while lying on your back, even if you tried, and that this insight might save many human lives.[46]

These opinions were not shared by everyone in Europe. The Italian mathematician Oronzio de Bernardi organized a large-scale experiment involving several hundred people in 1792 to resolve once and for all the issue of human weight. He came to the conclusion that in spite of all possible differences that might exist between individuals,

> human beings of every age and every body type from every region of the world ... [are] one eleventh lighter than rainwater and one tenth lighter than saltwater. If a person submerses himself in seawater, nine parts will sink and the tenth part of his body will protrude above the surface.[47]

The German philanthropist Johann Christian Friedrich GutsMuths disagreed. He wrote in 1798:

> My reservations about this claim concern first: its expansion to include all nations, second: to all individuals, regardless of their widely differing physical

---

vol. 11 (1765), article '*nager*', pp. 5–6.

[43]   Chapelle, *Traité*, p. 15.

[44]   Brisson, *Dictionnaire*, vol. 2, pp. 201–2.

[45]   Roger, *Méthode sûre*, p. 8; also p. 6. In addition, see Roger, *Essai*, p. 27 and pp. 29–30.

[46]   Thévenot, *L'art de nager* (1782), p. 133.

[47]   This is GutsMuths' summary of Bernardi's ideas (Johann Christian Friedrich GutsMuths, *Kleines Lehrbuch der Schwimmkunst zum Selbstunterrichte, enthaltend eine vollständige praktische Anweisung zu allen Arten des Schwimmens, nach den Grundsätzen der neuen italienischen Schule des Bernardi und der älteren deutschen bearbeitet* (Weimar, 1798), introduction, p. VIII): 'der Mensch von jedem Alter und jeder körperlichen Beschaffenheit aus jeder Weltgegend ... um ein Eilftel leichter als Regenwasser und um ein Zehntel leichter als Seewasser [ist]. Und wenn er sich hinein senkt, so werden nur neun Theile ins Wasser tauchen und der zehnte Theil seines Körpers wird über die Oberfläche hervorragen.'

constitutions 3) its specific and allegedly generally applicable expansion to 1/11 and in seawater 1/10 of absolute bodily weight.[48]

GutsMuths therefore concluded: 'It depends on the individual body.'[49] In his swimming manual he consequently proposed two different training methods for people with higher and lower specific weights. At this time people also spoke of the 'old German' and 'new Italian school' represented by GutsMuths and Bernardi respectively. Those who believed people to be heavier than water favoured a technique characterized by vigorous strokes against the water, while the other party, with its trust in the load-bearing capacity of the liquid element, advised gentler motions in the water instead.

Thus, swimming was seen less as an athletic activity than as a means of survival in an unpredictable element. In addition, the frequent emphasis on its military usefulness suggests the unspoken assumption that both readers and swimmers were male.[50] Only rarely were women addressed as a separate target audience, even though water posed the same dangers for them as for men.[51] For this reason the ideal swimmer was defined by pragmatics, not by artistry as in earlier swimming treatises, as Roger stated (1783) and many other authors repeated:

> The true swimmer is someone who can swim in all situations, who rests exclusively by changing his technique, and who – when he has to cover a great distance and fears he will get a cramp – varies his position in order to move those muscles that are in danger of becoming stiff.[52]

The ability to adapt to any given situation was the ideal that led Roger to declare hyperbolically: 'The most capable swimmer will use different techniques in each

---

[48]   GutsMuths, *Kleines Lehrbuch*, introduction, p. IX: 'Meine Bedenklichkeiten bey dieser Behauptung betreffen erstens: Ihre Ausdehnung auf alle Nationen, zweytens: auf alle Individuen, ungeachtet der verschiedensten körperlichen Constitutionen 3) Ihre bestimmte und allgemein gültig seyn sollende Ausdehnung bis auf 1/11 und im Seewasser bis auf 1/10 des absoluten körperlichen Gewichts.' See also pp. X–XII.

[49]   GutsMuths, *Kleines Lehrbuch*, preface, p. XIV: 'Es kommt auf den individuellen Körper an.'

[50]   See for instance the title page of the 1782 Thévenot edition: 'Ouvrage utile à tout le monde, & destiné particuliérement [sic] à l'éducation des jeunes Militaires du Corps Royal de la Marine.'

[51]   Roger, *Méthode sûre*, pp. 22–3; Roger, *Essai*, p. 45.

[52]   Roger, *Méthode sûre*, p. 10: 'Le véritable nageur est celui qui nage dans toutes les situations, qui ne se repose d'une manière que par une autre, qui, ayant beaucoup de chemin à faire, & craignant d'être saisi d'une crampe, variera ses attitudes pour donner de l'action aux muscles qu'il sent près de se roidir [sic].' See also Roger, *Essai*, pp. 31–2; and Thévenot, *L'art de nager* (1782), pp. 139, 145.

of these places: the Seine, the Rhine, the Rhône and the ocean.'[53] Using this logic, eighteenth-century authors re-interpreted artistic elements that were relics from much older swimming treatises.[54] In the 1782 edition of Thévenot, for example, the 'compass', a circular motion dating back to the sixteenth century, had now become a (somewhat complicated) method for extricating oneself from kelp – something mentioned so frequently that it suggests this was one of the greatest concerns of eighteenth-century authors on swimming.[55] The feat known as the 'goat leap' (see Figure 11.2) was no longer just the height of swimming artistry: it was functionalized, and became an agility training exercise for dangerous situations.[56]

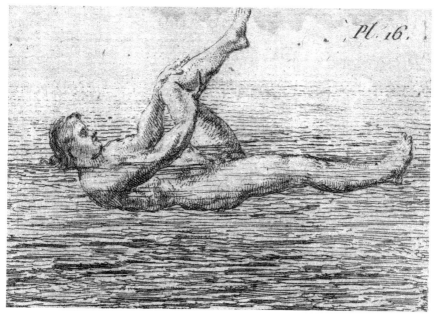

Figure 11.2   The 'goat leap' seen as the height of swimming artistry in the sixteenth and seventeenth centuries became an agility training exercise for dangerous situations in the more pragmatic late eighteenth-century swimming manuals

Source: Melchisedech Thévenot, *L'art de nager* (Paris, 1782). © Deutsches Schiffahrtsmuseum, Bremerhaven.

---

[53]   Roger, *Méthode sûre*, p. 30: 'le plus habile nageur emploie d'autres moyens sur la Seine, sur le Rhin, sur le Rhône & dans l'Océan.'

[54]   Thévenot, *L'art de nager* (1696) is actually a translation of a Latin swimming manual by Everard Digby from the year 1587. The modified illustrations were also taken from this sixteenth-century text.

[55]   Thévenot, *L'art de nager* (1782), pp. 139–41.

[56]   Thévenot, *L'art de nager* (1782), p. 151.

The number of swimming techniques discussed therefore tended to be lower in the eighteenth-century treatises than in earlier manuals, since in reality many feats were dispensable if usefulness was the most important factor. In 1783 Nicolas Roger wrote exclusively about the breaststroke, for example, though he listed many other techniques.[57] By merely *introducing* the art of swimming, keeping the scope of his pamphlet small and the price at 24 sous, Roger was the only author whose work actually did justice to the idea of an instructional manual on how to swim.[58] Admittedly, the price corresponded to a half or whole day's wages for workers and servants respectively,[59] but it was still far less expensive than the annual fee charged by the recently established Paris Swimming School. There, a first-class membership cost 96 livres and a second-class membership 48 livres per year, which was more than most residents of the city could afford. In the absence of an actual teacher but with at least a helping hand, these swimming manuals could serve as makeshift tutorials. But this was clearly not the best way to learn to swim.[60] In some cases the format of the text itself makes this project seem ludicrous. Even if the majority of the swimming manuals were published in a handy octave or duodecimal format, they were sometimes hundreds of pages long, and most contained no illustrations whatsoever. Those that were illustrated did not depict any motion sequences, even though instructional serial graphics had been common in military literature since the seventeenth century.[61] Instead, the manuals contained only individual images that could hardly be used as a basis for learning a sequence of movements.[62] Thus, the intentions and the practical use of the manuals often seem to be at odds, which leads us to ask if it really was the authors' primary goal to write instruction manuals for people who wished to learn how to swim.

---

[57] Roger, *Méthode sûre*, p. 29. Translated literally, he is teaching 'frog swimming', which in contrast to 'breaststroke' involved simultaneous movements of the arms and legs.

[58] Roger, *Essai*, Avis.

[59] Wolfgang Cilleßen, *Exotismus und Kommerz: Bäder- und Vergnügungswesen im Paris des späten 18. Jahrhunderts* (Frankfurt/M., 2000), p. 58.

[60] Thévenot/Poncelin therefore advises right at the beginning of the actual swimming manual that an experienced swimmer should be on hand to assist (Thévenot, *L'art de nager* (1782), p. 121).

[61] Janina Wellmann, 'Hand und Leib, Arbeiten und Üben. Instruktionsgraphiken der Bewegung im 17. und 18. Jahrhundert', in Rebekka v. Mallinckrodt (ed.), *Bewegtes Leben. Körpertechniken in der Frühen Neuzeit* (Wiesbaden, 2008), pp. 15–38 and pp. 249–59; Jörg Jochen Berns, *Film vor dem Film. Bewegende und bewegliche Bilder als Mittel der Imaginationssteuerung in Mittelalter und Früher Neuzeit* (Marburg, 2000), p. 97.

[62] Nicolas Roger (*Méthode sûre*, p. 30) said that there was no point in having illustrations, since they were unable to adequately depict all the variables involved.

Publish or Perish in the Eighteenth Century: The Authors and Publishers of Swimming Manuals

As early as 1971 Robert Darnton showed that the High Enlightenment in France produced two kinds of authors:[63] first, an established group of writers who could support themselves thanks to privileges and protection from the institutions of the Old Regime (and whose views were correspondingly kept in check); and second, a far greater number of hopeful young men who in many cases had come to the capital from the provinces to make their fortune in the relatively new profession of letters. In the final 25 years of the Old Regime Paris abounded with well-educated writers and jurists who had no jobs. At the same time, the developing literary market could not support this many authors even though the reading public had grown considerably in the course of the eighteenth century. One important reason was that the privileged book dealers and publishers still dictated the terms and paid poorly for manuscripts. Their precarious financial situation forced authors to make money from anything and everything: to publish on the widest variety of topics imaginable, to compile excerpts and anthologies and to re-publish other authors' texts – sometimes anonymously and at other times using their own name or a pseudonym, both in order to get around the publishing privileges and censors of the time and also simply to survive by using the sheer number and combination of different occasional jobs that were available. These authors also served as popularizers of the Enlightenment. As Darnton notes, their services were urgently needed by the *philosophes* who wished to have an effect outside the salons and influence public opinion.[64]

Darnton's thesis has seen some revision over the years, but even today it continues to inspire research, in some cases even more significantly than his later work. Jeremy Popkin and John Lough have shown that authors of the so-called 'literary underground' were far better connected than Darnton maintained, and were thus actually enmeshed in the system of the Old Regime.[65] Sometimes different factions at court even used these writings to influence public opinion.[66] Therefore pamphleteers did not automatically become vitriolic radical

---

[63]   This and the following from Robert Darnton, 'The High Enlightenment and the Low-Life of Literature', in Robert Darnton, *The Literary Underground of the Old Regime* (Cambridge, MA, 1982), pp. 1–40.

[64]   Darnton, 'Pamphleteer', pp. 71, 112.

[65]   Jeremy Popkin, 'Pamphlet Journalism at the End of the Old Regime', *Eighteenth Century Studies*, 22 (spring 1989): pp. 351–67; John Lough, 'The French Literary Underground Reconsidered', *Studies on Voltaire*, 329 (1995): pp. 471–82.

[66]   For this and the following see the essays by Jeremy D. Popkin, David A. Bell, Thomas E. Kaiser and Renato Pasta in Haydn T. Mason (ed.), *The Darnton Debate: Books and Revolution in the Eighteenth Century* (Oxford, 1998).

revolutionaries; instead, pre-revolutionary men of letters were situated all along the political spectrum. Neither were the distinctions between high and low literature or High and Low Enlightenment (abandoned later by Darnton himself) so clear and oppositional. Finally, historians note that Darnton's focus on the literary market, influenced by his work with publishers' archives, had led him to neglect Enlightenment ideas and ideals.

With all due respect to the explicit concerns of the Enlightenment, it appears that both the authors and publishers of late eighteenth-century French manuals on swimming belonged to the group of hack writers whose economic status was precarious. The identity of the authors is often unknown since they used pseudonyms or worked anonymously unless the text was a revised edition of an earlier work. In this case the original author's name was used as a trademark of sorts even if the actual content had been substantially changed as in the Thévenot text mentioned earlier. Other writers cannot be found in the common biographical reference works, that is, they were probably not among the illustrious scientists, publicists, teachers, doctors and military figures of the time. Even so, they were still men whose education and social standing had enabled them to work as writers in the first place. In two cases, though, both also highly influential works for French swimming literature in the eighteenth and on into the nineteenth century, it is possible to reconstruct the author's social profile more precisely. One of these was Gabriel Feydel alias Nicolas Roger,[67] who published swimming manuals in 1783 and 1787. The other was Poncelin de la Roche-Tilhac, publisher and editor of the radically expanded and revised Thévenot editions of 1781, 1782 and 1786. Their writings were not only republished many times, but also had influence in the form of tacit loans and compilations. In addition, both manuals were included in the 1786 volume of the *Encyclopédie méthodique* entitled *Arts académique. Équitation, Escrime, Danse, et Art de Nager*,[68] which meant that at least on paper, swimming was elevated to the canon of knightly exercises taught in the academies.[69] By this

---

[67] He himself indicates that it is a pseudonym in the anonymous second edition of the swimming manual: Roger, *Essai*, title page: 'Par l'Auteur des Préceptes publiés en 1783, sous le nom de Nicolas Roger, plongeur de profession, & insérés depuis dans l'Encyclopédie.' See also Roger, *Essai*, p. 22.

[68] *Encyclopédie méthodique* (206 vols, Paris, 1782–1832), here *Arts académiques. Équitation, Escrime, Danse, et Art de Nager* (1786), pp. 425–45. The only things omitted from the Thévenot edition of 1782 were the new editor's commentaries on the first Thévenot edition, a chapter on using oil during storms, passages about bathing and rescuing drowned people, the schedule of the swimming school and all pictures. In contrast, Nicolas Roger's *Méthode sûre pour apprendre à nager* of 1783 was included in its entirety.

[69] *Encyclopédie méthodique. Arts académiques*, Avertissement: 'On y joint l'Art de Nager, trop peu répandu parmi nous, & qui seroit si utile en un grand nombre de circonstances.'

integration into the *Encyclopédie*, both manuals achieved canonical status. Their authors doubtless aspired to a similar ascent themselves.

Like his father before him, Gabriel Feydel (1756–1840) initially embarked on a military career.[70] For the year 1776 he described himself as a 'jeune officier du Roi'. When submitting the design for a double axle (ostensibly his own invention) to the *Académie des sciences* in 1786, and again in 1787 in the *Journal général de France*, Feydel presented himself as an 'ancien lieutenant de cavalerie' and 'auteur de quelques pages de *l'Encyclopédie méthodique*'. He repeatedly advertised for himself in this manner by mentioning that his swimming manual had been included in the encyclopedia.[71] Here we also have a good example of the versatility of Enlightenment entrepreneurs who tried to earn both money and honour in a wide variety of fields.[72] Apparently Feydel had already left the military at this time.

His publishing career began with numerous, often polemical, letters to various periodicals and journals that included frequent critiques of the nobility during the pre-revolutionary period and were therefore occasionally censored. Feydel presumably had a classical education since he also reviewed works in Latin and took part in literary controversies. His publications all appeared between 1783 (the first swimming manual) and 1821. In other words, his texts on swimming were also his first publishing efforts. This may explain why the manuals of 1783 and 1787 appeared under the pseudonym Nicolas Roger. As we see from the title pages, by calling him a 'professional diver', he provided his fictive author with authority and expertise.[73] The swimming and diving instructions in both manuals were so precise, realistic and original that in all likelihood Gabriel Feydel knew how to swim. His claim that he was not working as a swimming instructor but only teaching his friends is also believable.[74] It is possible that he found such work beneath his dignity.

When publishing the second edition of his swimming manual Feydel apparently realized that this was a field where he might make a name for himself. Using his own name (Feydel) he shrewdly advertised in the 1787 *Journal de Paris* for the swimming manual he had published under the pseudonym 'Roger'.[75] The text accordingly became much more comprehensive, and included references to contemporary debates and scholarly publications. In addition,

---

[70]   This and the following: Nicole Brondel, 'Gabriel Feydel', in *Dictionnaire des journalistes (1600–1789)*, http://dictionnaire-journalistes.gazettes18e.fr/journaliste/303-gabriel-feydel [last accessed October 25th, 2015].

[71]   See for example Roger, *Essai*, title page.

[72]   Darnton, 'Pamphleteer', pp. 78, 108, 114.

[73]   Roger, *Méthode sûre*, title page; Roger, *Essai*, title page.

[74]   Roger, *Essai*, p. 23.

[75]   *Journal de Paris*, 1787, pp. 724–5, Variete. Aux Auteurs du Journal de Paris, le 27 Mai 1787, here p. 724: 'Les gens du métier en font l'éloge.'

Feydel inserted a new section about swimming in general before the largely unchanged centre section, and concluded with a plan for a swimming school. He now also promoted himself as a much sought-after specialist[76] whose entire brochure had been included in the *Encyclopédie*, though in somewhat garbled form due to printing errors and the carelessness of copyists (hence the need for a new edition).[77] If there was sufficient demand, he also declared himself willing to expand and re-publish his short text (which – according to his account – was only a substitute for a much more detailed version, unfortunately lost to fire).[78] Feydel was clearly trying to stoke the demand himself, but we know of no further edition.

The details of the printing history are interesting. The first edition of 1783 got neither the censors' endorsement nor a royal printing privilege. Both were actually necessary for a legal printing. That the second swimming manual was (allegedly) produced in London does not necessarily mean it was forbidden in France: it is possible that it had received only a *permission tacite* or a *simple tolérance*.[79] In fact, a red stamp on the title page indicates that the work was printed in London, but was also available at the Palais Royal. As the private property of the Duke of Orléans, the Palais Royal was largely beyond the control of the police, that is, it was a place where censorship could be bypassed, which is

---

[76] Roger, *Essai*, pp. 22–3: 'Des gens en place me firent l'honneur de me consulter sur la forme qu'on pouroit doner à des écoles de nâge. Des spéculateurs me consultèrent sur la possibilité d'en établir sans compromettre leur fortune. Diverses persones désirerent que je leur donasse des leçons; quelques'unes m'écrivirent des billets auxquels je n'ai point répondu. Je saisis l'occasion de leur en faire mes excuses: je ne donne de leçons qu'à mes amis.'

[77] Roger, *Essai*, p. 23.

[78] Roger, *Essai*, p. 63.

[79] *Permissions tacites* were granted for many books that were not banned outright, but whose publication should also not appear to have the support of the government. For this reason, a fictive foreign place of publication was invented (Gudrun Gersmann, *Im Schatten der Bastille. Die Welt der Schriftsteller, Kolporteure und Buchhändler am Vorabend der Französischen Revolution* (Stuttgart, 1993), p. 23). This was a very common practice as Raymond Birn states: 'between 1750 and 1789, perhaps one of every two new books circulating in the kingdom was either "tacitly permitted", produced abroad, or else was a clandestine production' (*Royal Censorship of Books in Eighteenth-Century France* (Stanford, 2012), p. 4). *Simples tolérances* were given by word of mouth and not recorded, the censor remained anonymous (Birn, *Royal Censorship*, pp. 24–5). There were furthermore *permissions 'très' tacites* and *approbations motivées* as categories between the two mentioned above (Birn, *Royal Censorship*, p. 69). In the years just before the revolution more and more books were approved by the censors that offered plans for public utility (Birn, *Royal Censorship*, p. 81), as was true also for the swimming tracts. For the complex interaction between pre-censorship and post-publication censorship, secret censorship and censorship 'à grand spectacle' that was exerted by different institutions of the Ancien Régime see also Barbara de Negroni, *Lectures interdites. Le travail des censeurs au XVIIIe siècle 1723–1774* (Paris, 1995).

why the Enlightenment camp also gathered there.[80] The title page says that people from the provinces who wish to obtain the booklet may turn to M. Biziaux, master bookbinder in the rue du Foin S. Jacques, n° 32. According to the BNF catalogue entry, however, this was a false address;[81] the parenthetical addition '*à l'anglaise*' which in other word combinations means 'secret' or 'clandestine' probably signalled that an underground printer was involved. As early as 1864 Emil Weller determined that the work had been printed in Paris.[82] 'London' may also have served as a symbolic location, since it was here that Frenchmen expelled from their own country congregated and produced pamphlets critical of the regime that were then smuggled back into France.[83] Even though clearly critical stances were taken in connection with swimming, the illegally produced works of the 1780s spoke a much clearer and more pointed language. It is therefore more likely that Gabriel Feydel lacked the connections and financial means needed to print legally in the Old Regime. As such, he was a typical representative of the 'literary underground' as described by Darnton.

Jean Charles Poncelin de la Roche-Tilhac (1746–1828), publisher of the Thévenot swimming manuals of 1781, 1782 and 1786, probably started off better situated than Gabriel Feydel. Poncelin was educated by the Jesuits and joined the clergy early. He became canon at Notre-Dame de Montreuil-Bellay in Anjou, and with his doctorate in law earned the position of *conseiller du Roi à la Table de marbre*, a post that gave him jurisdiction over the admiralty. Later he was *avocat au parlement*, relocated to Paris and worked on diverse historical texts. Since his *Recueil d'événements, ou Tableau de l'année 1781* was ostensibly published in Amsterdam (1782), and his *Histoire des révolutions de Taiti* (Paris, 1782) appeared under a pseudonym,[84] we can surmise that he was distancing himself from the Old Regime. Hoefer has documented that Poncelin borrowed heavily from other authors, which suggests that he wanted to publish as much

---

[80]   Tom Ambrose, *Godfather of the Revolution: The Life of Philippe Égalité duc d'Orléans* (London, 2008), p. 50; Jeremy D. Popkin, 'Robert Darnton's Alternative (to the) Enlightenment', in Haydn T. Mason (ed.), *The Darnton Debate: Books and Revolution in the Eighteenth Century* (Oxford, 1998), pp. 105–28, here p. 111.

[81]   http://catalogue.bnf.fr/servlet/biblio?idNoeud=1&ID=39317337&SN1=0&SN2=0 &host=catalogue [last accessed October 25th, 2015].

[82]   Emil Weller, *Die falschen und fingierten Druckorte. Repertorium der seit der Erfindung der Buchdruckerkunst unter falscher Firma erschienenen deutschen, lateinischen und französischen Schriften* (3 vols, 2nd edn, Leipzig, 1864–1867), vol. 2, p. 232.

[83]   Robert Darnton, 'A Spy in Grub Street', in Robert Darnton, *The Literary Underground of the Old Regime* (Cambridge, MA, 1982), pp. 41–70, here p. 62.

[84]   Jean Chrétien Ferdinand Hoefer (ed.), *Nouvelle biographie générale depuis les temps les plus reculés jusqu'à 1850–60. Avec les renseignements bibliographiques et l'indication des sources à consulter* (46 vols, Paris, 1852–1866, repr. Copenhagen, 1963–1969), vol. 40, pp. 737–8.

and as quickly as possible in order to turn a profit.[85] Robert Granderoute likewise describes Poncelin as more of a compiler than an author 'que guide souvent un esprit de spéculation commerciale'.[86] His choice of the Thévenot text fits into this strategy since it involved the re-publication of an older work, and in the new edition he also borrowed heavily from the writings of other authors.[87] Even so, Poncelin did publish legally. For the Thévenot edition of 1781 he obtained a licence from the censor Blin de Saint-Maure, and also secured a royal printing privilege for a five-year period (that is, no one else was allowed to print this text, sell it or import it from a foreign country). He immediately passed along the privilege to his publisher Lamy and was probably compensated in return. Why Poncelin de la Roche-Tilhac's name is only abbreviated on the title page, licence and privilege is unclear. But like Gabriel Feydel he was just at the start of his career in publishing, possibly trying to minimize his risk of public disgrace.

At the same time he hoped just as fervently as Feydel that his writings would bring him success. Thus Poncelin de la Roche-Tilhac criticized above all else the style and lack of method in the original Thévenot edition of 1696, no doubt in an effort to cast his own merits in a flattering light.[88] Gabriel Feydel found fault with both the old (1696) and new Poncelin (1782) versions equally as unrealistic: experienced swimmers would laugh at this work, which was also lacking in scientific method.[89] In the second expanded edition of his swimming

---

[85]   Hoefer, *Nouvelle biographie*, vol. 40, pp. 737–8.

[86]   Robert Granderoute, 'Jean Charles Poncelin de la Roche-Tilhac', in *Dictionnaire des journalistes*, http://dictionnaire-journalistes.gazettes18e.fr/journaliste/650-jean-charles-poncelin-de-la-roche-tilhac [last accessed October 25th, 2015].

[87]   At the end of the first part on the benefits of the baths, a new section added by Poncelin himself, he seems to have run out of steam, since after having just praised and given a detailed account of [Hugues] Maret, he quotes him for a total of 15 pages and then ends the chapter (Thévenot, *L'art de nager* (1782), pp. 97–112). His explanation for doing so occurs several pages later: 'La matiere m'a paru trop intéressante pour la soumettre entiérement [sic] à mes propres réflexions, ce sont les matériaux des autres, dont j'ai fait usage sans aucun scruple' (pp. 114–15).

[88]   Thévenot, *L'art de nager* (1782), pp. 112–14: 'Cet Opuscule, malgré la négligence du style, la monotonie des idées, & la confusion des principes, avoit eu le plus grand succès. La justesse des regles que l'Auteur y prescrit sur la natation, & le laconisme estimable qu'il a su mettre dans ses leçons, couvrent les défauts qu'une méthode plus éclairée eût pu éviter ... Je m'apperçus bientôt qu'il ne suffisoit pas de traduire le langage gaulois de Thévenot en un françois intelligible, pour donner à son Art de nager le degré de mérite dont il étoit susceptible.'

[89]   Roger, *Essai*, p. 19: '... mais tout l'effet de ce livre se réduisoit à faire rire les nâgeurs à qui par hasard il tomboit sous la main. Il faut être observateur pour découvrir des élémens, pour asseoir des principes, pour créer des préceptes raisonés; & l'auteur du livre atribué [sic] à Thevenot n'étoit rien moins qu'observateur. En mil sept cent quatre-vingt-deux, un écrivain aparament [sic] aussi bon citoyen que mauvais nâgeur, a cru rendre service au public

manual (1787) Feydel clearly expressed his lofty ambitions and correspondingly high hopes for fame as – in his view – he laid out the principles of a new art:

> The art of horsemanship was not yet imagined when the knight of Pluvinel set forth its basic principles in the sixteenth century; today, a knight of Pluvinel would need to ask us how to hold a bridle. As soon as academies for the art of swimming produce masters like Laguérinière, Nestier, Labie, d'Abzac, and Lambesc[90] and our cavalry fords a river as if marching down a broad street; and as soon as the swimming manuals published are as complete as those we have on riding, my writings will betray my inadequacy: yet perhaps one day people will recall that it was I who took the first step in this direction.[91]

Some authors of swimming tracts enjoyed considerable success both in terms of social status and economic profit. Oronzio de Bernardi, the Italian mathematician mentioned earlier, was accepted into several scientific academies after publishing his swimming manual. What is more, he received a medal and a lifetime pension from Ferdinand IV.[92] Both Gabriel Feydel and Jean Charles Poncelin de la Roche-Tilhac became highly successful publicists during the time of the Revolution, though ultimately they held completely different political views. We know nothing about the careers of most other authors who wrote on swimming, and yet, their influence on historiography has been so profound that even today our research in many cases starts from the premise that before these writers took up their pens, swimming in Europe was virtually unknown.

---

en ressuscitant ce livre. ... Quant au fond de l'ouvrage atribué [sic] à Thevenot, l'éditeur s'est contenté d'y changer quelques expressions, & d'allonger quelques phases, pour en rajeunir le stile, comme il dit.'

[90]   Antoine Pluvinel (1555–1620), François Robichon de la Guérinière (1688–1751), Louis Cazeau de Nestier (1686–1754) and Vicomte Pierre Marie d'Abzac (1744–1827) were all famous riding instructors who also wrote hippological works.

[91]   Roger, *Essai*, p. 64: 'L'art de monter un cheval étoit à peine soupçoné quand le chevalier de Pluvinel en vint poser les principes au seizieme siécle [sic]; aujourd'hui le chevalier de Pluvinel viendroit nous demander comment il faut empoigner la bride. Lorsque les académies de nâge auront produit des Laguerinière, des Nestier, des Labie, des d'Abzac, des Lambesc; lorsque notre cavalerie traversera un fleuve comme elle suit une grande route; lorsqu'on aura des traités de nâge aussi complets que nos traités d'équitation; alors mes essais décéleront mon impuissance: mais peut-être n'aura-t-on pas oublié que ce fut moi qui ouvris la carriere.' (final sentence of the text)

[92]   Camillo Minieri Riccio, *Memorie storiche degli scrittori nati nel Regno di Napoli* (Naples, 1844), p. 187; Carlo Villani, *Scrittori ed artisti pugliesi antichi, moderni e contemporanei* (Trani, 1904), pp. 129–30.

Chapter 12

Swordsmanship and Society in Early Modern Japan

Michael Wert

Martial arts were the first forms of native physical activity to become sports in Japan. The intellectual and cultural shifts in Japanese sport history paralleled developments in the West and did not suddenly become 'modern' after Japan's growing exposure to Western sports. The creation of swordsmanship as a cultural art in the seventeenth century established a precedent for teachers of other combat skills to transform their technical know-how into professionalized and commercialized art forms. By the nineteenth century, swordsmanship had fully emerged as a new field of knowledge that reflected the social, educational, political and economic changes in society, as had modern sports in the West. In tracing these changes through the lens of swordsmanship, I reject an argument popularized long ago by Allen Guttmann, that modern sport is uniquely Western. By liberating the definition of 'modernity' from modernization theory's superficial focus on technology and institutions, as it applies, in this case, to sport, it becomes possible to see modernity as a global historical moment not led by the West.

Allen Guttmann has applied modernization theory to Japanese sport, but because his paradigm, like modernization theory in general, is Eurocentric, it fails to provide a useful framework for understanding the transformations of physical culture in early modern Japan, roughly the late fifteenth to mid nineteenth centuries. Thompson and Guttmann's comprehensive *Japanese Sports: A History* displays an inherent tension between Guttmann's modernization theory paradigm and Japanese historical evidence that seems to undermine it.[1] Throughout the volume, Thompson, a Japan scholar, summarizes the Japanese-language scholarship on early modern sports, citing arguments that sport developments paralleled trends in European history. On one hand, Thompson and Guttmann, too, accept that premodern, or in this case, non-European sports, might display characteristics of modern Western sports.[2] They note, for example,

---

[1]   Allen Guttmann and Lee Thompson, *Japanese Sports: A History* (Honolulu, 2001), pp. 3–4.

[2]   Guttmann and Thompson, *Japanese Sports*, p. 4.

that Japanese sumo teachers founded a national sumo association in 1751, the first year that Great Britain developed its first national sports organization.[3] But elsewhere, they invent reasons for disqualifying non-European, and non-modern, examples that challenge the modernization paradigm. Thus, record keeping in Japanese archery during the early modern period, and the intense competition to break those records, is dismissed as not being rational because lords (*daimyō*) who encouraged their samurai to compete in archery, copied and rebuilt the temple shooting grounds of Sanjūsangendō, the main site for national archery competitions.[4] It is unclear whether Thompson and Guttmann deem the reproduction of the temple grounds irrational, or if the intermingling of religion with competition is at fault. Either way, the presence of sacred symbolism even in twenty-first-century Western sports is just as rational, or irrational, as it would have been in early modern Japan.

While modernization theory, and the concept of modernity, may provide a useful way for historians of Western Europe to describe a set of events that occurred at a particular historical moment, many similar characteristics of modernity happened elsewhere at the same time and even earlier.[5] The authors acknowledge the many criticisms levelled against modernization theory but continue to defend it as useful. Modernization theory was especially controversial in the Japanese studies field during the 1950s and 1960s, when Japan was held up as a successful example of modernization along Western lines.[6]

In general, writings about martial arts and sports in Japan tend to define modern sport as a post-Meiji Restoration (1868) phenomenon that owes much to the influence of the West. After the fall of the last samurai-dominated regime, the Tokugawa shogunate, the oligarchs in the new Meiji government accelerated a strategy begun under the previous regime – turning to Western experts for advice in reforming Japan's government and infrastructure. As the number of Westerners in Japan increased, they brought with them Western sports and ideas about physical education. Some Western sports, most notably baseball, became popular in Japan during an early stage of the Japanese–Western interaction, while native sports either 'modernized' and thrived, or only minimally changed to suit modern sensibilities, and thus failed to attract widespread attention.

---

[3]   Guttmann and Thompson, *Japanese Sports*, p. 23.

[4]   Guttmann and Thompson, *Japanese Sports*, p. 56.

[5]   For a cogent argument on this point, see Bin Wong, http://afe.easia.columbia.edu/chinawh/web/s2/.

[6]   Even then, defenders of modernization theory tried to decouple modernization from Westernization, an effort that ultimately failed. For more on modernization theory in Japanese studies see Sebastian Conrad, '"The Colonial Ties are Liquidated": Modernization Theory, Post-War Japan and the Global Cold War', *Past and Present*, 216/1 (2012): pp. 181–214.

Inoue Shun, for example, argues that judo was the first Japanese form of physical culture to modernize, becoming a model for other martial arts to do the same.[7] Judo's founder, Kanō Jigorō, possessed a unique background for this task. He was a practitioner of *jūjutsu*, an early modern martial art that emphasized grappling, and an educator who had studied Western physical education theories. In the decade immediately following the Meiji Restoration, samurai and martial culture were stigmatized as examples of an old, backwards Japan. Kanō hoped to rehabilitate *jūjutsu* by changing its techniques, practice and goals. Inoue identifies nine ways in which Kanō modernized *jūjutsu*: comparing and analysing techniques of various *jūjutsu* styles to systemize judo, creating ranks to motivate students, establishing rules for competition and judging, founding a modern organization to develop judo, emphasizing judo's educational value, promoting judo through literary means (lectures, publications, etc.), internationalizing judo, admitting and promoting women's participation in judo, and making judo a watchable tournament sport.[8]

Sport can be a useful lens for viewing the broad social and intellectual changes over time rather than limiting sport to the narrower technological and institutional changes that Guttmann's modernization theory version of sport confines it to. Instead, I appropriate Pierre Bourdieu's genealogy of sport history to trace the emergence of, and changes within, swordsmanship. While his study is also grounded in the Western European experience, and differences with Japanese history are to be expected, he analyses broad phenomena that are applicable to any society, early modern or modern. These include the relationship between learning and the body, the maintenance of elite privilege, and the growth of non-elite sport.

Bourdieu traces the rise of modern sports back to the moment when sports became a distinct field of knowledge. The shift from earlier, presumably non-sport games and combative techniques, occurred among the elite, who transformed play into sport in the same way that they transformed folk dances into a high-art form.[9] This transition, that Bourdieu associates with nineteenth-century modernity in particular, was accompanied by its own philosophy of character formation and other features of manliness that defined ideal, future leaders – sport was political.[10] This amateur elite ideal of sport, Bourdieu argues, was opposed to the 'victory at all costs' attitude of the plebeian. Practice became an end in itself.[11]

---

[7]   Inoue Shun, *Budō no Tanjō* (Tokyo, 2004).

[8]   Inoue, *Budō no Tanjō*, p. 9.

[9]   Pierre Bourdieu, 'Sport and Social Class', *Social Science Information*, 17/6 (1978): pp. 819–40, at p. 823.

[10]   Bourdieu, 'Sport and Social Class': p. 824.

[11]   Bourdieu, 'Sport and Social Class': pp. 824–5. Bourdieu also reminds us that many members of the first Olympic committee were from the nobility.

Both approaches to defining sport are important, but Bourdieu's methodology has broader implications for societal changes over time. As other scholars have noted, Guttmann's modernization paradigm does not describe a break with earlier physical, and I would add non-European, activities, but simply illustrates a difference of degree rather than substance.[12] The same is true for many of the categories that Inoue uses to describe judo's modernization. Kanō's innovations may reflect his study of Western physical education, but analysing and comparing techniques of different styles, writing about martial practice as a form of self-development, and awarding rank had been central features of martial practice, especially swordsmanship, since the seventeenth century.

Swordsmanship as a Cultural Art

The dominant narrative regarding the development of swordsmanship from the late sixteenth century to the end of the Tokugawa period (1600–1868), and commoners' involvement in swordsmanship, generally follows three stages.[13] In the first stage, during the early seventeenth century, swordsmanship consisted of a handful of styles (*ryūha*) that began, putatively, as effective combative arts forged from the experience of the Warring States period (1467–1568). As the name implies, Japan was divided into warring domains led by warlords who sought to advance their territorial claims. The 'three unifiers' gradually brought an end to the warfare, and the last unifier, Tokugawa Ieyasu, founded a samurai-dominated regime, the Tokugawa shogunate. Except for a few violent events during the seventeenth century, Japan entered into a relatively peaceful era, creating an identity crisis for samurai whose role shifted from warrior to bureaucrat, a process referred to by one scholar as 'taming of the samurai'.[14]

In the second stage, from roughly the late seventeenth into the eighteenth century, those styles gradually became commercialized art forms, and began featuring abstract concepts and mysticism to attract customers.[15] Tokugawa period commentators bemoaned this transition as a weakening of combat skill. Intellectuals at the time referred to this new type of swordsmanship as 'flowery swordsmanship', an interpretation that has continued into the modern

---

[12] Ben Carrington, *Race, Sport and Politics: The Sporting Black Diaspora* (London, 2010), fn. 14, p. 16.

[13] For a summary of Japanese secondary literature on early modern swordsmanship and archery, and their transition from combat skill to rule-bound sport, see Cameron Hurst, *Armed Martial Arts of Japan: Swordsmanship and Archery* (New Haven, 1998).

[14] Eido Ikegami, *Taming of the Samurai: Honorific Individualism and the Making of Modern Japan* (Cambridge, 1995). See chapter 7 in particular.

[15] John Rogers, *The Development of the Military Profession in Tokugawa Japan* (PhD Diss. Harvard, 1998), p. 155.

era.[16] During this stage, scholars note an increase in the number of non-warrior practitioners of swordsmanship. As John Rogers argues, after the early 1700s, most of the eight or so styles of swordsmanship that existed in the first stage, stagnated, as the demand for swordsmanship among samurai elites saturated. Teachers of the most prominent styles opened their schools to non-warriors, saving those styles from obscurity. Moreover, during the third stage, from about the mid-eighteenth century, swordsmanship, which presented few opportunities for competition other than outright duelling, developed free-style fencing methods within the community of elite commoners and low-ranking warriors.[17] In the nineteenth century, this group pushed changes in equipment and established commonly accepted rules for fencing competitions; the forerunner of modern *kendō*.

I argue that swordsmanship was never meant, primarily, to impart combat skill. For millennia, warfare was conducted without well-defined weapon styles, famous teachers, or esoteric martial treatises. While some primary sources from the sixteenth century suggest that a few men became well known as sword teachers, there is little evidence that they chose to articulate their art – swordsmanship was not yet a field of knowledge. The first writings about swordsmanship from the seventeenth century employed the vocabulary and pedagogy common among other cultural arts, like Noh theatre, tea ceremony and flower arrangement. Only then did swordsmanship as a martial *art* come into existence, through the propagation of, and competition among, distinct styles.[18] Reversing the narrative of swordsmanship from battle-tested skill, to commercialized cultural art, to sport, swordsmanship began, primarily, as an art used to accrue social and cultural capital and, while retaining those features, also developed ludic and competitive characteristics as it spread, becoming both a sport and method of self-defence.

---

[16] These critiques were a familiar lament by contemporary writers who idealized samurai of the Warring States. For examples of such complaints, see Kengo Tominaga, *Kendō Gohyakunenshi* (Tokyo, 1972), pp. 267–8.

[17] Scholars typically argue that the shogunate prohibited inter-style competition but there is no primary source evidence for this. However, there was also no official edict concerning *kenka ryōseibai*, the punishment for both parties involved in a fight. Also, such free-style competition was often forbidden by swords teachers themselves.

[18] Even in Noh, which influenced the earliest writings on swordsmanship, practitioners did not use the term 'style' or 'school' (*ryū*) until the late sixteenth century. See Eric Rath, *The Ethos of Noh: Actors and their Art* (Cambridge, 2004), p. 134. Before the Tokugawa period, there was little effort to intellectualize combat, and although many Tokugawa period writings about swordsmanship claim that certain styles were invented before the seventeenth century, there is, frankly, little evidence to support this.

Thus, swordsmanship was, to borrow Bourdieu's phrase, 'an activity with no purpose'.[19] The earliest styles, like the *Yagyū Shinkage-ryū* and *Ittō-ryū*, that still exist today, catered mostly to the elite among the samurai status: the ruling shogun, lords and high-ranking samurai advisors. These styles appealed to intellectual interests as well as physical development. For example, the shogun's swordsmanship tutor, Yagyū Munenori, published an influential text called the *Family-Transmitted Book on Swordsmanship* (*Heihō Kadensho*, 1632), a work that drew from a variety of sources, including Zen and Noh.[20] For elite amateur participants, physical activity was an end in itself. Free-style fencing was not practised among the samurai elite; they made no effort to hold matches, or become professionalized experts. A typical practice session might include engaging in predetermined attack and defence drills with wooden swords, and repetition of basic movements. Swordsmanship may have had practical applicability, and there were stories of duels to the death using swords, but this was not its primary purpose – most samurai could reasonably expect never to have to draw upon their acquired skills. Neither the shogun nor the roughly 250 lords would have needed, or have been expected, to defend themselves with a sword.

But swordsmanship was not useless. Samurai elite accumulated social and cultural capital proscribed from the uninitiated: knowledge of etiquette, bodily comportment and behaviour. Swordsmanship, practised in a controlled manner with wooden swords, allowed men to interact through a physical activity that strengthened their identity as warriors of a similar status. Recreation as status reinforcement existed elsewhere in the early modern world. French aristocrats often practised *paume*, an early form of tennis, as an end unto itself, for the health of the practitioners, or for social capital – an excuse to interact with other nobles.[21]

Fuse Kenji argues that martial art training, an obligation of all warriors, became the site of daily status discrimination.[22] His study of the structure of martial art training within two early modern territories, the Kawagoe and Maebashi domains, illustrates a basic feature of martial art practice in other domains; namely, that for much of the Tokugawa period, low-ranking, marginal warriors would not have trained alongside their superiors.

---

[19]   Bourdieu, 'Sport and Social Class': p. 824.

[20]   For more on the connection to Noh, and on esotericism on Yagyū Shinkage-ryū see Morinaga Maki, *Secrecy in Japanese Arts* (New York, 2005). For more on the influence of Zen on the Yagyū family writings, see Peter Haskel, *Sword of Zen: Master Takuan and his Writings on Immovable Wisdom and the Sword Taie* (Honolulu, 2013).

[21]   Corry Cropper, *Playing at Monarchy: Sport as Metaphor in Nineteenth-Century France* (Lincoln, 2008), pp. 12–13.

[22]   Fuse Kenji, *Kakyū Bushi to Bakumatsu Meiji: Kawagoe Maebashihan no Bujutsu Ryūha to Shizoku Jusan* (Tokyo, 2006), p. 38.

Martial arts and swordsmanship styles, practised differently by different warrior status groups, had an inverse relationship between cultural capital value and combat efficacy. The more abstract the style, the less useful it would be for combat but the more desirable it became as a pursuit for elites. Lords lent official support to certain martial art styles based upon the art's pedigree and the status of its students. In the Kawagoe domain, swordsmanship teachers of officially sanctioned styles were chosen from middle-ranking samurai (the elite never became teachers). They required permission from the domain to teach, received a stipend for their services, and could appoint assistant teachers. Samurai who trained in these styles often received money to pay for their equipment and training. In the last month of the year, advanced students in each official style were awarded cash for their efforts, and once a year, members of each style demonstrated their techniques in front of the shogunate's senior councillors.

Combat efficacy became the defining characteristic of martial arts among low-ranking swordsmen because, using Bourdieu's logic, they were not separated from the everyday life and work of these lower status groups. Low-ranking warriors trained in styles that, although recognized by the domain, did not receive official sanction. Unofficial styles received no financial support from the domain nor did their low-ranking warrior pupils receive payment for training or equipment, further burdening those already strapped for resources. However, low-ranking warriors who used the arts directly in their duties received some compensation. This occurred among foot soldiers who, in many domains, occupied a status lower than warrior, and studied arresting techniques or staff fighting, skills used in their policing roles.[23] Unlike their social betters, practitioners of these styles did not demonstrate in front of top officials. High-ranking samurai could learn unofficial styles or arts devoted to skills used by low-ranking warriors, but they did so privately and voluntarily.

Throughout the early modern period, it became an obligation of all warriors to learn swordsmanship, but non-warriors also trained in the art despite repeated efforts to discourage commoner practice. Theoretically, warriors, who comprised roughly 8 per cent of the total Japanese population, monopolized all means of violence after the Warring States period. The so-called 'sword hunts' of the sixteenth century did not remove all weapons from the countryside, and many urban residents carried short swords, especially during travel. Their participation in martial art practice is typically thought to be a phenomenon of the early or late Tokugawa period, when the putatively strict status system that separated warriors from commoners, had either yet to take shape, or was collapsing. Commoners trained in swordsmanship for a variety of reasons throughout the Tokugawa period; as a source of cultural and social capital, method of self-defence, and form of play. At the same time, fencing as a sport developed, an activity that was

---

[23] Fuse, *Kakyū Bushi*, pp. 54–5.

more socially accessible than older swordsmanship, and provided opportunities for competition. But fencing did not completely replace swordsmanship as a cultural and social art.

The Growth of Fencing

For the first half of the Tokugawa period, free-style fencing was not only uncommon, it was mostly forbidden. Written oaths signed by pupils newly admitted to a style, typically forbade students from engaging in matches of any sort, threatening expulsion and divine punishment from a host of Shinto and Buddhist gods. Although there is no clear evidence that the shogunate issued any edicts against competitive fencing, Tokugawa period commentators blamed the decline of martial arts on the outlawing of inter-style matches (*taryū jiai*).[24] The reasons for this are not hard to imagine; for one, authorities wanted to discourage any possible conflicts that might arise among samurai that could turn violent, especially if samurai from multiple domains became involved – the shogunate wanted to avoid another Warring States period. Second, poor performance in competition would have damaged the style's reputation, and thus, the livelihood, of sword teachers. Finally, competition would have been extremely dangerous before the eighteenth century, when proper equipment had not yet allowed for safe, full-contact training.

The development of fencing, especially competitive fencing among different swordsmanship styles, represented a watershed moment in the relationship among people of different statuses. Most styles of swordsmanship throughout the eighteenth century continued to emphasize training that focused on the repetition of predetermined attack and defence sequences between two people using wooden swords. There was little opportunity to experience free-style fencing. The development of armour and bamboo swords wrapped in leather in the early eighteenth century, allowed practitioners to attack each other using full force. These equipment changes began in private sword academies in the capital city, Edo. As the popularity of swordsmanship grew, styles that employed this equipment and emphasized fencing, outnumbered schools that refused to adopt the new practice. Inter-style fencing became popular among warriors and commoners alike, but styles dominated by the low-ranking warriors, and commoner elites, eclipsed older styles that catered to high-ranking samurai. With little salience of samurai authority in rural culture, and the broad appropriations of martial practice in the countryside, competitive fencing styles were predisposed to commoners rather than samurai.

---

[24]   Tominaga, *Kendō Gohyakunenshi*, pp. 272–3.

Swordsmanship as Commoner Status Symbol

The commoner swordsmanship boom began with decrees in 1721 and 1733 that allowed 'landed samurai' (*gōshi*) to use surnames and carry swords which led to a dramatic rise in the number of landed samurai wanting to learn swordsmanship.[25] Depending upon the domain, 'landed samurai' was either a self-appointed title by rural elite commoners, often village officials, who claimed to descend from warrior stock. At other times, 'landed samurai' was an official title awarded to rural elites by a local lord in exchange for money or some other extraordinary work performed. Exactly because the landed samurai title was ambiguous, it was not enough to simply wear two swords as a marker of status, landed samurai had to embody their claimed past. In so doing, rural elites tried to convince themselves, and others, that their warrior lineage was legitimate. Robert Nye points to a similar phenomenon to explain the popularity of honour, duelling and masculinity in early modern France, by invoking Bourdieu: 'The body believes in what it plays at: it weeps if it mimes grief. It does not represent what it performs, it does not memorize the past, it *enacts* the past, bringing it back to life. What is "learned by the body" is not something that one has, like knowledge that can be brandished, but something that one is.'[26]

Economic prosperity for rural elites in the eighteenth and nineteenth centuries allowed them to engage in cultural pursuits that helped them network with other elite commoners and warriors. Rural entrepreneurs pushed economic development with encouragement from lords who hoped to borrow more money and collect more tax.[27] Wandering samurai in the mid-eighteenth century took advantage of this newfound rural market for education and cultural arts.[28] Experts, too, added new features to their art to profit from the rise of commoner students. Teachers of tea ceremony and incense appreciation standardized their teachings and created grading systems in response to the booming amateur market.[29] Even cuisine schools began to impart licences of mastery, allowing students to wear coloured trousers, with each new colour signifying a promotion to a new rank within the school.[30]

---

[25] Takahashi Satoshi, *Kunisada Chūji no Jidai: Yomi, Kaki to Kenjutsu* (Tokyo, 1991), p. 256.

[26] Pierre Bourdieu, *Logic of Practice* (Stanford, 1990), p. 73, emphasis in the original. Robert Nye, *Masculinity and Male Codes of Honor in Modern France* (New York, 1993), p. 6.

[27] Edward Pratt, *Japan's Protoindustrial Elite: The Economic Foundations of the Gōnō* (Honolulu, 1999), p. 15.

[28] Brian Platt, *Building and Burning: Schooling and State Formation in Japan, 1750–1890* (Cambridge, 2004), p. 38.

[29] Rath, *The Ethos of Noh*, pp. 193–4.

[30] Eric Rath, *Food and Fantasy in Early Modern Japan* (Berkeley, 2010), p. 41.

With fewer limitations placed upon rural martial practice than in warrior swordsmanship, important differences emerged that explain why rural swordsmanship developed free-style fencing, and how that practice was eventually encouraged by local authorities. Wada and Enomoto assert that martial arts in the countryside retained characteristics of medieval martial arts, namely the inclusion of esoteric Buddhist practices, such as the use of spells, which filtered into rural ceremonies, festivals and even theatre.[31] In the Owari and Mikawa regions of Aichi Prefecture, peasants held ceremonies using staves (*bō no te*) where they performed stylized two-person drills, a practice also found in swordsmanship, in order to predict the weather, and they engaged in faux matches (*shiai*) to predict the future. Villagers organized their teachings into styles, imitating martial arts by awarding scrolls that imparted secret teachings and designated rank.[32]

In nineteenth-century Kawasaki City, several wandering, masterless samurai (*rōnin*) who taught swordsmanship in the Kaga domain, also opened a school in town where they taught various martial arts to be used in local lion dances. Other sword teachers followed suit, creating performance-based styles that taught the use of staves, swords, halberds and even sickles connected to chains. These innovations provided a sizeable profit, and hybrid martial art-performance groups continued well into the Meiji period (1868–1912).[33] The use of mock and real weapons in this mix of ludic martial activity affected how commoners consumed and appropriated martial arts differently than samurai. Martial themes appeared throughout rural culture. Plays that featured martial valour, with large casts that involved youth associations where everyone could be involved, were popular in the countryside because they broke the monotony of everyday life.[34]

Martial arts play extended to archery as well. In Shizuoka Prefecture, peasants practised *Heki-ryū Insai-ha* archery for use in competitions and religious ceremonies.[35] In the second month of 1741, for example, villagers held

---

[31]   Enomoto Shōji and Wada Tetsuya, 'Kinsei Sonraku ni okeru Bujutsushi Kenkyū no Genjō to Wadai', in Watanabe Ichirō sensei koki kinen ronshūkai (ed.), *Budō Bunka no Kenkyū* (Tokyo, 1995), pp. 134–47, at pp. 140–41.

[32]   For more on this folk art, and efforts to preserve it, see Owari Ashi-shi-shi, *Bunkazaihen* (Owari Ashi-shi, 1980), pp. 235–323.

[33]   Kanazawashi-shi hensan iinkai, *Kanazawashi-shi Shiryōhen* (19 vols, Kanazawashi, 1996), vol. 14, pp. 463–9.

[34]   Anne Walthall, 'Peripheries: Rural Culture in Tokugawa Japan', *Monumenta Nipponica*, 39/4 (1984): pp. 380–82.

[35]   As Morgan Pitelka noted, Ihara Saikaku listed archery as one of the 'arts of play' (*yūgei*) enjoyed by commoners as early as the late seventeenth century. See Morgan Pitelka, *Handmade Culture: Raku Potters, Patrions, and Tea Practitioners in Japan* (Honolulu, 2005), p. 92.

a five-day archery contest to bring good crops and ward off harm.[36] One member of the local elite lamented in 1835 that commoners were receiving rank in *Heki-ryū* and calling what they did 'the art of archery', but were really just meeting to gamble on competitions. He felt that this would hurt the reputation of *Heki-ryū* and respectable people would stop sending their young to study the art.[37]

The multifaceted practice of archery, as both a cultural martial art and as a source of bawdy gambling, also has implications for rural swordsmanship. Wada argues that martial-like activities were less rigid than warrior-dominated urban swordsmanship because rural arts incorporated rural culture, religion and recreation.[38] This might help explain why competitive fencing flourished among rural commoner practitioners and the low-ranking warriors who were more likely to interact with them.

Martial art training excursions became popular among warriors and, like religious pilgrimages, also provided commoners with an excuse to travel. Many travelling swordsmen were practitioners of new fencing styles, such as *Shintō Munen-ryū* and *Jikishin Kage-ryū*. They trained wherever and with whomever would have them, domain schools, private schools and other travelling swordsmen encountered on the road. Upon visiting a new school, swordsmen might simply learn whatever was being taught at the time, and if allowed, would engage in a fencing match. Some swordsmen recorded their visits and even asked training partners, or school managers and teachers, to sign a passbook like those used for temple pilgrimages. One Saga domain warrior, who received permission from the domain to spend two years training on the road, kept a record of places visited, people encountered and rumours about happenings in society, such as the arrival of Western ships. He mostly trained in domain schools with other warriors, but he also wrote about encounters with swordsmen of other statuses, including a landed samurai who was travelling to train in swordsmanship.[39]

By producing texts related to their travels, these men contributed to social networks of martial artists of all statuses, especially through the production of texts. They even published lists of notable swordsmen (*eimeiroku*). One such list, compiled in 1860 by two warriors, records 633 names, many of them commoners, and most from newer fencing styles like *Shintō Munen-ryū* and *Hokushin Ittō-ryū*.[40]

---

[36] Nishiyama Matsunosuke, *Iemoto no Kenkyū* (Tokyo, 1982), p. 289.

[37] Original reproduced in Iwasaki Tetsushi, 'Kinsei Tōkaido no Shukueki Bunka Tōtōmi Heki-ryū Insaiha kessha no tenkai', *Shizuoka Daigaku Kenritsu Gakutanki Daigakubu Kenkyū Kiyo*, 12/1 (1998): pp. 1–60, at p. 7.

[38] Enomoto and Wada, 'Kinsei Sonraku', p. 141.

[39] Muta Bunnosuke, 'Shokoku kaireki nichiroku' (1855), in Mori Senzō et al. (eds), *Zuihitsu Hyakkaen* (15 vols, Tokyo, 1979), vol. 13, pp. 217–403, at p. 270.

[40] For an in-depth study of this *eimeiroku* see Watanabe Ichirō, *Bakumatsu Kantō Kenjutsu Eimeiroku no Kenkyū* (Tokyo, 1967).

Swordsmanship and Unrest: A Nineteenth-Century Fencing Boom

Rural instability also pushed greater numbers of commoners into swordsmanship. In the eighteenth century, famine, increasing numbers of wandering people, and the inability of local authorities to provide adequate stability, forced rural elites to protect themselves. This trend continued into the nineteenth century as peasant protests grew in frequency and intensity. Young men began to break from earlier forms of peasant protest in which harm against individuals and arson had been avoided. Protests often involved destruction of property rather than targeting people. But in the mid-nineteenth century, groups of young men referred to by other rural commoners as 'evil bands', began carrying weapons, stealing, setting fires and attacking other peasants.[41]

Rural elites took it upon themselves to defend against the increasing violence in the countryside by sending their sons to train in martial arts which facilitated the spread of martial art styles. In one rural style, *Nen-ryū*, the number of students newly enrolled in the nineteenth century rose during the peak years of 'smashings' (*uchikowashi*).[42] This enabled the custodians of martial arts in the countryside to secure their positions by increasing the number of students from elite families. In exchange for loyalty and patronage, advanced pupils, often of privileged background whose presence had been socially advantageous for the style, were allowed to form their own sword subgroups. *Honma Nen-ryū*, for example, was an offshoot of *Nen-ryū* formed in the late eighteenth century by an advanced practitioner and relatively wealthy commoner named Honma Sengorō.

By the late 1790s, the carrying of swords by unauthorized persons from common travellers to unregistered wanderers was enough of a problem to cause comment among samurai officials. One samurai bureaucrat complained, 'In the Kantō region, there are many vagabonds who travel together carrying swords and making trouble'. Referring to another domain in Kantō, he stated, 'the ruler of this region allows too many people to use surnames and carry swords, even people coming into his territory from other domains are doing so'.[43] It is no surprise that the shogunate tried to prohibit the practice of rural swordsmanship. It issued edicts against rural theatre, dance and elaborate festivals, hotbeds of wandering troublemakers.[44]

---

[41]   Suda Tsutomu, *Akutō no Jūkyūseiki: Minshu Undo no Henshitsu to 'Kindai Ikoki'* (Tokyo, 2002).

[42]   A chart listing the numbers of enrolled practitioners and new pledges can be found in Takahashi, *Kunisada Chūji no Jidai*, p. 254. I compared this with a list of *uchikowashi* in the region found in Michio Aoki and Tadao Yamada, *Tempōki no Seiji to Shakai* (Tokyo, 1981), p. 114.

[43]   Takahashi Satoshi, 'Bakuhanseika Sonraku ni okeru "Bu" no Denshō: Nōmin Kenjutsu no Kyo to Jitsu', *Kikan Nihon Shisōshi*, 29 (1987): p. 61.

[44]   Walthall, 'Peripheries': p. 372.

At the turn of the nineteenth century the shogunate issued what became a series of edicts banning commoners from practising martial arts. The first such prohibition, from 1804, stated:

> Each of the four statuses has a separate occupation, but recently people have been setting up training areas in their houses or adding them to their houses, and teaching non-samurai and townsmen martial arts.[45] This is not a proper art for those of townsman status, and naturally they lose their occupations. Moreover this is insolence. If one hears of such activity report it to an official ... the practice of martial arts by townsmen is strictly prohibited.[46]

The success of commoners who established training areas in Edo offended the shogunate's sense of control over space. These privately built schools acted as meeting places for men of all statuses. Less than a year later, in the fifth month of 1805, the shogunate shifted its attention to the Kantō countryside and banned peasants from practising swordsmanship:

> We have heard that in this region there are unemployed samurai wandering about. Peasants are learning martial arts and gathering together for practice which might cause them to ignore their agricultural work. They forget their status and become uppity. They should be told to stop and martial art instructors should not introduce their arts to the villagers.[47]

The shogunate saw the connection between growing disorder and martial arts practice. Its newly created Kantō Regulatory Patrol issued warnings about commoners betting on rifle and archery shooting in the Kiryū area of Gunma Prefecture. The same prohibition, verbatim, was issued again in 1831, 1839 and 1867. A similar document was sent to the shogunate inspectors in 1843 asking that townsmen not be allowed to practice martial arts.[48] In the latter case, the offence was directed at sword teachers who 'awarded townsmen with rank certificates'.[49] These certificates acknowledged the recipient's accumulated cultural capital. Rank dissemination among commoners diluted their symbolic value for the samurai who once monopolized them.

---

[45] The 'four statuses' refers to a Confucian ideal about hierarchy in society where people belonged to one of the following groups: warrior, peasant, artisan or merchant.

[46] Shinzo Takayanagi and Ishii Ryosuke (eds), *Ofuregaki Tempō Shūsei ge* (Tokyo, 1941), pp. 440–41.

[47] Saitamaken (ed.), *Shinpen Saitamaken-shi Shiryōhen* (26 vols, Saitamaken, 1980), vol. 12, pp. 742–3.

[48] Ishii Ryōsuke and Harafuji Hiroshi (eds.), *Bakumatsu Ofuregaki Shūsei* (7 vols, Tokyo, 1992), vol. 5, p. 113.

[49] Tōkyōshi (ed.), *Tōkyōshi Shikō: Shigaihen* (176 vols, Tokyo, 1985), vol. 40, p. 550.

Not only were these hortatory proclamations unenforceable, but officials directly and indirectly encouraged commoner swordsmanship. The shogunate began to depend on rural martial power, thereby loosening its monopoly over violence. It had already overreached its policing ability and cooperated with rural commoner elites to control groups of indigents roaming throughout the countryside. The Kantō Regulatory Patrol had to rely upon rural elites for information on wanderers and criminals, the most frequent topic found in letters between village officials and the patrol.[50] Villages formed leagues centred on larger, wealthier villages that hosted criminal holding centres. League members practised swordsmanship for its practical use and to strengthen internal social cohesion.

As the number of commoner swordsmen increased, especially in the countryside, the competition between older swordsmanship and new fencing styles became potentially violent. Teachers often erected dedication panels at local Shinto shrines to enforce group identity, receive blessings from the local spirits, and advertise. During the Ikaho Incident (1822), students of a famous Edo-city sword teacher, Chiba Shūsaku, tried to erect a panel at the Ikaho Shrine located in a resort town in present-day Gunma Prefecture. Students and supporters of *Nen-ryū*, a popular style in the Gunma area, packed the inns to stop the dedication from occurring. To avoid a showdown, Chiba and his students backed down and prevented a confrontation. Such early modern tension might not have reached the degree of twenty-first-century football hooliganism, but the intersection of sport celebrity, rivalry and violence was not an entirely Western or modern phenomenon as is often assumed.

Fencing as a Modern Field of Knowledge and Competition

The growth of fencing as a modern sport could not have occurred without the gradual standardization of equipment and customs that allowed for free-style competition. But these superficial changes only reflected deeper and broader social transformations that allowed fencing to become a new field of knowledge. Fencing, as a field of knowledge, was a site for competition over expertise and celebrity, and a source of tension between older, elite forms of physical culture, and commoner sport.

Not everyone was enamoured with the rise of fencing over earlier forms of swordsmanship. Some felt that wearing armour and using a light bamboo sword did not reproduce realistic combative conditions, as fencing advocates had argued. Some fencers created bamboo swords that were longer than real ones in order to defeat opponents by taking advantage of greater reach. Still others

---

[50]   Iwata Miyuki, *Bakumatsu no Jōhō to Shakai Henkaku* (Tokyo, 2001), p. 22.

complained that swordsmanship was losing its role as an activity to cultivate the self. One critic argued that focusing one's training on simply winning a match might be sufficient while still young, but once a swordsman reaches 40 or 50 years of age, their skill will worsen because they focused too much on training the body, but never perfected the 'art', nor trained the heart and mind (*kokoro*).[51]

This critique reflects two phenomena in the emergence of modern sport as described by Bourdieu. First, in modern sport, members of the working class engage in sport mostly while they are young, when the focus is on competition rather than self-development. The elite, for whom self-development is the primary goal, continue to practise into old age. Second, the criticisms of the swordsmanship commentator above echo what Bourdieu sees as the origin of modern sport: the moment when sport as a field of knowledge itself became a site of competition. Despite many complaints, the fencing styles dominated. New types of publications appeared that listed the names of highly skilled fencers, famous matches held and their results. Swordsmanship had made the transition from physical culture to sport, a phenomenon pushed by commoners.

Non-warrior fencers never consciously challenged the status system; they articulated swordsmanship as a way to reinforce economic class differences between the elite and non-elite. Fencing experts did not aspire to samurai status, but many wanted to differentiate themselves from poorer commoner neighbours. Rural elites tried to convince local lords that granting privileges typically reserved for warriors, such as wearing swords, using a surname, or practising swordsmanship, helped them govern the countryside.

Changes in mid-nineteenth century military structure presented some commoners with opportunities to cross status lines that separated them from the warrior status group. As Western ships appeared in East Asian seas with greater frequency in the late eighteenth and nineteenth centuries, the Japanese shogunate pushed lords to embark on military reforms, especially coastal defence. Many reforms centred on Western military science; translating texts, buying Western ships, replacing archery with Western gunnery. To reinvigorate warriors, some lords changed their domain's martial art curricula by encouraging cross training and forcing warriors of all ranks to train in what lords believed to be more realistic forms of swordsmanship – the rough and tumble freestyle fencing that could prepare warriors for the physical strain of real combat. Commoner fencing experts, like Ōkawa Heibei, even received samurai status in order to train local warriors.

---

[51] Yamaga Motomizu, 'Bubunbi no Kan narabi Gakkō', reprinted in Sumita Shōichi (ed.), *Nihon Kaibō Shiryō Shōsho* (10 vols, Tokyo, 1932), vol. 1, p. 310. For more on Yamaga's attitudes towards fencing in general see Abe Hiroo, 'Kinsei Goki no Bugeikan ni kansuru Kenkyū: Satō Nobuhiro, Yamaga Motomizu wo chūshin ni', *Kokugakuin Daigaku Kiyo*, 48 (2010): pp. 1–28.

Ōkawa is an example of how status, modernity and sport intersected. He used his appointment to warrior status in the Kawagoe domain as a vehicle to promote his style, *Shintō Munen-ryū*.[52] He believed in the efficacy of his style because it emphasized practical training unlike the older styles already employed by domain. Before becoming a servant of the domain, Ōkawa had travelled throughout the Kantō Plain training at other schools and engaged in inter-style matches on his own, becoming famous in 1836 for defeating a practitioner of the rival *Kogen Ittō-ryū*. The *Shintō Munen-ryū* was well known for encouraging such competition, which it conducted by hosting students from other schools or allowing its own members to travel and train in various styles. Even as a guard working for the domain, Ōkawa received permission to use his free time to travel throughout the Kantō Plain for the purpose of training. Domain officials accepted Ōkawa's promotion of inter-style competitions among lower-ranked warriors who trained in *Shintō Munen-ryū*, allowing his students to engage in matches outside of Kawagoe and welcoming visitors into Kawagoe to do the same.

The fall of the Tokugawa shogunate and the collapse of the early modern status system fundamentally changed swordsmanship in Japan by separating what had once been a multifaceted activity. First, swordsmanship no longer existed as a form of self-defence. Several years after the Meiji Restoration (1868), the status system and warrior privileges were abolished; swords could no longer be carried legally. Second, modern *kendō* fencing followed the initiatives begun with the changes in older *jūjutsu* to judo: incorporating *kendō* into the school system, standardizing rank and competition rules, forming a national association, etc. Some of these trends were new, others, such as the ideal of martial virtue, or notions of self-development, built upon early modern swordsmanship. Some early modern styles of swordsmanship that eschewed competitions, like *Yagyū Shinkage-ryū* or *Ittō-ryū*, continue to exist in the twenty-first century, separately from modern *kendō*, and define themselves as cultural arts or realistic combat systems in contrast to what they see as the overly 'sportive' *kendō*. Third, and perhaps most importantly, however, swordsmanship fell into decline because it was no longer a source of cultural or social capital. Commoners no longer appropriated swordsmanship to differentiate themselves from those of a lower economic class. Nevertheless, *kendō* in the late nineteenth- and early twentieth-centuries adopted an invented martial ideal, *bushidō*, which granted practitioners a sense of warrior ancestry and national pride buoyed by the military victories of imperial Japan.

---

[52]   Yamamoto Kunio, *Saitamaken Kenkaku Retsuden* (Tokyo, 1981), p. 246.

Index

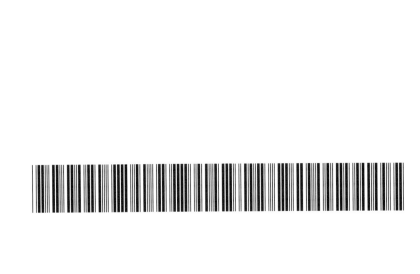